TRAUMA MANAGEMENT
Volume VI

Series Editors

F. William Blaisdell, M.D.
Professor and Chairman
Department of Surgery
University of California, Davis
Sacramento, California

Donald D. Trunkey, M.D.
Professor and Chairman
Department of Surgery
The Oregon Health Sciences University
Portland, Oregon

EXTREMITY TRAUMA

James P. Kennedy, M.D.
Instructor of Orthopedic Surgery
Northeastern Ohio Universities
College of Medicine
Rootstown, Ohio

F. William Blaisdell, M.D.
Professsor and Chairman
Department of Surgery
University of California, Davis
Sacramento, California

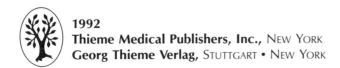

1992
Thieme Medical Publishers, Inc., NEW YORK
Georg Thieme Verlag, STUTTGART • NEW YORK

Thieme Medical Publishers, Inc.
381 Park Avenue South
New York, New York 10016

EXTREMITY TRAUMA
James P. Kennedy
F. William Blaisdell

Library of Congress Cataloging-in-Publication Data

Kennedy, James P.
  Extremity trauma / James P. Kennedy, F. William Blaisdell.
    p.   cm.—(Trauma management : v. 6)
  Includes bibliographical references and index.
  ISBN 0-86577-420-X (Thieme Medical Publishers).—ISBN
3-13-776101-8 (G. Thieme Verlag)
  1. Extremities (Anatomy)—Wounds and injuries. I. Blaisdell, F.
William (Frank William), 1927–   . II. Title. III. Series.
  [DNLM: 1. Extremities—injuries.   2. Wounds and Injuries—
diagnosis.   3. Wounds and Injuries—therapy.   WO 700 T766 1982,
v. 6]
  RD551.K36   1992
  617.5'8044—dc20
  DNLM/DLC
  for Library of Congress   92-339
                                                                CIP

Important note: Medicine is an ever-changing science. Research and clinical experience are continually broadening our knowledge, in particular our knowledge of proper treatment and drug therapy. Insofar as this book mentions any dosage or applications, readers may rest assured that the authors, editors, and publishers have made every effort to ensure that such references are strictly in accordance with the state of knowledge at the time of production of the book. Nevertheless, every user is requested to carefully examine the manufacturers' leaflets accompanying each drug to check on his own responsibility whether the dosage schedules recommended therein or the contraindications stated by the manufacturers differ from the statements made in the present book. Such examination is particularly important with drugs that are either rarely used or have been newly released on the market.

Some of the product names, patents, and registered designs referred to in this book are in fact registered trademarks or proprietary names even though specific reference to this fact is not always made in the text. Therefore, the appearance of a name without designation as proprietary is not to be construed as a representation by the publisher that it is in the public domain.

Printed in the United States of America.

5   4   3   2   1

TMP ISBN 0-86577-420-X
GTV ISBN 3-13-776101-8

To my parents—who tolerated without complaint the long years of my irregular hours and the demands of medical school and residency. Without them I could never have achieved what I have.

—*J.P.K.*

Contents

Contributors vi

Foreword   *H. David Moehring, M.D.* vii

Preface   *Michael W. Chapman, M.D.* ix

Acknowledgments x

1. **Initial Assessment and General Management** 1
   James P. Kennedy, M.D., and F. William Blaisdell, M.D.

2. **Soft Tissue Injury** 16
   James P. Kennedy, M.D.

3. **Splinting and Immobilization** 29
   James P. Kennedy, M.D.

4. **Upper Extremity Vascular Injury** 40
   F. William Blaisdell, M.D.

5. **Lower Extremity Vascular Injury** 60
   F. William Blaisdell, M.D.

6. **Extremity Nerve Injury** 82
   Lawrence H. Pitts, M.D., and F. William Blaisdell, M.D.

7. **Open Fractures and Dislocations** 98
   James P. Kennedy, M.D.

8. **Fractures and Dislocations of the Shoulder; Scapula and Clavicle Injuries** 115
   James P. Kennedy, M.D.

9. **Fractures of the Humerus and Forearm; Elbow Fractures and Dislocations** 136
   James P. Kennedy, M.D.

10. **Wrist Fractures and Dislocations** 162
    James P. Kennedy, M.D.

11. **Hand Injury** 185
     Eugene Kilgore, M.D.

12. **Management of Specific Hand Injuries** 198
     Eugene Kilgore, M.D.

13. **Pelvis Fractures** 214
     James P. Kennedy, M.D.

14. **Acetabulum Fractures and Hip Dislocation** 240
     James P. Kennedy, M.D.

15. **Hip Fractures** 261
     James P. Kennedy, M.D.

16. **Femur Fractures** 276
     James P. Kennedy, M.D.

17. **Fracture and Dislocation of the Knee and Patella** 287
     James P. Kennedy, M.D.

18. **Fracture of the Tibia/Fibula Shaft and Pilon Fracture** 304
     James P. Kennedy, M.D.

19. **Fractures and Dislocations of the Ankle and Foot** 322
     James P. Kennedy, M.D.

20. **Compartment Syndrome** 344
     James P. Kennedy, M.D.

21. **Traumatic Amputation** 358
     James P. Kennedy, M.D.

     Index 368

Contributors

F. William Blaisdell, M.D.
Professor and Chairman
Department of Surgery
University of California, Davis
Sacramento, California

Michael W. Chapman, M.D.
Professor and Chairman
Department of Orthopedics
University of California, Davis
Sacramento, California

James P. Kennedy, M.D.
Instructor of Orthopedic Surgery
Northeastern Ohio Universities
    College of Medicine
Rootstown, Ohio

Eugene Kilgore, M.D.
Clinical Professor of Surgery
University of California, San Francisco
San Francisco, California

H. David Moehring, M.D.
Assistant Professor of Orthopedic Surgery
University of California, Davis
Sacramento, California

Lawrence H. Pitts, M.D.
Professor of Neurosurgery
University of California, San Francisco
San Francisco, California

Foreword

Despite improved safety standards in the auto industry, workplace, and sports arena, extremity trauma remains a continuing problem in our active, modern society (Figure 1). It is interesting to note that in an 1847 survey of 2,328 fracture patients admitted over eleven years at l'Hôtel Dieu, Joseph-François Malgaigne found only 30 with more than one fracture.* Today, multiple fractures for the polytraumatized patient are the norm.

This treatise is an attempt to succinctly address the diagnosis of these injuries and discuss contemporary treatment rationale. The material presented should be of value to family practitioners, emergency physicians, general surgeons, and all ancillary medical personnel who are involved in the initial care, transport, and treatment of extremity injuries. Prompt diagnosis and emergent treatment of extremity trauma is crucial to the outcome. It is important to recognize the potential for associated complications and pitfalls in diagnosis. In this regard, occult and/or frequently missed injuries are noted in each section. Treatment of open fractures and the early detection of neurovascular injury and compartment syndrome are addressed in separate chapters. The reader is referred to a selected bibliography for an in depth focus on areas of particular interest.

This past decade has seen continuing advancement regarding the treatment of extremity trauma. While minor soft tissue injuries and simple fractures are adequately treated nonoperatively, advancing methodology and surgical techniques have resulted in improved treatment of major soft tissue and bone pathology. Exposed bone, neurovascular, and tendinous structures are more aggressively treated by early coverage with local muscle flaps, skin grafts, or remote microvascular grafts. From an orthopaedic aspect, aggressive treatment of intra-articular fractures and modern implant technology have resulted in shortened healing times and improved results. The data from modern trauma centers have clearly shown the advantage of surgical stabilization of multiple fractures in the polytraumatized patient. This treatment allows the patient to be free of cumbersome casts or traction, to be nursed more easily and humanely, and, most importantly, improves respiratory function through early mobilization. A significant portion of the aggressive approach to orthopaedic injuries can be attributed to technological advances in patient monitoring, resulting in safer anesthesia and improved postoperative care.

Often, surgical treatment of complex intra-articular and certain long bone fractures is the only way to meet the standard of care and current patient expectations. Nevertheless, surgical treatment is not without some inherent risk, and thus appropriate judgement, timing, and patient selection are of vital importance to minimize the potential for

---

*Malgaigne JF. *A Treatise on Fractures, Translated from the French with Notes and Additions by John Packard*. Philadelphia, Pa: JB Lippincott, Co., 1859.

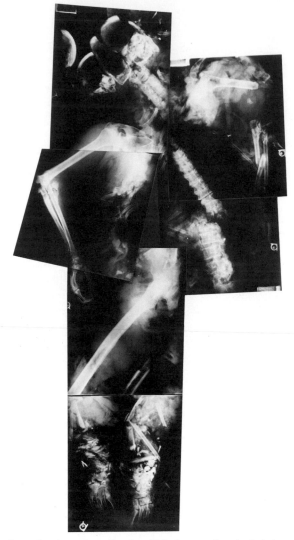

Figure 1. Composite photo of patient who suffered multiple fractures in a fatal airplane crash.

complications. Recently there has been a resurgence of emphasis on the biology of fracture healing, which entails careful handling of the soft tissue, avoidance of unnecessary bone stripping, or excessive metal fixation. In this regard the use of the image intensifier and arthroscope have made possible indirect reduction and closed treatment of certain fractures and related articular pathology.

While modern fracture fixation devices and related technical improvements continue, available systems are more than adequate to meet fixation requirements. The next decade will see greater focus on the biological aspect of soft tissue and fracture healing as more is learned about the multiple factors involved in this process. The anticipated development of healing accelerants and adjuvants to this complex unfolding biological montage will hopefully result in improved limb salvage, function, and reduction of disability.

H. David Moehring, M.D.

Preface

Major injuries to the extremities can result from blunt or penetrating trauma. The former most commonly involves fractures, the latter, soft tissues, including nerves and blood vessels. Of all the trauma specialists, the orthopaedic surgeon is most commonly involved because blunt trauma is far and away the most common cause of major extremity injury. Nonetheless, certain of these injuries, particularly those about the knee and elbow, may be associated with limb-threatening vascular and neurologic injuries which stress the expertise of multiple surgical specialists. When penetrating trauma is involved, the most common lesions which are associated with disability or potential limb loss consist of vascular and neurologic injuries.

This book is designed to lay out priorities for the management of the patient with multiple systemic injuries or with injuries limited to the extremities. This involves the general assessment of the patient and the conduction of the specific examination of the injured extremity. It includes principles in the management of vascular, neurologic, bony, and ligamentous injuries. There is emphasis on management of fractures since these constitute the vast majority of these challenging major injuries. Moreover, initial stabilization by internal or external fixation of these injuries has constituted the most recent significant advance in trauma management.

The orientation of the book is toward all physicians in training and those specialists who have occasion to see and participate in the management of trauma.

Michael W. Chapman, M.D.

Acknowledgments

I would like to acknowledge the assistance of all those who both directly and indirectly assisted in the publication of this book. Of inestimable value were the orthopaedic residents on the Trauma Service at the University of California Davis Medical Center. Their expertise, willingness to work, and diligence in patient care permitted me the time to prepare this text, and their enthusiasm, good natures, and inquisitiveness made our long hours of work short.

To F. William Blaisdell, M.D., I owe my deep indebtedness for providing me the opportunity to produce this work. He and his office staff were endlessly patient and understanding of my naiveté in such endeavors. Along with Jim Costello from Thieme Medical Publishers, he gave invaluable assistance to this novice author on the mechanics of putting all of this information together on paper.

Steve Lippitt, M.D., graciously provided the illustrations even though this took valuable time away from his family and career demands. His expert orthopaedic knowledge permitted him to produce clear drawings to convey concepts with nary a revision.

The medical photography departments at both the University of California, Davis and Akron General Medical Centers produced excellent work and were patient without end with my demands for reproductions. Mike Smith, M.D., Jeff Albert, M.D., and Walter Johnson graciously gave their assistance in the production of the photos as well.

My orthopaedic mentors were instrumental in teaching me not only orthopaedics, but also that this knowledge is most valuable when it is given to somebody else. I especially would like to acknowledge Buel S. Smith, M.D., under whose excellent tutelage high-caliber orthopaedists are consistently produced, and Harry O'Dell, M.D., who still teaches me something every day and who epitomizes the physician and gentleman we all strive to be, but few become.

Finally, but most importantly, Michael W. Chapman, M.D., and H. David Moehring, M.D., gave me the opportunity to gain the experience in treating the polytrauma patient that made the writing of this book possible. Dave could always be counted on to eloquently provide an eclectic viewpoint of the problem at hand. Mike's organizational abilities, endless energy supply, and innovative ideas were nothing less than awe-inspiring. I am forever in their debt for the unselfish offering of their valuable time, clear insight into complicated problems, and willingness to come to the operating room in the middle of the night to help the sometimes haggard trauma fellow. Although I know I can never repay that debt, if the reader gets a small fraction from this book of what their experience gave me, at least the first installment on that debt can be made.

James P. Kennedy, M.D.

Initial Assessment and General Management

JAMES P. KENNEDY, M.D.
F. WILLIAM BLAISDELL, M.D.

HISTORY: Until well into the twentieth century the evaluation of wounds of the extremities and fractures was through mechanical and direct means. This consisted of observation, palpation, and manipulation of the involved limb—basic techniques which are still appropriate today, but to which have been added other, indirect means, such as the various imaging modalities. In instances of penetrating trauma, probing the wound with the ungloved finger was the definitive means of assessing the injury.[1] This permitted the more definitive evaluation of comminuted fractures, the determination of the degree of soft tissue injury, and the presence of foreign bodies such as wood, dirt, or fragments of clothing. When the wounding object was a bullet or metallic fragment, removal was considered essential. Sophisticated devices including porcelain probes which revealed the presence of lead, grooved directors, and grasping forceps were developed.[2] Most of these latter techniques have been abandoned in favor of radiographs, arteriograms, CT scans, and MRI imaging.

INTRODUCTION

Extremity injuries fall into two basic types: blunt and penetrating with crush injury perhaps constituting a third category. These can vary from minor skin and soft tissue injuries to fractures of all types involving major and minor bones, vascular, and neurologic injuries. Injuries to extremities constitute by far the largest percentage of bodily injuries which present to emergency rooms. Most of the injuries are minor and are not life threatening, but the morbidity which results is the primary cause of disability following trauma. High-speed motor vehicle accidents, falls from heights, or athletic injuries constitute the most common cause of limb damage. The most frequent serious fractures are those related to the pelvis, femur, and tibia.

INITIAL SURVEY

The initial survey of the patient should be made quickly for the more immediate life-threatening injuries involving head, neck, chest, and abdomen.[3] Following airway assessment and stabilization, bleeding and circulation are next in priority. Bleeding constitutes the foremost immediate emergency and is primarily a complication of penetrating trauma. This can be controlled by direct pressure over or within the bleeding site in almost all instances. When bleeding involves the forearm or lower leg, temporary application of a tourniquet may permit the wound to be explored locally and the bleeding point definitively secured.

Finally, the adequacy of the circulatory system needs assessment. If the patient is hypotensive, or peripheral perfusion is poor, immediate vascular access is necessary for fluid administration. Urinary output should be monitored with a bladder catheter and a chest x-ray obtained. If the patient does not respond immediately to resuscitation, intra-abdominal bleeding is the most likely source in the absence of other causes of overt hemorrhage. In this circumstance immediate laparotomy is indicated.

SECONDARY SURVEY-SPECIFIC EVALUATION

The entire body must be visualized not only from the standpoint of identifying possible injuries, but also for surgical planning. This includes log-rolling the patient to inspect the spine and sacral areas. Many a physician has been chagrined when lacerations or contusions are discovered in the operating room converting what was thought to be a closed fracture into an open one, or when such lesions foil the planned operative approach. Once this has occurred, it is easy to understand why one must be compulsive about following protocol.

Palpation of all areas can be done along with inspection. Hands can quickly be run up and down the extremities, pelvis, and spine assessing for areas of tenderness. Axial percussion of the heel or extended wrist[4] is another useful technique for gross localization of extremity fractures in the conscious patient.

Vascular Assessment

Examination of the radial and ulnar pulses in the upper extremity and the dorsalis pedis and posterior tibial pulses in the lower extremity is the initial screening maneuver for vascular injury. In all instances, when distal pulses are diminished, the proximal major pulses should be checked: in the upper extremity the brachial, axillary, and subclavian; in the lower extremity the femoral and the popliteal. Decrease in any of these compared to the opposite side demands further investigation. A cool extremity with slightly diminished pulses is often said to be due to "spasm" of the blood vessels. "Spasm" implies a reflex phenomenon in an injured limb; the implication is that this is a physiologic response. The presence of spasm, however, is indicative of some type of vessel injury. This can range from a minor stretch injury with minimal disruption of arterial integrity to major injuries such as thrombosis of a vessel segment but with pulse and flow maintained by collaterals. Spasm demands specific investigation unless it involves a noncritical vessel, that is an isolated injury of a radial or ulnar artery, or one of the three lower leg vessels. In these instances, the significance may be minimal since the remaining vessel(s) usually is (are) capable of providing protective collateral circulation. In most instances, where possible, restoring all vascular continuity is appropriate. This is especially true when patients may be exposed to cold climates as cold exposure may compromise collateral flow and be associated with morbidity.

If there is a possibility of injury in a proximal large vessel, distal blood pressures in the limbs can be compared. In lower extremities, it usually averages 10 to 15 mm Hg higher than the upper extremities. The assessment of distal systolic pressure at the foot and ankle level is greatly facilitated by the use of a Doppler probe.[5] Additional evaluation should include auscultation along the course of the vessel. The presence of a systolic bruit localizes the site of injury. A systolic-diastolic murmur is a manifestation of an arteriovenous communication.

Any suggestion of vascular injury requires angiography. Certain lesions at high risk for arterial injury, such as knee dislocation, should also be so assessed.[7,9]

The presence of stocking or glove anesthesia in association with paralysis in a cool limb is a manifestation of profound ischemia and constitutes the one major extremity emergency other than bleeding as noted previously.

Fracture Assessment

The limbs should be inspected for deformity. The skin and subcutaneous tissue should be assessed for evidence of loss of integrity or for soft tissue swelling, or lack of symmetry. Careful palpation in the obtunded or uncooperative patient can identify areas of bony deformity or crepitation. Pain with passive range of motion suggests injury and dictates x-ray evaluation.

Open fractures are defined as any break in the integrity of the skin, no matter how minor, in association with underlying fracture. Even an abrasion can become secondarily infected and lead to metastatic infection at the fracture site. Small wounds usually are a sign that the skin has been punctured by a fragment of bone. With reduction of the fracture, the end of the bone responsible may be some distance from the site of skin perforation and may contain not only bacterial contamination but foreign material such as dirt. Open fractures constitute an orthopaedic emergency and require treatment prior to the onset of bacterial invasion, ideally within six to eight hours and mandatorily within 12 hours of injury. Open fractures are classified by the size of the wound, the amount of injured tissue, the degree of contamination, and the extent of the bony injury[6] (Table 1–1).

Serial examinations of the patient are crucial during the initial period of observation.

Table 1–1 Classification of Open Fractures

Type I—fracture is a low energy injury which is relatively clean and with a skin laceration less than 1 cm. Presumably, if due to blunt trauma, the bone is passed from the inside out. There should be minimal soft tissue damage.

Type II—injury results from a moderate force which usually results in comminution of the bone and a skin laceration greater than 1 cm. There is a moderate amount of adjacent skin contusion and muscle damage.

Type III—injury results from a high energy force and produces a significantly displaced fracture pattern with severe comminution, segmental fractures, or a bone defect. There many be extensive skin loss, muscle damage, and damage to other deep structures.

Most trauma patients are not fully cooperative and are often not fully conscious during the initial exam. Also, severe pain from long bone or pelvis fractures will mask relatively minor injuries. It is not at all unusual to discover minor fractures or sprains upon examining a patient two or three days after initial injury. In fact, it is so common that the patient and family should be initially made aware of this so that they will bring these minor "aches and pains" to the attention of the physician.

Dislocation Assessment

Dislocation of a joint is most often manifest by deformity, pain with motion, and swelling. Palpation may often reveal bony protuberances in abnormal locations. In some instances, the dislocation spontaneously reduces, which makes diagnosis more difficult. Instability of the joint may be present which can be confirmed by stress films. The importance of making a diagnosis of dislocation cannot be overemphasized, since failure to do so may result in serious long-term disability or loss of limb. An example is dislocation of the knee which has a high incidence of associated popliteal artery injury.[7] Dislocation of the hip constitutes an orthopaedic emergency. Failure to recognize and promptly reduce this injury risks avascular necrosis of the femoral head.

Neurologic Assessment

A thorough distal neurovascular exam is required of all four extremities with detailed peripheral nerve assessment of an injured area. A rectal exam is mandatory for assessment of the sacral nerve roots. Unfortunately, patients who are obtunded often cannot be given an adequate peripheral neurologic exam.[4] In these cases, the presence of reflexes and withdrawal from pain are helpful when present. Serial peripheral neurologic exams are important in cases of spinal cord injury as progressive spinal cord lesions must rapidly be decompressed. Partial cord lesions may sometimes also be given a relatively high surgical priority as the neurologic deficit may improve with decompression. Peripheral nerve lesions that are not in danger of progressing are a relatively low priority in the trauma patient. Most cases can be adequately treated on a delayed basis.[8] Examination of the peripheral nerves is discussed in Chapter 6.

RADIOLOGY

Penetrating wounds vary in the need for x-rays. Simple stabbings or penetrating wounds may require local x-ray evaluation if there is a possibility of vascular injury (angiography), joint penetration, or if a foreign body is present in the wound. All gunshot wounds should have x-rays to locate the foreign body if no exit wound is evident or to assess for bony injury or bullet fragments if through and through injury is present.

Standard x-rays are part of the protocol for evaluation of the multiple trauma patient to rule out orthopaedic injury. These include a complete C-spine series and AP pelvis films. Generally, a cross-fire portable C-spine is obtained in the emergency department, followed by the completion of the exam in the radiology department. It is important that all of C7 is visualized.[3,4] In some instances it may be appropriate to include routine x-ray exam of the dorsal and lumbar spine as well, due to the high incidence of injuries at these locations. Films of the complete spine are required if one spinal fracture is found, as there is 20% incidence of multiple spinal fractures if one fracture is detected.[10]

In obtunded blunt trauma patients with a Glasgow Coma Scale of 10 or less there can be a 31% incidence of major orthopaedic injury.[11] This includes a 14% incidence of axial spine injuries, a 10% incidence of pelvic fracture or hip dislocation, and a 15% incidence of femur and tibia/fibula fractures. So if injuries to these areas cannot be ruled out by examination of a cooperative patient, and the mechanism of injury is suggestive, radiographs of the entire axial spine, pelvis and lower extremity long bones are indicated. In addition to the standard films, x-rays are ordered of all areas that are questionable based on the physical exam.

In obtaining films, the general rule is to be sure to include all of the bone in question including the joint above and joint below to avoid the embarrassment (not to mention morbidity to the patient) or missing a related injury such as the hip fracture associated with an ipsilateral femoral shaft fracture.

Other x-rays will be warranted based on the mechanism of injury or the discovery of one injury that is commonly associated with other injuries. For example, forehead lacerations suggest the possibility of cervical spine injury. Dashboard injuries may result in patella fracture or laceration, knee ligamentous injury, hip dislocation, and/or posterior acetabular fractures (Figure 1-1, A & B). Children hit by a car can receive Waddell's triad[12] consisting of a tibia or femur fracture from the bumper, a chest injury from the hood, and a closed head injury from striking the pavement. Falls from a height in patients landing on their feet commonly result in the "Lover's Triad" (named because of rapid escapes out of second floor bedroom windows) of calcaneus, tibial plateau, and spinal compression fractures.

Some occult fractures, such as nondisplaced scaphoid and femoral neck fractures, can present initially with normal radiographs. If an x-ray is negative, but the history, physical exam, and mechanism of injury lead to suspicion for a fracture, the patient should be immobilized as if a fracture were present. The presence of an occult fracture can then be ruled out with scintigraphic bone scanning or tomography.

GENERAL MANAGEMENT

The problems presented by penetrating and blunt trauma are different and each poses a different set of problems for the trauma surgeon. Penetrating trauma problems are likely to cause vascular and neurologic injury while blunt trauma results primarily in fractures and dislocations.

PENETRATING TRAUMA

Superficial lacerations of the upper extremities are common following household accidents. Most penetrating wounds other than gunshot wounds or blast injuries are relatively benign. The most common serious problems caused by penetrating trauma are vascular—injury to superficial veins or major arteries—or neurologic, with damage to major nerves.

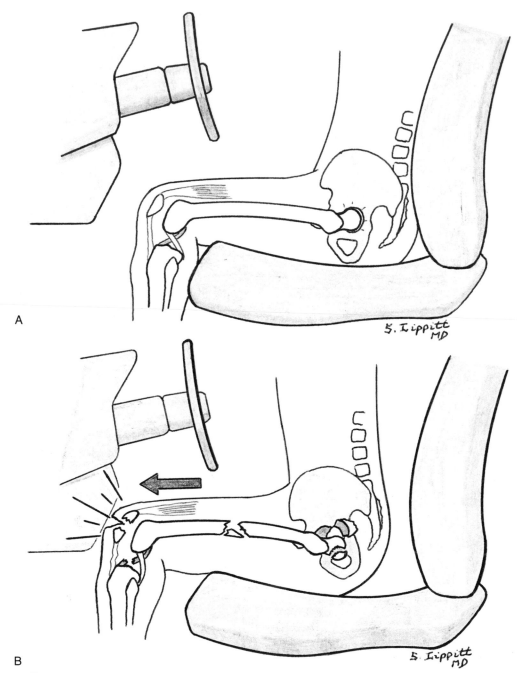

A

B

Figure 1–1.   A, B: Dashboard Injury Mechanism. An axial load is applied from the knee striking the dashboard at the time of impact. The force is directed up the femur. Lacerations over the knee, patellar fractures, knee ligamentous injuries, fractures of the femoral shaft or head, posterior hip dislocation, and posterior wall acetabular fractures are commonly seen alone or in combination with this mechanism of injury. When a soft tissue injury is seen over the knee, or with the knowledge that a dashboard injury has occurred, the physician should seek out these associated injuries in the automobile accident victim.

Since the mass of the thigh is considerably greater than that of the arm, the chances of major vascular and neurologic injury are less than that of the upper extremity. However, because the collateral circulation is less adequate, the consequences of vascular injury, when it occurs, are usually more severe in the lower as opposed to the upper extremity.

With penetrating trauma the wound should be examined and can be probed with an applicator stick to determine its direction. Exit wounds should be noted and x-rays obtained to look for foreign bodies, for bullet fragments, or fragments of bone which should indicate the possibility of secondary missile tracks.

Vascular

Large expanding arterial hematomas require immediate operation not only to decompress the hematoma, but also to ligate the bleeding vessel and rule out major vascular injury. Active bleeding or expanding hematomas should be tamponaded with direct pressure over the wound site, or if the wound is larger, the gloved finger can be inserted to compress the bleeding vessel in the depth of the wound. The patient can then be taken to the operating room for direct exposure and repair of the injured vessel which is usually arterial. Distal arterial injuries in the forearm or lower leg can be controlled in the emergency room. A proximal tourniquet briefly can be placed to ensure a dry field for local wound exploration. It is imperative not to aggravate the problem by blindly clamping bleeding vessels deep to the fascia since major nerves are associated with major blood vessels and permanent disability may result from inadvertent nerve damage. Following control of bleeding with a clamp or ligature, the patient can be taken to the operating room for definitive treatment.

If there is no active bleeding, further vascular assessment should be carried out as a first priority. If the limb is cooler than the opposite limb, and an injury involving the upper extremity is at or above the elbow, arteriography is usually indicated to establish the presence or absence of injury. If the injury is below the elbow and is limited to the radial or ulnar artery, observation may be appropriate since one normal lower arm vessel is capable of compensating for the other in most instances.

Regarding the lower extremity, management differs whether the thigh or the lower leg is involved. The tibial tubercle marks the location at which the popliteal artery has usually given origin to the three vessels of the lower leg. Injuries above this level carry a much more severe prognosis whether blood vessels, nerves, or bones are involved. Injuries distal to where the popliteal artery is presumed to have already divided into the anterior tibial, posterior tibial, and peroneal arteries present a less severe problem. Vascular injuries at this level rarely result in severe vascular compromise. The three vessels in the lower leg provide collateral for one another. Thus injury to any one is not necessarily associated with risk of severe ischemia, even though extensive thrombosis occurs. Secondary hemorrhage from these vessels which are four millimeters or less in diameter is rare, and, therefore, even a missed injury does not necessarily lead to serious consequences.

The general principles of treatment of penetrating extremity injuries are as follows. If there is no active bleeding, routine x-rays should be taken to establish the presence or absence of foreign bodies and to rule out bullet fragments and secondary missiles such as bone. If it can be established that the path of the wounding object does not pass near major vessels, and there are no neurologic changes distal to the injury and no pulse changes or major bleeding, the wound can be observed after it has been cleaned, debrided, and dressed.

When the wound tract passes in proximity to major vessels, particularly when gunshot wounds are present, arteriography or exploration should be carried out, depending upon the accessibility of the presumably injured vessel and the presence or absence of hematomas or vascular changes. A bullet passing an inch away from the vessel can, by the shock induced, produce intimal damage which may result in secondary thrombotic problems.

Venous injuries often accompany arterial injuries, but are often missed and as such, are not associated with risk of secondary complications. They rarely are associated with secondary hemorrhage but may rarely result in thrombosis and/or embolism from the injured vessel. These injuries are most commonly noted at the time of exploration for arterial injury, and if simple lacerations are present, the vessels should be repaired if possible.

Neurologic

As opposed to blunt trauma, evidence of injury to a nerve from penetrating trauma usually dictates repair unless the wound is dirty or contaminated or other injuries are present. An exception is the gunshot wound where the extent of the injury may be difficult to assess. Most lacerations result in minimal damage other than that immediately related to the nerve end. The sharply divided nerve can be debrided and repair done under magnification.

Orthopaedic

Orthopaedic injuries are relatively uncommon following most penetrating trauma; exceptions are traumatic arthrotomies and gunshot wounds which, when the bone is hit, result in comminuted fractures if the bullet is travelling at high velocity. These often require open debridement of the wound, with reduction of fracture fragments, and may or may not lend themselves to internal fixation depending upon the degree of tissue devitalization or contamination.[10]

BLUNT TRAUMA

Fractures and soft tissue injuries are the primary problem when dealing with blunt trauma. Vascular and neurologic injuries do occur in association with fractures and when there is the possibility of vascular injury; this often takes priority over orthopaedic problems.

Vascular

Following blunt trauma, the most common injury to blood vessels is a stretch type injury. This results in thrombosis rather than hemorrhage. Sharp bone fragments can produce lacerations of major vessels. Fractures and dislocations which have an especially high incidence of vascular injury are those about the elbow and knee. If examination discloses signs of vascular injury, then arteriography should be carried out to determine the nature of the arterial injury. If the limb is acutely ischemic, arteriography, if necessary to document the location of the injury, is best carried out in the operating room before or after exposure of the presumed site of injury. The result of vascular repair in this instance is directly related to the duration of ischemia before vascular repair is completed. When the limb is viable, arteriography can be carried out in the radiologic suite. If there is no overt damage to the vessel and no obstruction or clot visible on the x-ray, then that extremity can be observed. If the vessel is normal on arteriographic examination, then treatment should be as related to soft tissue and orthopaedic injuries.

If the arteriogram shows evidence of intimal defects, intravascular clot, or obstruction of the vessel, then immediate exploration is indicated. The collateral circulation of the lower extremity is not as good as the upper extremity and thrombosis tends to be progressive. This may result in an initially viable limb becoming a nonviable one. Unless the limb can be kept under direct observation, it is imperative that partially occlusive injuries be corrected. When there is good distal flow, no "spasm," pulse deficiency, or coldness in the limb, minor lesions which have been picked up incidentally may be observed.

Venous injuries which are associated with blunt trauma are recognized primarily when arterial injuries are being exposed. These are shearing, tearing, type injuries and rarely lend themselves to simple repair.

Neurologic

Loss of motor or sensory function in the anatomical area consistent with injury to a major nerve does not necessarily require immediate investigation. These are often contused injuries and function may return spontaneously. Should exploration of the wound be carried out, the exact extent of the injury may be difficult to assess. If a divided nerve should be encountered at operation, primary repair may be performed if the wound is clean and the patient stable. For dirty wounds, or unstable patients, the nerve ends are best approximated, stabilized to the surrounding soft tissues, and marked with nonabsorbable suture to facilitate subsequent identification. Repair is then best deferred until the wound has healed or the patient can tolerate the procedure.

Fractures

For closed fractures, immediate reduction and immobilization is often appropriate. Most fractures of the femur and tibia are now being treated by internal fixation which has resulted in a marked decrease in morbidity. External fixation represents an alternative if there is extensive soft tissue contamination or damage.

If open or compound fractures are present, it is imperative to debride the wounds within six to twelve hours of injury. This involves extending the wound longitudinally from normal tissue above to normal tissue below. The wound tract and all nonviable tissue should be excised and all gross foreign material debrided. The fracture site and the wound should then be irrigated with copious amounts of saline. High-pressure irrigators facilitate this maneuver. Following irrigation and debridement, appropriate fixation of the extremity should be carried out.

If the open fractures are seen and treated early and contamination is minimal, internal fixation may be appropriate treatment for some injuries. External fixation or traction is utilized in the remaining instances.

Dislocations

An immediate emergency is hip dislocation, as avascular necrosis may result with even an hour delay in reduction. This is because the only collateral to the head of the femur is through the capsule of the joint. Dislocation stretches and renders the capsule ischemic and thrombosis of the feeding vessels may occur. Reduction of hip dislocations can even go on as resuscitation is being instituted. Reduction can be done within a matter of minutes immediately following induction of anesthesia for other procedures, such as laparotomy for urgent bleeding.

Knee dislocation constitutes another special problem. The dislocation can be anterior, posterior, lateral, or rotatory. Since most dislocations occur with auto accidents, dislocation of the distal leg is usually posterior. All of these dislocations stretch the popliteal artery with high probability of damage. One of the commonest medicolegal problems results from failure to promptly recognize popliteal artery injury. Ischemic consequences of unrecognized injury may well develop when the knee is immobilized in plaster or not monitored closely. If the injury consists of a simple intimal tear, flow may well proceed past the area of injury and result in what appears to be normal distal perfusion. With the passage of hours, particularly if the knee is absolutely immobilized, there may be a progressive buildup of platelet thrombus with ultimate obstruction of the popliteal artery and resultant distal ischemia. The collateral about the knee joint, particularly in a patient with a major knee injury, such as dislocation, is usually marginal; so thrombosis of the main artery under these circumstances results in severe ischemia of the distal leg. For this reason, popliteal dislocations, whether or not pulses are normal, should have arteriography if possible. This can be done in the operating room with needle puncture of the common femoral artery and appropriate time delay to allow the dye to reach the popliteal region or can be done in the x-ray suite utilizing a multiple film changer. Should the intimal tear detected be so minor that there is no decrease in pulse or evidence of ischemia or intravascular thrombus, then it may be observed. Any change in pulse status or limb perfusion should result in immediate operation. All lesions associated with compromise of the lumen, whether from intimal disruption or from thrombus, should be operated on immediately.

Hand Injuries

Because of the intricate nature of the hand and because injuries of the hand result in significant disability, meticulous treatment is required. Emergency management involves immobilization of the hand in the position of function, that is, with the wrist dorsiflexed, the thumb abducted and slightly flexed, and the fingers slightly flexed (the football throwing position).

Hand injuries can involve the soft tissues, the tendons, the nerves, and, of course, the bones. Most blunt trauma problems involve fractures. These, for the most part, carry less morbidity than corresponding tendon or nerve injuries as the vascularity of the hand assures good healing, the primary exception being carpal injuries such as the navicular.

PEDIATRIC FRACTURES

In adults, many isolated fractures are stabilized via surgical methods to permit rapid mobilization of the limb and better functional recovery. With a few exceptions such as hip fractures, most isolated fractures in children can be handled nonoperatively.

The trauma victim with open growth plates is different. Although not universally handled the same as the adult, the two are very similar.[14] Often the child is more resistant to the complications that occur in adults at long-term bedrest with multiple system injury, but no childhood immunity to these complications exists. Therefore, the pediatric trauma victim is to be approached with the same treatment philosophy of rapid mobilization as for the adult.[12,13,18] Although the same philosophy is used, different treatment techniques may be required to attain the goals of this philosophy.

Many fractures in the pediatric polytrauma victim require the same stabilization procedures that are used in these fractures in adults (such as pelvis, femur, and tibia fractures as well as most open fractures)[18] to allow early mobilization for the prevention of systemic complications.[14]

Fractures that involve displacement of the growth plates (Salter-Harris III and IV lesions), more than any other fracture, demand anatomic reduction[12] to prevent subsequent growth deformity whether they occur as isolated injuries or in the trauma victim. Many of these will require forms of internal fixation to stabilize them.

Operative treatment can interfere with subsequent growth if the surgery violates the growth plate. In such instances, special operative techniques are required such as the use of thin smooth pins that are removed after a few weeks instead of plates and screws. Alternatively, fixation devices may be placed in such a way so as to avoid the growth plate. Otherwise, the potential growth deformity that can result from standard adult fixation techniques may be worse than those that might occur from not operating on the fracture.

Due to the rapid healing powers in children, the goal of early mobilization can often be reached with closed treatment of some of the less severe fractures such as ankles and tibias. In the younger child especially, early bone healing and stability may occur within the first couple of weeks. The child is also very resilient to immobilization of the extremities. The stiffness found in adults after weeks of joint immobilization is rarely encountered in children.

PRIORITIZATION OF FRACTURES

When multiple orthopaedic injuries are present coupled with other major system trauma, priorities must be developed for the order in which these should be handled. Listing all potential combinations would be encyclopedic, yet still inadequate. There is no formula for "the only way to do it." However, by using the basic philosophy outlined on approaching orthopaedic trauma, and the details from the ensuing chapters, a sound plan of management can be arrived upon.

Obviously, the issues that must be first dealt with are those that are life threatening. By and large, these are nonorthopaedic injuries involving the head and trunk. Occasionally the orthopaedist is called upon to intervene in some life-threatening situations. These include exsanguination from fracture lacerations of major vessels or from severe pelvic fracture, and massive crushing injuries such as traumatic near-hemipelvectomy or forequarter amputation. Here the massive tissue trauma contributes to hemodynamic instability or coagulopathy and requires completion of the amputation to reverse these processes.

Once it is clear the patient is stable after the acutely life-threatening injuries are taken care of, the limb-threatening injuries can be addressed.[16] The time when the patient's life is no longer acutely threatened by the injuries can be difficult to clearly delineate. The orthopaedic injuries influence the overall status of the patient and vice versa. Because of this, the operative care of fractures in the polytrauma victim is often more aggressive than that used for the same fracture occurring as an isolated injury.[14–16] Operative stabilization of fractures prevents ongoing tissue injury, modifies blood loss, permits the patient to be mobilized, and by so doing prevents or modifies pulmonary and thromboembolic complications. The patient is rarely a more favorable candidate for surgical treatment than in the first 24 to 36 hours following injury and following initial stabilization.

The musculoskeletal injuries should be classified as emergent, urgent, semi-elective, or elective, and then addressed surgically on this basis (Table 1–2). This is a relative scale and does not mean that the patient's emergent injuries are operated immediately, and then he is returned at a later date to operate on the elective injuries. Every injury is best treated as soon as possible, and the classification is only to decide the order of addressing the patient's injuries—ideally all at the same sitting.

The emergent injuries threaten the survivability of the limb, or indirectly, that of the patient, and therefore must be addressed immediately. This often requires working on an extremity while the general surgeon is doing an abdominal procedure. The treatment of life-threatening injuries such as traumatic amputations or near-amputations causing massive hemorrhage and the crush injuries leading to coagulopathy already mentioned take precedence over any other orthopaedic injuries.

The first limb-threatening issues dealt with are the ischemic limbs with vascular compromise.[16] This includes lesions to the vessels themselves, indirect vessel lesions due to compression from displaced fractures or dislocated joints, and the compartment syndromes.

Joint dislocations must be reduced as soon as possible, but certainly within the first six

---

Table 1–2   Injury Prioritization

Emergent	**Semi-Elective**
Life threatening	Fractures preventing patient mobil-
Exsanguinating injuries	ization
Traumatic amputations	Lower extremity
Near amputations	Acetabulum
Pelvic crush fractures	Minor pelvis
Massive crush causing coagulopathy	Major upper extremity
Limb threatening	Open soft tissue injuries
Vessel injuries	Lacerations
Vessel compromise from fractures or dislocations	Tendon and ligament lacerations
Compartment syndrome	**Elective**
Joint dislocations	Minor upper extremity fractures
Progressive neurologic lesions	Minor foot and ankle fractures
Urgent	"Non-operative" fractures oper-
Open fractures	atively stabilized to ease nursing
Traumatic arthrotomies	care
Fractures contributing to ARDS, fat embolism,	Closed soft tissue injuries
hemorrhage	Ligament and tendon tears
Long bones	
Major pelvic disruptions	
Fractures associated with massive swelling	
Fractures at risk for avascular necrosis	

hours of injury. All will do best when reduced in this initial emergent period. The sooner the joint is reduced, the easier and less traumatic the reduction and the quicker the restoration of normal circulation to the periarticular structures. A closed reduction can be performed in a matter of minutes and thus will not delay any other necessary procedures.

Other emergent injuries are those where a partial neurologic lesion is present and is in danger of progression. These are primarily situations where pressure is present on the nerves due to displaced fracture fragments or a dislocation, or a compartment syndrome, and rapid decompression is required. Decompression can often be done by simply reducing the dislocation or grossly aligning the fracture fragments. Progressive neurologic lesions from spinal cord injury fall into this category as well.

The next group, the urgent injuries, include fractures that are best treated early before their natural course of development causes complications that might preclude a good local result. These injuries are treated within the first six hours, and certainly no later than twelve hours postinjury. As a rule, once the patient has been stabilized, the sooner any injury is treated the better, no matter what its prioritization. Thus, injuries in the emergent category take precedence over those in the urgent. If no emergent injuries are present, one proceeds directly with the urgent injuries without delay.

The most common urgent injuries are open fractures and open dislocations, and traumatic arthrotomies. The treatment of these injuries is more thoroughly discussed in Chapter 7. If the survivability of a limb is not in question, open injuries should be addressed before any others as the incidence of infection rises with the length of time before irrigation and debridement can be carried out. Major fractures, such as long bone and pelvic injuries, which require stabilization to prevent systemic complications such as continued hemorrhage or pulmonary compromise, should be treated at this stage as well.[16,17]

Other urgent injuries include cases where massive swelling is expected, such as pilon fractures of the distal tibia and the Lisfranc injuries to the midfoot. Some fractures and dislocations by their nature compromise the blood supply to vital areas of the bone or joint. These include fractures involving the femoral, radial, and humeral heads as well as talar fractures. Prompt treatment of these injuries may prevent avascular necrosis and a poor result.

The next group of injuries, the semielective, when occurring by themselves, can often be treated just as effectively on a delayed basis, but should be treated in a timely fashion in the multiple trauma victim. These are generally the injuries which interfere with mobilization of the patient. Although their presence may not directly threaten the patient's condition initially, and prompt intervention is not mandatory for a good functional result, treating them on a timely basis will help to improve the patient's overall status. The patient with multiple injuries is generally in his best medical condition early on, and prompt treatment may be associated with the best overall chance to lower morbidity and decrease the risk of possible mortality. Stabilizing the lower extremity fractures (such as femoral condylar and tibial plateau fractures) and the acetabular and more minor pelvic fractures will allow the rapid mobilization of the patient and prevent pulmonary and thromboembolic problems.

The last group of fractures requiring treatment, the elective fractures, are those that do not interfere with mobilizing the patient. Examples would include minor upper extremity fractures, and lesser fractures about the foot and ankle. If these need operative fixation, they have the last priority. On occasion, an intraoperative event may occur and cut short the time available to treat the patient. At such times, the important procedures will have been completed and the more minor ones can be done later on a delayed basis.

SUMMARY OF GENERAL PRINCIPLES

When there has been a major vascular injury and the limb is ischemic, every attempt should be made to restore blood flow within 6 to 8 hours of injury. This appears to be the golden period for vascular ischemia since major masses of muscle are lost if revascularization is not carried out in this period and the reperfusion of profoundly ischemic limbs with damaged muscle can result in loss of life. Moreover, if revascularization is carried out so late that major muscle masses have been lost then further attempts to salvage the limb should be abandoned since a prosthesis often promises a more prompt and complete rehabilitation. Therefore, emphasis must be on screening immediately for vascular injuries and even subtle changes should be taken seriously. Arteriography should be used liberally to evaluate the blood vessels of the extremity.

Most injuries related to blunt trauma consist of fractures. These far and away result in most of the morbidity in the trauma victim, since soft tissue injuries, blood vessel injuries, and all but nerve injuries heal promptly. Fractures, however, can result in disabilities lasting for months, and if major joints are involved, often result in permanent disability.

Ordinarily, when the bone is broken, the endosteum and periosteum are torn and the surrounding soft parts are damaged to a greater or lesser extent. As a result of ruptured blood vessels and lymphatics, the tissues become hemorrhagic, indurated with blood lymph, and exudate. This results in progressive swelling, pain, and local circulatory disturbances, all of which are increased by handling the extremity and motion of the bone fragments.

Damage to the associated soft tissues progress in the first 24 hours, and at the end of this time muscles and other soft parts have become edematous and indurated. Bullae or blisters may form within the skin. Satisfactory reduction of fractures attempted at this point in time is more difficult to accomplish, produces further soft tissue damage, and has a higher risk of infection. There is no question that the best time to treat fractures is within the first 24 hours following injury. Reduction and fixation of these fractures stabilize the area of injury, prevent further soft tissue damage, lower secondary morbidity from multiple organ failure syndromes, and actually decrease the risk of infection both locally and systemically.

Traction may be necessary to manage certain injuries that cannot be reduced, fixed, and stabilized initially. Inevitably, fracture fragments move within the traction device which slows local fracture healing, particularly in the restless, agitated patient, and may result in progressive soft tissue damage.

Because of excellent vascularity, upper extremity fractures and dislocations, as a rule, tend to do well unless vascularity has been compromised through vascular or extensive soft tissue injury. The upper extremity is more easily immobilized, stresses during healing of the fracture are less, and prognosis for most fractures is excellent. Hand injuries can vary from simple to complex. The more complex injuries are then related to crush, or those related to flexor tendon or nerve injury. Every effort should be made to save as much tissue as possible with badly injured upper extremities. This should be carried to the point where traumatic amputations, particularly those distal to the forearm, should have an attempt made at replantation should this service be available. Every bit of tissue in the upper extremity is important for function. Salvage of fingers, portions of hand, or as much length of the extremity as possible decreases the severity of the subsequent disability.

Attempts to maximize the salvage of tissue in the lower extremities is not so important since function is far less specialized and a prosthesis readily substitutes for loss of a limb, particularly when the amputation is carried out at the below-knee or more distal level. Limitation caused by below-knee amputation is negligible compared to the morbidity of ill-advised attempts to salvage anesthetic limbs to which there has been extensive bony damage.

Lower extremity fractures and dislocations, particularly those which involve the hip, the knee joint, and the ankle joint, can produce prolonged morbidity. When joints are involved, internal fixation with precise realignment of fractures markedly lessens morbidity. Internal or external fixation of long bones which is sufficient to produce good stabilization and permits early mobilization lessens morbidity.

Neurologic injuries, particularly those involving proximal nerves, remain the major unsolved problem. The more distal the nerve injury, the better the prognosis following repair. Proximal lesions involving the brachial plexus, the lumbosacral plexus, or the sciatic nerve carry a poor prognosis. Muscle atrophy is profound before reinnervation of muscles occurs. The use of magnification techniques to properly align nerve bundles combined with meticulous suturing technique have markedly improved the prognosis of neurologic injuries.

Microvascular techniques have progressed to the point where replantation following clean amputation of hand or digits are associated with a relatively good prognosis. Lower extremity replantation is less successful than those related to the upper extremity. As previously noted, prosthetic rehabilitation is usually more satisfactory than replantation.

Excellent results in the management of extremity injuries require a smooth functioning team and close working relationships between the various specialties involved in trauma, including orthopaedists, hand surgeons, and general and vascular surgeons.

REFERENCES

1. Gross SD. *A Manual of Military Surgery*. San Francisco, Calif: Norman Publishing Co; 1990.
2. Dammann G. *Civil War Medical Instruments and Equipment*. Missoula, Mont: Pictorial Histories Publishing Co; 1963.
3. Committee on Trauma, American College of Surgeons. *The Early Care of the Injured Patient*. Philadelphia, Pa: WB Saunders; 1972.
4. Shaftan GW. The initial evaluation of the multiple trauma patient. *World J Surg*. 1983;7:19–25.
5. Andersen RJ, Robsen RW, Lee BC. Reduced dependency on arteriography for penetrating extremity trauma: influence of wound location and noninvasive vascular studies. *J Trauma*. 1990;30:1059.
6. Gustillo RB, Mendoza RM, Williams DN. Problems in the management of Type III (severe) open fractures. *J Trauma*. 1984;24:742.
7. Peck JJ, Eastman B, Bergan JJ, Sedwitz MM, Hoyt DB, McReynolds DG. Popliteal vascular trauma: a community experience. *Arch Surg*. 1990;125.1339.
8. Sunderland S. *Nerves and Nerve Injuries*. New York, NY: Churchill Livingstone; 1978.
9. Cone JB. Vascular injury associated with fracture-dislocations of the lower extremity. *Clin Orthop*. 1989;243:30–35.
10. Chapman MW, ed. *Operative Orthopaedics*. Philadelphia, Pa: JB Lippincott Co; 1988.
11. Mackersie RC, et al. Major skeletal injuries in the obtunded blunt trauma patient: a case for routine radiologic survey. *J Trauma*. 1988;28:1450–1454.
12. Rang M. *Children's Fractures*. 2nd ed. Philadelphia, Pa: JB Lippincott Co; 1983.
13. Allgöwer M, Border J. Management of open fractures in the multiple trauma patient. *World J Surg*. 1983;70:88.
14. Loder RT. Pediatric polytrauma: orthopaedic care and hospital course. *J Orthop Trauma*. 1987;1:48–54.
15. Myers MH. *The Multiply Injured Patient with Complex Fractures*. Philadelphia, Pa: Lea & Febiger; 1984.
16. Tscherne H, et al. Osteosynthesis of major fractures in polytrauma. *World J Surg*. 1983;7:80–87.
17. Bone L, Bucholz R. The management of fractures in the patient with multiple trauma. *J Bone Joint Surg*. 1986;68–A:945–949.
18. Weber BG, Bruner Ch, Freuler F, eds. *Treatment of Fractures in Children and Adolescents*. Berlin, Germany: Springer–Verlag; 1980.

2
Soft Tissue Injury

JAMES P. KENNEDY, M.D.

HISTORY: The treatment of wounds likely began when man first injured himself. However, the first recorded documentation of wound management was in the Edwin Smith papyrus (1650 BC), which discussed the management of a gaping wound of the shoulder. The recommendation was that "thou shouldst bind it with fresh meat the first day." If on the second examination "thou findest a wound, its flesh laid back, thou shouldst draw together for him its gash with two strips of linen over that gash; thou shouldst treat it afterwards with grease, honey, and lint every day until he recovers."[17]

Although the Hippocratic legacy left much to be desired in its recommendations regarding wounds, the Greek emphasis on cleanliness and generous affusions with wine were a discovery which survived the ups and downs of history. Later, the subsequent bleedings, starvings and purgings that were the standard during the Middle Ages for the treatment of wounds spread over the Western world and more than undid the positive recommendations of the Greeks.[17]

INTRODUCTION

Soft tissue injuries in the polytrauma victim are often initially overlooked due to more serious life- or limb-threatening injuries that take precedence in treatment. Although most of the soft tissue injuries don't require emergent attention, it is important to recognize such injuries and address them after the patient is stabilized and when the other more important injuries have been treated. Doing so will result in fewer complications and a better end result.

The presence and location of such injuries as scratches, abrasions, contusions, lacerations, and avulsions will not only provide a clue that underlying injury may be present, but also will influence how the underlying vascular, neurological, and musculoskeletal injuries can be treated.

16

EXAMINATION

Examination of soft tissue injuries is crucial to determine their nature and severity as well as to rule out the presence of injury to underlying tendons, arteries, or nerves. It must also be determined whether the soft tissue envelope about a fracture site or joint has been violated.

Unfortunately, it is not always possible to have the luxury of examining a cooperative patient and getting an unequivocal exam. Adequate systemic or local analgesia is often necessary to examine these injuries. After preparation with an antiseptic solution, the entire area should be thoroughly examined visually and by palpation to determine its depth and direction. In order to perform this, the traumatic wound must generally be extended in order to obtain proper exposure. The exploration is done keeping in mind the wounding mechanism and the position of the extremity at the time of injury.

Patients are rarely injured in the supine position in which they are routinely examined. A laceration over the patella may reveal intact fascia with the knee in extension, but with the knee flexed (as it was at the time of injury), the "hidden" infrapatellar tendon laceration can be found (Figure 2–1A, B).

All structures coursing beneath the skin at the level of injury are also functionally examined—even if the wound appears small. Knives, especially, are notorious for causing a small, innocent-looking entrance wound, yet producing significant internal injury at a site distant from their entrance.

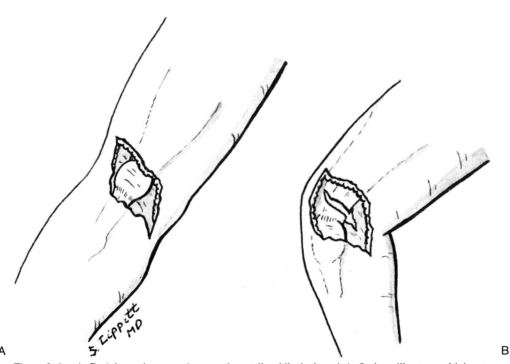

A   B

Figure 2–1. **A, B:** A laceration occurring over the patella while the knee is in flexion will not reveal injury to deep tissues if examined in extension. When examined in the position which the injury occurred, a laceration to the quadriceps tendon may be found.

Nerve injury is determined by two-point sensory exam and motor testing of each respective peripheral nerve. Tendons are individually examined by active range of motion. These tests must not be resistive as this will cause pain and, more importantly, may convert a partial tendon laceration into a complete one. The presence of gentle active movement is sufficient to confirm an intact motor nerve-muscle-tendon unit. The vascular exam consists of noting whether palpable pulses are present distal to the laceration as well as documenting the status of distal perfusion.

If examination cannot confirm the presence of normal underlying structures, surgical exploration may be indicated. This is especially true when lacerations are found about joints. The management of traumatic arthrotomies are discussed below.

Whenever examination reveals that a break in the skin has occurred, tetanus prophylaxis is instituted based on the patient's immunization history (Table 2–1). Minor clean lacerations without other associated injury require only prompt debridement and irrigation without the use of systemic antibiotics. Traumatic arthrotomies, grossly contaminated lacerations, cases in which treatment is delayed, or those that have significant soft tissue devitalization are given prophylactic perioperative systemic antibiotics. Lacerations involving fracture sites are treated by the open fracture protocol (see Chapter 7).

ABRASION

Abrasions are generally minor nuisances, but as such, are at risk for being ignored. The location of an abrasion must always be noted, as any planned operative approach should avoid this area if at all possible to decrease risk for infection.

Abrasions are cleaned with an antiseptic solution. A soft brush used on "road rash" will remove grit and dirt. Application of a brush early will prevent complications and help avoid tattooing from intradermal foreign material. An occlusive nonadherent dressing such as petroleum jelly-impregnated gauze, or an antibiotic ointment with gauze will promote healing and ease the pain of dressing changes.

CONTUSION

Contusions are a result of blunt trauma to the soft tissues with resultant hemorrhage and edema. Any area with visible signs of contusion is at risk for more significant underlying

Table 2–1   Tetanus Prophylaxis Regimen

IMMUNIZATION HISTORY	IMMUNOGLOBULIN (HYPERTET)	TOXOID (dT)
None		
Unknown	250 mg	.5 cc
No booster for more than 10 yrs		
Last booster between 5 and 10 yrs	—	.5 cc
Last booster less than 5 yrs	—	—

injuries. In the uncooperative or unconscious patient this means radiographic studies are required to rule out underlying fractures.

With more significant contusion and bleeding, hematoma may develop. Usually treated symptomatically, only cases of large hematomas which produce pressure on and functional impairment of neurovascular structures require surgical decompression. Large intramuscular hematomas may not be completely resorbed, and can become fibrotic or be converted into cartilaginous tissue.[29]

Intramuscular hematomas sometimes ossify to form myositis ossificans, also known as myositis ossificans traumatica,[29] in a process similar to the formation of fracture callus.[8] Myositis ossificans itself is pain-free unless pressure on surrounding tissues occurs, the lesion is in a location making it susceptible to repetitive trauma, or irritation from surrounding muscle or tendon motion leads to bursitis.

Irritation through excessive use or repetitive trauma may increase the amount of bone that ultimately forms.[15] This commonly occurs in the case of a football player who receives repetitive helmet blows to his thigh during the course of the season. Similarly, premature excision of the lesion during its active phase may lead to recurrence.[8]

Restricted joint motion or pain may be such to warrant excision of the lesion. Radiographic studies will help judge the maturity of the lesion for the proper timing of surgery.[22] Inactive myositis ossificans will have the trabecular pattern of mature, remodeled bone. Technetium bone scans are more accurate in assessing maturation. Other helpful studies include erythrocyte sedimentation rate and alkaline phosphatase levels.

LACERATION

Lacerations range from simple full thickness skin injuries to deep complex lacerations into subcutaneous tissue, fascia, or muscle. Flap avulsions with extensive subcutaneous undermining and complete avulsions with skin and subcutaneous loss are higher grades of laceration.

Simple superficial skin and subcutaneous lacerations can generally be treated in the emergency department, especially if they are clean, sharp lacerations without surrounding soft tissue damage. Following cleansing, a minimal sharp debridement is done to freshen up the skin edges if needed. Epinephrine in the locally infiltrated anesthetic is helpful with hemostasis. If the wound is promptly seen and treated, it may be sutured closed primarily. When a delay of more than 6 to 8 hours is encountered, however, it is best to leave the wound open and allow closure by secondary intention if it is small, or to perform a delayed primary closure when it is large.

More significant lacerations involving deep fascia and muscle require exploration, irrigation, and debridement in the operating room as they cannot be adequately explored without proper anesthesia, hemostasis, lighting, and surgical instruments. More than one patient has developed clostridial infection, acute osteomyelitis, or a septic joint from closing what appeared to be an innocent laceration in the emergency room, but what in fact was a deeper injury with devitalized tissue, retained foreign material, or communication with a fracture or joint.

After the surgical prep and removal of any gross foreign material, surgically extend the wound as needed for adequate exposure and exploration. The tourniquet is used here only if necessary for an adequate exploration. As soon as the hemorrhage is controlled, the tourniquet is deflated. Carefully inspect the tract of the wound for damage to vital structures in the region. The exploration is carried out in this fashion in all directions from the wound tract until normal tissues are encountered. If the wound is found to be in contact with a fracture, the protocol for open fractures is followed (see Chapter 3). Copiously irrigate the wound with a pulsatile lavage system to dilute the bacterial load and flush foreign material from the wound.

Following copious irrigation, all devitalized and contused skin, subcutaneous fat, muscle, and fascia are excised back to normal tissue. Damaged structures requiring treatment are repaired at this time. Vascular repair is generally performed initially to reperfuse the extremity. Sometimes it is helpful to obtain bony stability first to prevent damage to the vascular repair during the fracture fixation. This can be rapidly and temporarily done with an external fixator which is revised to a definitive fixation once the extremity is no longer ischemic.

Small fascial defects secondary to clean lacerations and not associated with soft tissue damage may be closed for cosmetic reasons to prevent muscle herniation. Large fascial defects generally should not be closed, especially when associated with other soft tissue or bony injury, or if one expects subsequent swelling. Compartment syndrome can be precipitated in such instances.[19]

Repair of muscle lacerations is tenuous due to the friable nature of muscle tissue, and fraught with difficulty.[7] For this reason, muscle bellies are generally not repaired unless a complete disruption of a functionally important muscle occurs. In these instances, an epimysial repair can be undertaken. Sutures can also be placed into fibrous septa within the muscle if possible.[8]

After muscle laceration, degeneration and necrosis of the damaged fibers will occur,[24] followed by repair and regeneration to some extent, with intermixed residual fibrosis. Such healing and regeneration takes six weeks, so muscle repairs should be protected for this length of time[29] through splinting or casting. The residual function of a repaired muscle depends largely upon whether it has been denervated by the injury.

Partial muscle belly lacerations can either be splinted without repair to protect the muscle from complete rupture until sufficiently healed, or an epimysial repair of the lacerated area can be performed.

If the deeper, complex lacerations not involving a fracture or extending into a joint are addressed early with aggressive treatment, they too can be closed primarily over a drain. If any delay is encountered, the wound should be left open to allow drainage with one or two loose sutures to prevent retraction of the wound margins. It is also helpful to loosely close soft tissue over any exposed vital structures such as tendon, nerves, or vascular structures to prevent their dessication or breakdown.

Suture is a foreign body and can contribute to infection. With traumatic wounds, the amount of nonabsorbable suture material used should be kept to a minimum. Synthetic sutures show a lower infection rate and monofilament is preferable to braided and multifilament materials.[26] Of the synthetic monofilaments, polydiaxanone appears superior in that it demonstrates the lowest affinity toward adherence of *Staphylococcus aureus* and *Escherichia coli*.[5]

Complex lacerations are generally benefited by the short use of a splint during the healing phase. Immobilization of the soft tissues will decrease pain, swelling, and inflammation, and promote healing.

AVULSIONS

Avulsions represent those lacerations with the most significant damage. When flap avulsions (Figure 2–2) occur, shearing forces widely undermine the skin and subcutaneous tissues causing extensive devascularization, especially in distally based flaps.

As a rule, proximally based flaps do relatively well as arterial inflow and especially venous drainage are adequate. Large, distally based flaps or degloving injuries rarely will heal due to edema and devascularization of subcutaneous tissues. Avulsed skin can sometimes be defatted and used as a full-thickness graft if the wound base is clean and the skin is not crushed or otherwise damaged.

These avulsion injuries are surgically handled just as the deeper complex lacerations are; however, a more extensive debridement is required due to the necessity of removing devitalized skin. This usually results in the wound not being able to be closed due to tissue loss. Flaps should be loosely tacked down to prevent their retraction. Suction drains are useful under the flap to eliminate dead space. A second debridement is often required as flaps demarcate.

Once the wound is clean with a good base and it is certain any flaps are surviving, closure of the remaining wound can be done. Based on its size and location, it can be left to spontaneously close by secondary intention; or skin grafts, or local or distant flaps can be used to close the defect.

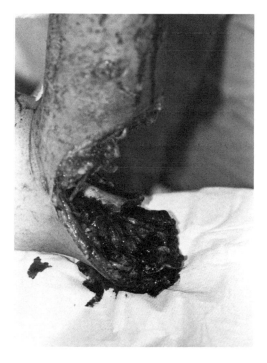

Figure 2–2. Flap avulsion of elbow resulting in near-amputation of the extremity. Humeral articular surface has been lost. Note exposed ulnar nerve at corner of wound.

TRAUMATIC ARTHROTOMY

Any laceration in the vicinity of a joint should raise the possibility of a traumatic arthrotomy. Long knife blades, shards of glass, or jagged pieces of metal can travel a great distance under the skin from the point of their entrance to penetrate into a distant joint.

Probing a wound with a gloved finger may confirm but does not rule out joint penetration. Often the capsular laceration is too small to allow the probing finger to identify it. Radiolucency of an air density within a joint cavity on radiographs (Figure 2–3) confirms that an arthrotomy has occurred and no further investigation is necessary. If air is not noted on the films, further work-up is required.

To identify a traumatic arthrotomy, or rather to confirm the absence of one, a saline, or preferably methylene blue, arthrogram must be performed. Using sterile technique and an entrance point away from the traumatic wound, a needle is placed into the joint. Fluid is injected until resistance is met. If the injected fluid is seen expressing itself from the wound, an arthrotomy has been confirmed. Saline leaking out of a bloody wound is easier to visualize if it has been tinged with methylene blue (Figure 2–4). Traumatic arthrotomy can also be confirmed in the x-ray department by an arthrogram, in which contrast material will be seen leaking out of the joint on the x-ray.

Once an arthrotomy has been confirmed, the patient should be started on the protocol for open fractures as described in Chapter 7. All of these steps are begun in the emergency room. An irrigation and debridement of the wound and joint is then performed on a timely basis in the operating room. After copious irrigation of the joint, an intra-articular drain is placed and the capsule is closed to prevent articular cartilage dessication.[23,28] The traumatic

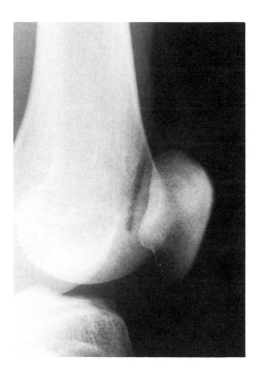

Figure 2–3. Traumatic arthrotomy resulting in air arthrogram. Note air density between patella and femur, and in the suprapatellar pouch.

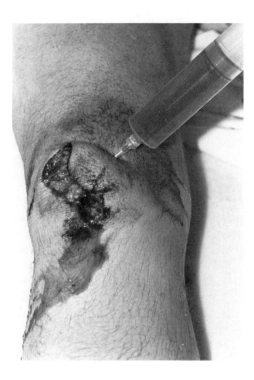

Figure 2–4. Traumatic arthrotomy demonstrated by methylene blue solution leaking out of wound after injection into joint.

portion of the wound is left open and the drain is pulled at 36 to 48 hours. The traumatic wound is then handled the same as for an open fracture (see Chapter 7).

Joints may be arthroscopically irrigated in the appropriate circumstances. With only a small violation of the capsule, the joint can be arthroscopically irrigated and inspected for intra-articular damage without a formal arthrotomy. This will save the patient a lengthy and more painful postinjury rehabilitation. If the capsule is widely open more than 2 to 3 cm, it will be difficult to maintain fluid insufflation sufficient enough to allow adequate inspection of the joint arthroscopically. Enlarging an arthrotomy of this size for direct inspection causes little further morbidity.

HEMARTHROSIS

Acute joint effusions (within 6 to 8 hours of injury) are generally hemarthroses. Sympathetic effusions of synovial fluid take 24 to 36 hours to develop postinjury. The presence of a hemarthrosis can be confirmed by joint aspiration. Such collections of blood can be as large as 300 cc mL. Such large effusions are quite painful[8] and can on occasion precipitate neurovascular compromise of surrounding structures. For these reasons, repeated aspiration of these tense hemarthroses may be required.

Blood, combined with synovial fluid, will produce an intense synovitis, contributing to the joint pain.[29] Although repeated hemarthroses (such as those that occur in hemophiliacs) will lead to eventual total arthritic destruction of the joint,[1] it is generally felt that a single isolated hemarthrosis will cause no long-term damage.[29] Therefore, most hemarthroses can be treated by bulky compressive dressings, ice, elevation, and rest until they resolve.

There are relatively few structures within the joint that can bleed, and the differential diagnosis is limited to damage of the vascular structures which include: anterior and posterior cruciate ruptures, peripheral meniscal tears (in the vascular zone), capsular tear or laceration, osteochondral fractures, or spontaneous bleeding diatheses such as seen in hemophilia or platelet disorders.

SWELLING SYNDROMES

The most important of these is the compartment syndrome discussed in Chapter 20. A condition less well known outside orthopaedic circles is fracture blistering. Although these do not compromise the limb as much as the compartment syndrome, fracture blisters do affect the type of treatment possible for the underlying fracture. If the fracture blisters are not treated appropriately, infection can occur.

Fracture blistering occurs from soft tissue swelling. Increased pressure within the dermis causes exudation of fluid resulting in the blistering which can occur rapidly after injury. Most commonly these blisters are small, few in number, and generally occur in areas without significant subcutaneous tissue such as the ankle. Severe cases can also occur (Figure 2–5), usually in conjunction with distal tibial pilon and tibial shaft fractures. The anticipation of the development of blistering will prompt the decision for early operation

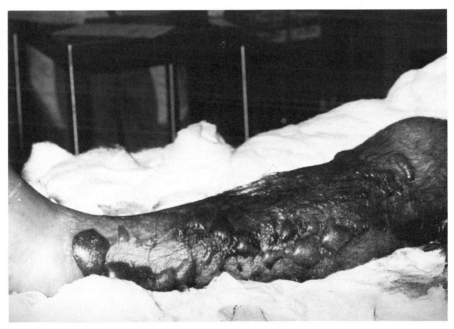

Figure 2–5.   Severe fracture blisters following tibial fracture.

before they occur. The operative incision will decompress the limb and often prevent later blistering, much as a fasciotomy decompresses a compartment syndrome.

Although it may be possible to operate through blisters after prepping the leg to break the blisters, debriding them, and reprepping, without increased incidence of infection,[13] most surgeons feel that the risk of infection is too high to permit placing an incision in an area of fracture blisters.

SPRAINS AND STRAINS

Sprained ligaments and strained muscles rarely if ever need to be addressed acutely in the polytrauma patient. Often the diagnosis is not immediately apparent, and may be delayed several days or even weeks until after the patient begins to recover from his severe injuries and notices a sore ankle. The knowledge that these "trivial" injuries often occur in the polytrauma victim will prompt the physician to look for them with serial exams and to warn the patient that additional minor injuries may be discovered late.

Sprains and strains are graded I, II, and III.[8] Grade I implies stretching and injury to the ligament or muscle without laxity or failure. Grade II describes a structure that is partially incompetent with laxity but without loss of continuity. Grade III injuries are those in which complete disruption and gross incompetency of the tissue has occurred. Grade III sprains may be associated with a joint dislocation.

In the trauma patient, the more minor Grade I and II injuries are treated symptomatically with elevation and immobilization. More severe injuries may need early operative intervention on occasion. These would include the Grade III sprains that are associated with joint dislocation. The treatment of dislocations and need for urgent or emergent relocation is discussed further in the chapters on individual anatomic areas. Surgical repair of Grade III sprains is generally not acutely indicated in the polytrauma victim.[8] If an open surgical procedure is being performed in the area of the injured ligament for other reasons, and if additional surgical time poses no added risk to the patient, primary ligamentous repair of Grade III lesions may be undertaken in selected patients. Otherwise, delayed reconstruction can be performed if late instability ensues.

HETEROTOPIC OSSIFICATION

Heterotopic ossification is the formation of bone in soft tissues or around a joint usually secondary to injury. The elbow, shoulder, and hip are the most frequently involved joints.[12] Risk of heterotopic ossification is present following soft tissue injury, burns, fracture, joint dislocation, or extensive surgical exposures of periarticular areas.[4] The risk of severe heterotopic ossification is increased in the polytrauma patient, especially if a head or spinal cord injury has occurred.[10] Heterotopic ossification is found in 11% of head-injured patients, and in 20% of those with spinal cord injury.[12] In these instances, heterotopic ossification can occur even in the absence of injury about the joint (Figure 2–6).

Although usually asymptomatic unless bursae form about the bone mass or surrounding structures are impinged upon, heterotopic ossification can lead to severely restricted joint motion or even ankylosis due to a mechanical block. For this reason, measures to prevent this condition are best undertaken for those patients at risk.

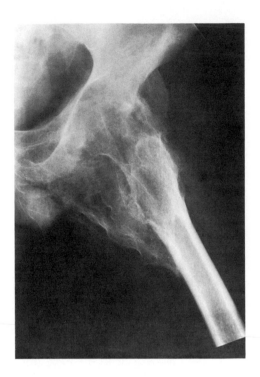

Figure 2–6. Severe heterotopic bone about hip joint. The patient suffered a head injury; the hip was not injured. The patient recovered, but was left with a bony ankylosis of his hip.

Various methods for the prevention of heterotopic ossification have been used in the past. Diphosphonates have been shown to inhibit mineralization, but osteoid will still form and will subsequently ossify with cessation of the diphosphonate[21] treatment.

Indomethacin has been shown to be effective in the prophylaxis of heterotopic ossification.[20] Recently, a protocol of indomethacin 25 mg given three times daily for the first six postoperative weeks was proven to give good results[25] in total hip patients. This regimen has proven equally effective following operative fixation of acetabular fractures.[18] Though not yet proven efficacious in generalized posttraumatic heterotopic ossification, it seems logical to assume that it will be effective in these instances as well.

Unfortunately, in many cases the polytrauma patient is unable to take oral input because of internal injuries. Although it is possible to administer the indomethacin via a rectal suppository, this method has not been used in clinical trials, and there is still concern about the development of a stress ulcer regardless of the route of administration.

For patients unable to tolerate oral prophylaxis, radiation has been shown to be helpful in the prevention of both posttraumatic heterotopic ossification,[4] and that associated with total hip arthroplasty.[2] Ionizing radiation will suppress the formation of heterotopic bone if given before the fourth postoperative day.[2] Radiation therapy is not without risks such as the induction of malignancy, sterility, and genetic mutation.[4] Although it is generally felt that divided doses of less than 3000 total rads are safe,[14] it seems logical to deliver the lowest possible effective dose. The standard protocol for the prophylaxis of heterotopic ossification has been 1000 rads in divided doses of 200 rads each.[2,4]

Although this regimen has been proven useful for total hip arthroplasty patients, it is logistically almost impossible to transport a critically ill patient for five consecutive days to the radiation therapy unit which is often ill-equipped to handle such unstable patients. Investigation is underway to see if single doses of radiation will be effective. Early results using a single 700 rad dose in total hip patients has been shown to be effective,[16] but this has yet to be proven useful for posttraumatic heterotopic ossification.

In the instances where for whatever reason the patient cannot be subjected to prophylaxis, early range of motion of the extremities must be diligently performed to minimize the subsequent loss of motion if heterotopic ossification occurs.

If the amount of motion obtained is not acceptable, the heterotopic ossification may be excised. The excision of these lesions is handled similarly to that of myositis ossificans, in that one must wait for the lesion to mature before attempting to remove it, or else recurrence will be a problem.[11] Just as for myositis ossificans, bone scans and alkaline phosphatase are helpful in gauging the maturity of the bone[9,11] for the timing of excision. Following the excision, the patient must be prophylaxed or the ossification is assured to recur.

REFERENCES

1. Arnold WD, Hilgartner MW. Hemophilic arthropathy. *J Bone Joint Surg*. 1977;59–A:287.
2. Ayers DC, et al. The prevention of heterotopic ossification in high-risk patients by low-dose radiation therapy after total hip arthroplasty. *J Bone Joint Surg*. 1986;68–A:1423–1430.
3. Benjamin JB, et al. Efficacy of a topical antibiotic irrigant in decreasing or eliminating bacterial contamination in surgical wounds. *Clin Orthop*. 1984;184:114–116.
4. Bosse MJ, et al. Heterotopic ossification as a complication of acetabular fracture: prophylaxis with low-dose radiation. *J Bone Joint Surg*. 1988;70–A:1231–1237.
5. Chu C, et al. Effects of physical configuration and chemical structure of suture materials on bacterial adhesion. A possible link to wound infection. *Am J Surg*. 1984;147.197–204.
6. Crenshaw AH, ed. *Campbell's Operative Orthopaedics*. 7th ed. St. Louis, Mo: CV Mosby Company; 1987.
7. Epps C Jr, ed. *Complications in Orthopaedic Surgery*. Philadelphia, Pa: JB Lippincott Co; 1978.
8. Evarts, CM, ed. *Surgery of the Musculoskeletal System*. New York, NY: Churchill Livingstone; 1983.
9. Furman R, et al. Elevation of the serum alkaline phosphatase coincident with ectopic-bone formation in paraplegic patients. *J Bone Joint Surg*. 1970;52–A:1131–1137.
10. Garland DE, et al. Periarticular heterotopic ossification in head injured adults: incidence and location. *J Bone Joint Surg*. 1980;62–A:1143.
11. Garland DE, et al. Resection of heterotopic ossification in the adult with head trauma. *J Bone Joint Surg*. 1985;67–A:1261–1269.
12. Garland DE. Clinical observations on fractures and heterotopic ossification in the spinal cord and traumatic brain injured populations. *Clin Orthop*. 1988;233:86–101.
13. Johnson KD. Personal communication. 1988.
14. Kim JH, et al. Radiation-induced soft tissue and bone sarcoma. *Radiology*. 1978;129:501–508.
15. Lipscomb G, et al. Treatment of myositis ossificans trauma in athletes. *Am J Sports Med*. 1976;4:111–120.
16. Lo TC, et al. Single dose postoperative hip irradiation in the prevention of heterotopic bone formation. *Radiat Oncol Biol Phys*. 1986;12(suppl 1):131–132.
17. Majno G. *The Healing Hand: Man and Wound in the Ancient World*. Boston, Mass: Harvard University Press; 1975.
18. McLaren AC. Prophylaxis with indomethacin for heterotopic bone. *J Bone Joint Surg*. 1990;72–A:245–247.
19. Mubarak SJ, Hargens AR. *Compartment Syndromes and Volkmann's Contracture*. Philadelphia, Pa: WB Saunders; 1981.
20. Nillson OS, et al. Influence of indomethacin on induced heterotopic bone formation in rats. *Clin Orthop*. 1986;207:239–245.
21. Nollen AJG. Effect of ethylhydroxydiphosphonate (EDHP) on heterotopic ossification. *Acta Orthop Scand*. 1986;57:358–361.
22. Norman A, Dorkman H. Juxtacortical circumscribed myositis ossificans. Evolution and radiographic features. *Radiology*. 1970;96:301–306.

23. Rockwood, CA Jr, Green DP, eds. *Fractures in Adults*. 2nd ed. Philadelphia, Pa: JB Lippincott; 1984.
24. Saunders JH, Sissons HA. Effect of denervation on regeneration of skeletal muscle after injury. *J Bone Joint Surg*. 1953;35–B:113.
25. Schmidt SA, et al. The use of indomethacin to prevent the formation of heterotopic bone after total hip replacement. *J Bone Joint Surg*. 1988;70–A:834–838.
26. Sharp WV. Suture resistance to infection. *Surgery*. 1982;91:61–63.
27. Sunderland S. *Nerves and Nerve Injuries*. London, Engl: Churchill Livingstone; 1978.
28. Tscherne H, Brüggemann H. Die Weichteilbehandlung bei Osteosynthesen, insbesondere bei offenen Frakturen. *Unfallheilkunde*. 1976;79:467.
29. Turek SL. *Orthopaedics*. 4th ed. Philadelphia, Pa: JB Lippincott; 1984.

3

Splinting and Immobilization

JAMES P. KENNEDY, M.D.

HISTORY: The earliest form of splints were sticks or pieces of wood wrapped with linen bandages to bind the fracture to reduce pain. This technique was used by the ancient Egyptians. Hippocrates advocated stiffening the bandages with lard mixed with wax, rosin, or pitch.[1] Fractures would often heal in a malaligned position. Later, through trial and error, various types of splints were discovered that improved functional results upon healing. Variations of these are still used today throughout Asia. A very effective means of treating forearm fractures is to firmly bind padded wooden splints over the interosseous membrane (Figure 3–1). The pressure causes the radius and ulna to diverge, tightens the interosseous membrane, and thus immobilizes the bones.

With time, attempts were made to obtain better immobilization and maintenance of anatomic positions through better fitting devices. Albucasis in the 10th century[2] used an early form of cast by stiffening bandages with egg whites.[3] Later, the Arabs placed limbs in molds which were then filled with plaster.[4] However, the modern cast as we know it today was not developed until the 1800s. From experience gained in the French Revolution and Napoleonic Wars, Dominique Jean Larrey began treating open fractures with rigid dressings made from bandages soaked in camphorated alcohol, lead acetate, and egg whites.[5] This was subsequently improved by Louis Jean Seutin, chief surgeon of the Belgian Army at the Battle of Waterloo. Seutin used cardboard splints and bandages soaked in laundry starch which he termed "bundage amidonnée."[6] Unfortunately, the bandage amidonnée took up to three days to dry.

The use of plaster of Paris or gypsum was first made known to the Western world in the early 1800s when a British diplomat saw the ancient Arabic technique of poured plaster being used in Turkey.[1] Casting techniques as we know them today were developed in 1851 when a Dutch military surgeon, Antonius Mathijsen,[7] began treating fractures with linen bandages into which dry powdered plaster of Paris had been rubbed. The bandages were moistened with a sponge or brush as they were applied, then rubbed until they hardened.[1]

At about the same time, Nikolai Ivanovitch Pirogov, professor of surgery at the Academy of Military Medicine in St. Petersburg, began using casts made from bandages which had been dipped into liquid plaster of

Paris[8] after seeing a sculptor use this technique to make models. Pirogov used these casts extensively during the Crimean War, and felt that all fractures from missile wounds should not be evacuated from the forward aid stations until immobilized in a proper cast.[1]

INTRODUCTION

Various forms of splinting can be used to immobilize extremities depending upon the purpose the splint is to serve. This can range from temporary immobilization to allow x-rays all the way to definitive treatment.

Splints that are applied in the emergency department must immobilize the injured extremity. This can adequately be done only by preventing movement at the joint above and below the injured area. For example, a tibia fracture must be splinted from the toes up to the proximal thigh. Temporary stability of the fracture will make the patient more comfortable and easier to transfer during his trip to the x-ray department. Also, immobilizing long bone fractures will prevent further soft tissue damage and help decrease the incidence of fat embolism. These splints must allow clear radiographic visualization of the injury. Generally, plaster splints will obscure radiographic detail and are applied after x-rays are obtained.

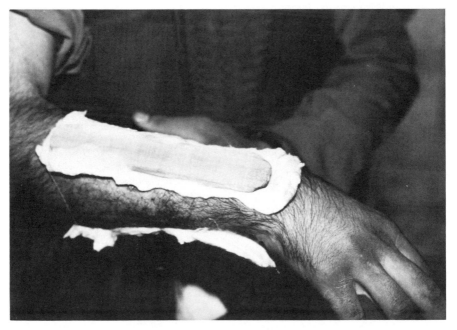

Figure 3–1.   Padded wooden splints placed over the interosseous membrane and wrapped snugly to immobilize a both-bone forearm fracture. This patient, treated by a local bone setter in Afghanistan, healed with an excellent functional result.

TYPES OF SPLINTS

For femur fractures, the Hare splint (Figure 3–2) is ideal. It permits x-rays to be taken and immobilizes the fracture through traction. Other fractures can be handled through "generic" splints. Various forms of prefabricated aluminum splints are available (Figure 3–3) that do an adequate job of immobilization and permit x-ray penetration. An ideal splint is the "cardboard box" made out of corrugated cardboard bent in the form of a "U" (Figure 3–4). These are inexpensive, strong, lightweight, disposable, simple to apply, easily trimmed with scissors, and radiolucent.

Once x-rays are obtained, a more permanent plaster splint can be applied. These mold and conform to the limb affording a greater degree of immobilization and therefore comfort. They can also be combined with the Robert Jones compressive dressing described below.

In general, the initial splint is purely an immobilizing splint pending definitive reduction and stabilization of the injury. However, the patient will be more comfortable and neurovascular function is improved if gentle traction is used to restore gross axial alignment prior to this initial splinting.

Width of splints are chosen appropriate for the size of the extremity. Precut slabs can be used, or these can be made by unrolling plaster rolls. A generous thickness of plaster is used to prevent breaking at points of stress. Short arm splints generally are 10 to 12 thicknesses; long arm splints need to be 15 to 20 to prevent breakage at the elbow. Short leg splints work well with 15 thicknesses whereas a long leg splint needs to be 20 or even 25 thicknesses. The splints must be very well padded, especially at their edges and at bony prominences to prevent abrasions, pressure sores, and burns from the heat that develops

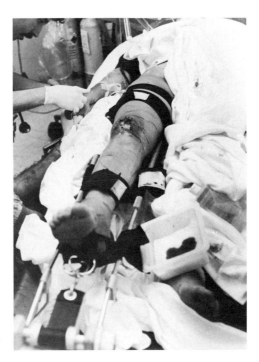

Figure 3–2. Hare splint to temporarily immobilize a femur fracture for transport.

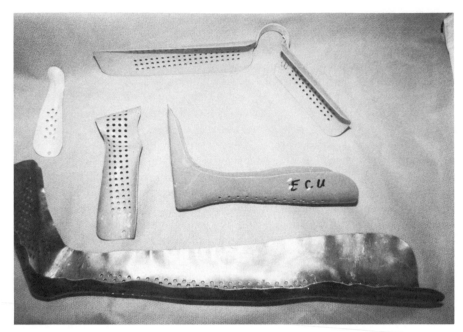

Figure 3–3. Various radiolucent aluminum splints for immobilization.

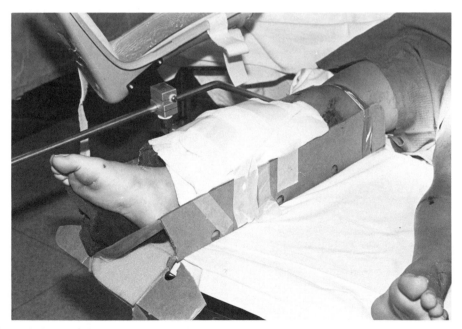

Figure 3–4. Cardboard box "U" splint to immobilize an open tibial fracture.

during the exothermic chemical reaction of the plaster hardening. If sufficient help is available, it is appropriate to apply a layer of padding to the extremity as well. The splint is applied to the extremity with bias-cut stockinette, Ace wrap, or Kerlix wrapped in such a fashion so as to prevent constriction.

Prepadded splints should not be used for anything other than temporary immobilization. Their foam rubber padding will become wet during the activation of the plaster. The authors have seen several cases of skin maceration and breakdown from this wet foam lying against the skin. In addition, they cannot be molded as a "custom" splint is.

APPLICATION

The initial "immobilization" splint used in the emergency room setting can be applied in any number of ways. In the lower extremity, it is good practice to try to place all ankles in as close to a neutral position as possible to prevent equinus deformity. This is especially true if the splint will not be changed to reposition the ankle within 24 hours. The neutral position can be achieved through a posterior splint bent at 90°, or a "U" or sugar-tong splint extending up the medial and lateral sides of the leg (Figure 3–5). For long leg splints, the knee should be gently flexed.

Splints in the upper extremity can be applied using the "resting position" of 20° of wrist extension, gentle flexion of the phalangeal joints, and abduction of the thumb (Figure 3–6). An easy way to remember this position is to imagine that the hand is in the drinking position holding a beverage can. The resting position should only be used for a short time,

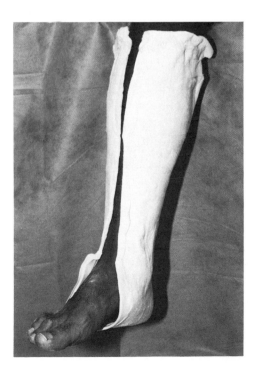

Figure 3–5.   Sugar-tong splint.

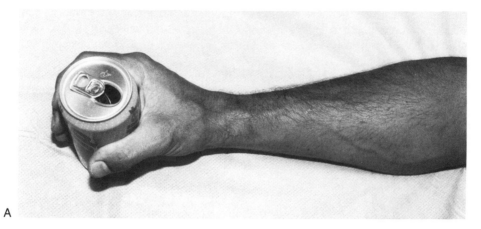

A

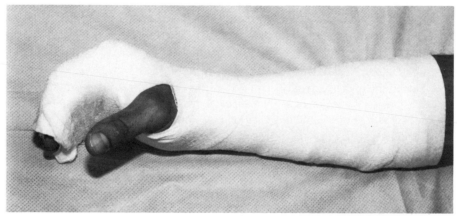

B

Figure 3–6.   **A:** The "beverage can" position for the resting hand. **B:** Resting hand splint.

and must not be confused with the "functional position" used for long-term immobilization to prevent joint contractures.

The *Robert Jones dressing* is a very useful all-purpose compressive dressing to be used acutely or following surgery (Figure 3–7). It immobilizes the injury, helps control swelling, and prevents circulatory compromise that might follow the application of tight fitting casts applied in the face of increasing swelling. A single layer of cast padding is applied to the skin to prevent irritation. Next, a layer of cotton batting is applied and then overlayered with Kerlix in some compression. The batting may be applied circumferentially or longitudinally. The author prefers the longitudinal method as it is quicker, easier for the surgeon to apply and remove, less painful for the patient, and less binding about the ankle. One or two layers of batting are applied in this manner. A splint is then applied and maintained in place with either bias or an Ace wrap. With one assistant and gentle technique, a long leg Robert Jones can be applied without undue patient discomfort even in the face of long bone fractures.

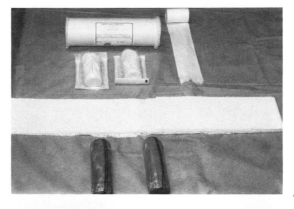

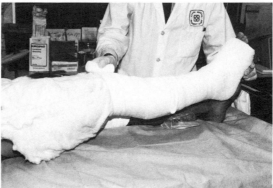

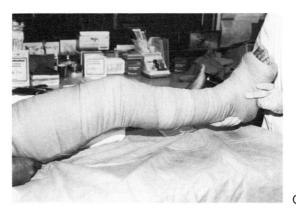

Figure 3–7. **A:** Materials needed for Robert Jones dressing. **B:** Snugly applying roller cotton batting. **C:** Robert Jones dressing finished off with splint and Ace bandage.

TRACTION

Initially described in the 1300s by Guy de Chauliac[1] who hung a weight from a cord attached to the leg over a pulley, traction changed little over the next 500 years. Starting in the 1800s, traction became more sophisticated through the use of various splints, frames, or slings in an attempt to better position fracture fragments. Skin traction uses tension on the skin for stabilization of a fracture. Popularized by Gurdon Buck who used it for femoral fractures during the Civil War,[9] Buck's traction is still the standard today for temporary immobilization of adult intertrochanteric hip fractures, and is frequently used for the definitive treatment of isolated pediatric lower extremity fractures or disorders of the hip.

TRACTION PRINCIPLES

Various forms of traction can be applied either through the bone with skeletal pins, or through the soft tissue with skin traction. It is important to know the various types (eg, Bryant's, Russel's, split Russel's, Dunlop, well-leg, balanced suspension, Apley's, Neufeld roller, Perkins, 90–90, etc.) if one plans to definitively manage fractures with traction. More simply, traction consists of applying a tension force either through the skeletal or soft tissue structures to the desired anatomic area to immobilize and prevent shortening prior to definitive fracture treatment.

For skin traction in adults, a maximum of only five pounds of weight can be used without fear of skin slough from ischemia secondary to shearing forces, and even less weight can be used for children. For this reason skin traction cannot be used in adults where there is risk of shortening at the fracture site requiring strong forces to overcome muscle pull.

The most convenient way to apply Buck's traction is to wrap the extremity with one layer of cast padding, then to apply a ready-made foam boot to which the weight is attached. An alternative is Buck's original method of fastening two strips of foam rubber or moleskin to the leg which has been painted with tincture of benzoin, then secure them with an Ace wrap. With either method, the skin must be inspected daily under the device to check for problems.

Most major fractures are best managed today utilizing skeletal traction. Traction applied directly through the skeleton permits better control of the fractured bone, allows visualization of the extremity, and allows the possibility for much greater amounts of weight to be used to reduce the fracture. Prior to the era of sterile technique, various pins had been used in an attempt to manipulate fracture fragments, but the first real use of skeletal traction was in 1903 by Codivilla who introduced the technique of pins and plaster.[10] With this method, skeletal pins are inserted into the bone and then incorporated into a cast which maintains the pins in position. This concept was expanded in 1907 by Steinmann who attached weights to through-and-through pins which permitted mobilization of the leg during traction.[11]

To employ skeletal traction, either large Steinmann pins with a traction bow, or small Kirschner wires with a clevis can be used (Figure 3–8). A large Steinmann pin is generally preferable. To prevent bowing, the thin Kirschner wire must have tension applied across it with the clevis (much as a bicycle spoke) to increase its resistance to bending. However, small wires can tend to cut out of the bone, especially if it is osteoporotic, when large traction forces are applied. Traction pins should always be inserted with a hand drill to prevent osteonecrosis from the heat generated with high-speed power drilling (Figure 3–9). An area of osteonecrosis about the pin can lead to premature loosening and an increased chance of a ring sequestrum and infection.

One has the choice of smooth, threaded, and hybrid pins. Each has its advantages. Smooth pins are easier to insert, but can tend to shift from side to side with long-term use.

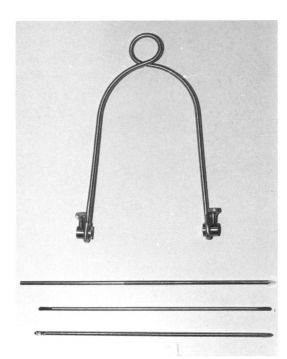

Figure 3–8. Traction bow for Steinmann pins. Hybrid, smooth, and threaded pins are pictured.

In most patients, the pin will not be present long enough to loosen, and if a large pin is chosen, it will be held tightly in the bone. (Compare the difference in ease of removing a small finishing nail versus a large spike from a piece of hard oak.) A threaded pin will not shift from side to side, but requires more force to insert or remove. A theoretical increased chance for infection exists if the skin does not seal tightly about the irregular surface of the threaded pins. If a pin is to be left in for any significant length of time, the best choice is the hybrid. This has a threaded intraosseous midsection to prevent sliding, but each end is smooth for better skin sealing. The most important factor for avoiding skin irritation and subsequent infection is tension on the skin. Tension will result in skin necrosis and irritation. Relaxing incisions to release the tension solve the problem but give the patient an ugly scar and are a poor remedy for poor technique.

The pin should be inserted from the most dangerous side to the least dangerous. Greater control is possible over where the pin goes in than where it will come out. Tibial pins are inserted from the lateral side to make sure that they do not pass posteriorly so as to interfere with the peroneal nerve. Distal femoral pins should be inserted medially so as to avoid injuring the femoral artery. Olecranon pins are inserted from the medial side where the ulnar nerve runs, and calcaneal pins are best inserted medially to avoid the posterior tibial neurovascular bundle.

Common insertion sites for pins include the proximal tibial pin at a distance of 1 to 3 cm below the anterior tibial tubercle, and the distal femoral pin just proximal to the condylar flare. During insertion of this latter pin, care must be taken so as not to violate the knee capsule and joint. Calcaneal pins through the posterior tuberosity are used fairly commonly as well. Skeletal traction can be utilized through any bone so long as the insertion of the pin

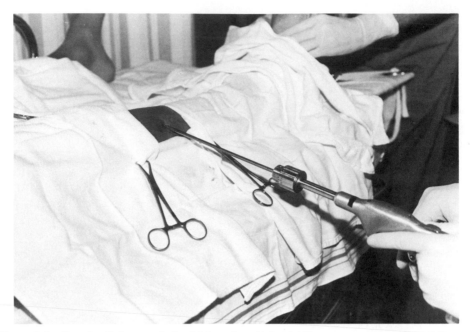

Figure 3–9. Inserting Steinmann pin for tibial traction with hand drill.

avoids vital structures. Many forms of traction used in the past have been made obsolete by internal fixation methods. Today in the multiple trauma patient there is probably little call for overhead olecranon traction for supracondylar humerus fractures, digital traction for phalangeal fractures, or side traction from the greater trochanter for acetabular fractures. The principal exception is the few instances in which the patient is too unstable to withstand surgery, forcing the physician to begin nonoperative management of the injuries. With modern anesthesia techniques and monitoring, these instances should be rare.

MANAGEMENT

The insertion of any pin is done with sterile technique using gloves and a sterile hand drill. The area is shaved if necessary, and prepped with antiseptic solution. The entrance site is chosen carefully so there will be no tension on the skin. A large wheal is raised at the entrance and exit sites with local anesthetic if the patient is not already under a general anesthetic. The soft tissues down to bone, and the periosteum especially, should be anesthetized as well. A small stab incision is necessary for the large Steinmann pins. The incision should be small enough so that the skin seals comfortably around the pin. The pin is then inserted without drilling to bone which can be palpated with the tip of the pin to choose the proper entrance site. Steady firm pressure is applied as the pin is advanced through both cortices with the drill. As the pin is advanced through the soft tissue on the far side, the skin will tent. Small pins can be popped through the skin; larger ones will require a second small stab incision at the site of exit. The pin is then advanced to the desired position and trimmed to its proper length. The sharp ends should be covered with caps or corks to prevent injury. A Betadine dressing can be applied initially to the pin site, but no further attention or dressing is required once the skin seals about the pin.

The patient can now be placed in traction. The amount of weight used depends on the size of the patient and the muscle forces that must be overcome. Simple immobilization of the extremity requires less weight than that needed to maintain a reduced position. More proximal fractures require more weight than distal fractures. For the average sized adult, pelvic and acetabular fractures generally require 20 to 30 pounds, femur fractures 15 to 20 pounds, and tibial fractures 10 to 20 pounds. Weight is gradually added in five-pound increments over the course of several minutes to allow the patient to adjust to the force. It is preferable to use the least amount of weight necessary, and add to it if it is insufficient.

Radiographs of the fracture are obtained after 8 to 12 hours of traction. This period allows for soft tissue relaxation and dissipation of muscle spasm. The alignment and amount of traction is then adjusted as needed based on the position of the bone.

REFERENCES

1. Peltier LF. *Fractures*. San Francisco, Calif: Norman Publishing; 1990.
2. Garrison FH. *History of Medicine*. Philadelphia, Pa: WB Saunders; 1929.
3. Rockwood, CA Jr, Green DP. *Fractures in Adults*. 2nd ed. Philadelphia, Pa: JP Lippincott; 1984.
4. Cimino WR, Skinner HB. The stiffness of cylindrical casts enforced with splint laminations: biomechanical considerations. *J Orthop Trauma*. 1989;3:338–344.
5. Larrey DJ. Mémoire sur une nouvelle manière de réduite ou de traiter les fractures des membres compliqueé de plais. *J Compl Dict Sci Méd*. 1824;20:193.
6. Seutin LJG. *Du Bandage Amidonnée*. Brussels, Belg: Société Encyclographique des Sciences Médicales; 1840.
7. Mathijsen A. New method for application of plaster of Paris bandage. *Clin Orthop*. 1965;38:3.
8. Pirogov NI. Der Gypsklebeverband bei einfachen und complicierten Knochenbruchen; *Klinische Chirurgie: Eine Sammlung von Monographin über die wichtigsten Gengenstande der prakitschen Chirurgie, II*. Leipzig, Ger: Breitkopf & Hartel; 1854.
9. Buck G. An improved method of treating fractures of the thigh illustrated by cases and a drawing. *Trans N Y Acad Med*. 1861;2:232–250.
10. Codivilla A. Sulla correzione della deformita da frattura del femore. *Bull Sci Med Bologna*. 1903;8:246–249.
11. Steinmann F. Eine neue Extensionsmethode in der Fracturenbehandlung. *Zentralblau für Chirurgie* 1907;34:938.

4

Upper Extremity Vascular Injury

F. WILLIAM BLAISDELL, M.D.

HISTORY: According to Hughes,[1] the first successful documented vascular repair was that of Hallowel acting on the suggestion by Lambert. In 1759, he repaired a wound of the brachial artery by placing a pin through the arterial walls and holding the edges in that position by applying a ligature in a Figure of Eight fashion about the pin. This technique (known as the Farrier's stitch) had been utilized by veterinarians but had fallen into disrepute following unsuccessful clinical experiments. In 1894, Heidenhain closed by catgut suture a one-centimeter opening in the axillary artery made accidentally while removing adherent carcinomatous glands.[1] The patient recovered without any circulatory disturbance. In Germany, in 1907, Lexer first used the saphenous vein as an arterial substitute to restore continuity after excision of an aneurysm of the axillary artery.[1] Carrel and Guthrie, around the turn of the century, established the feasibility of arterial anastomoses in numerous experiments in animals.[2] However, vascular repair was tried intermittently in World War I and most of the attempts to suture blood vessels were associated with disaster. This was because of the high frequency of infection and secondary hemorrhage which complicated the repair.

Ligation remained the standard of treatment through World War II and the experiences with vascular injuries were reported by DeBakey and Simeone in 1946.[3] There were 2471 arterial injuries, and almost all were treated by ligation with a subsequent amputation rate approximating 49%. There were only 81 repairs attempted, 78 by lateral suture and three by end-to-end anastomosis. One of the major contributions of the Korean War to medicine was the introduction of vascular repair. This was due to the improvements in anesthesia, blood transfusion, and the advent of antibiotics. In this experience with 300 arterial injuries, 269 were repaired and 35 ligated. The overall amputation rate was 13%, in marked contrast to that of 49% in World War II.[1]

INTRODUCTION

Those injuries to the subclavian and innominate arteries have been dealt with elsewhere. Injuries discussed in this chapter will be confined to the axillary, brachial, radial, and ulnar arteries. These represent nearly a third of all vascular injuries seen in American trauma centers at the present time. As opposed to other vascular injuries, the results of treatment, due to excellent collateral, have always been quite good, even though the routine repair of blood vessels is of very modern vintage.

The most optimum military medical organization came in the Vietnam War which involved rapid evacuation by helicopter to base hospitals. This permitted early definitive treatment and the management of the vascular injury left little to be desired. The amputation rate following all extremity vascular repairs fell to approximately 8%.[1] The amputation rates for axillary and brachial injuries fell to minimal levels with only one amputation in 42 axillary and brachial injuries recorded by the Vascular Registry.[1] At the present time, in most civilian practices, vascular repair is highly successful. Most upper extremity amputations, when they occur, are usually related to massive tissue injury or to associated neurologic injury rather than failure of the vascular repair.

INCIDENCE

Although the upper extremities constitute only 10% of the total body mass, injuries to upper extremity blood vessels are extremely common. They represent nearly a third of all major vascular injuries in the experience of most trauma centers, and close to half of the injuries involving the upper or lower extremities.[4–6] Drapanas noted in his review of recent conflicts of this century, World Wars I, II, the Korean War, and the Vietnam War combined, that the upper extremity vascular trauma incidence was 33% of all vascular injuries.[5]

In all trauma centers, even those in which blunt trauma normally predominates, the highest incidence of vascular injury is that associated with a penetrating trauma. The location of the injuries is most commonly radial and/or ulnar arteries, followed by the brachial artery, with the axillary artery the lowest in incidence. The incidence parallels the length of the artery exposed to trauma so that radial and ulnar artery injuries approximate 45%, brachial artery 35%, and axillary artery less than 20%.[5]

As regards blunt trauma, most of the vascular injuries occur about the elbow—either being associated with supracondylar fractures, with elbow dislocation, or, to a lesser degree, with infra-articular fractures of the radius and ulna.[4] It is probable that injuries to the upper extremity vessels are underdiagnosed because of the excellent collateral. Blunt reported an incidence of only 3% for vascular injuries associated with 89 supracondylar fractures and no vascular injuries associated with 108 humeral fractures.

Hardin et al found an incidence of associated vein or nerve injuries in 90%.[7] Visser found that 71% of upper extremity vascular injuries were associated with nerve injury.[8] All authors have found that associated nerve injury far more often than the vascular injury determined the ultimate functional result.[7,9,10]

ANATOMY

The *axillary artery* is approximately 14 to 16 cm in length. The junction with the subclavian artery arbitrarily starts at the lateral border of the first rib and ends at the inferior border of teres major muscle, where it becomes the brachial artery (Figure 4–1). The axillary artery is composed of three parts. The first part lies between the edge of the first rib and the proximal

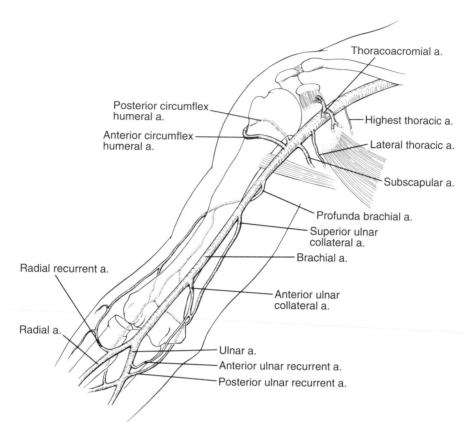

Figure 4–1.   Arteries of the upper arm.

edge of the pectoralis minor tendon; the second part underlies this muscle; and the third part extends from the lateral edge of the pectoralis minor to the teres major. There is only one small branch of the first portion of the axillary artery—the highest thoracic, a one-millimeter branch. Should ligation be required, this is the optimal location since there is major collateral circulation from the subclavian to the more distal branches of the axillary artery. There are two major branches of the second portion of the axillary artery, the thoracoacromial and the lateral thoracic arteries. The thoracoacromial, emerging anteriorly, is an important collateral branch which divides almost immediately into four branches which supply the deltoid muscle, the pectoral musculature, and the infraclavicular region. The second branch, the lateral thoracic artery, emerges from the inferior aspect of the distal part of the second portion of the axillary artery and travels along the lower border of the pectoralis minor muscle to the chest wall. The third portion of the axillary artery has three branches. The first, the subscapular, is the largest branch of the axillary artery. It emerges posteriorly and inferiorly from the artery and descends along the lower border of the subscapular muscle and scapula to the muscles of the posterior chest wall. The other branches of the third portion of the axillary artery are the anterior and posterior circumflex humeral arteries, which form an arterial ring around the neck of the humerus. Both passing in the direction named and take origin from the superior and anterior portion of the artery.

These numerous branches provide excellent collateral about the shoulder. So much so that there may still be an excellent collateral pulse with short occlusions of the axillary artery.

The *axillary vein* corresponds in course to the axillary artery, passing anterior and slightly inferior to the axillary artery. The axillary vein usually consists of a single trunk which, in its lower portion, is composed of the confluence of the basilic vein plus the one or two brachial veins which are associated with the brachial artery. The cephalic vein pierces the infraclavicular fascia and joins the axillary vein just before it passes under the clavicle.

The primary anatomical problem relative to the axillary artery is its intimate relationship with the brachial plexus. In the proximal third of the artery, the plexus lies laterally and superiorly, whereas in the distal third of the axillary artery, the three cords of the plexus virtually surround the artery. This results in an extremely high incidence of nerve injury associated with both blunt and penetrating axillary artery traumas. The posterior cord lies posterior and inferior to the second and third portion of the artery. The medial cord lies anterior and inferior to the artery. The lateral cord is superior and distally anterior to the artery, joining anteriorly with the branch of the medial cord to form the median nerve lying on the anterior portion of the first portion of the brachial artery. In slightly built patients the axillary artery can be palpated infraclavicularly at the junction of the medial and middle third of this bone as it emerges from under the clavicle. With the arm elevated, the third portion of the axillary artery can be palpated high in the center of the axilla—the root of the upper arm.

The *brachial artery* is a continuation of the axillary artery, arbitrarily originating at the lower border of the teres major muscle. It leaves the axilla medially, deep to the median nerve and it courses distally in a lateral direction, gradually becoming anterior to the humerus and posterior to the bicipital fascia at the elbow. As the brachial artery passes downward it gradually moves in front of the humerus and at the bend of the elbow lies midway between the two condyles. The artery remains rather superficial throughout its entire length, being covered in front by the integument of the superficial and deep fascia. The bicipital fascia separates it opposite the elbow from the median basilic vein; the median nerve crosses it at the elbow. Behind, starting above, it is separated from the long head of the triceps by the radial nerve and the superior profunda artery. It then lies upon the inner head of the triceps and next to the insertion of the coracobrachialis. Lastly, above the elbow, it lies on the brachialis muscle.

The *basilic vein* lies on the inner side of the artery but is separated from it in the lower part of the arm by the deep fascia. The brachial artery is accompanied by two venae comitantes which lie in close contact with the artery being connected at intervals by short transverse communicating branches. There are three major branches taking origin from the brachial artery and a number of smaller inconsistent muscular branches. The largest of the three major branches is the profunda brachial artery which arises as the first branch from the upper portion of the brachial artery. Occasionally it originates as high as the teres major muscle but usually two or three finger breadths to a hand's breadth below. It is a companion vessel of the radial nerve and it passes downward, backward, and outward between the medial and long head of the triceps muscle. It is an important collateral with branches to both the axillary artery and to collaterals about the elbow. The second main branch of the brachial artery is the inferior profunda artery (superior ulnar collateral artery). This vessel follows the course of the ulnar nerve and, after the vessel originates from the brachial artery at approximately the middle of the arm, it passes behind the medial epicondyle and anastomoses with the ulnar recurrent artery. The last main branch of the brachial artery is the anterior ulnar collateral artery which anastomoses with the rich collateral above the elbow. It arises from the brachial about 5 cm above the elbow joint and passes transversely inward upon the brachialis muscle, piercing the internal intermuscular septum and winds around the back of the humerus between heads of the triceps, forming an arch above the olecranon fossa. The median nerve is closely related to the brachial artery throughout its entire course down the arm, whereas the radial nerve is associated only with the proximal portion of the artery, and the ulnar nerve separates from the artery approximately in the middle of the upper arm.

While there is no major *brachial vein*, the two venae comitantes pass upward on either side of the artery and are joined at varying levels in the upper arm by the basilic vein. The major superficial veins of the arm, the basilic and the cephalic vein, can be ligated with impunity. Their anatomical location should be known, partially because they provide a means of vascular access in emergency circumstances. The *cephalic vein* is formed by the union of the median, cephalic, and radial forearm veins, and courses along the outer border of the biceps muscle lying in the same groove with the upper external cutaneous branch of the radial nerve. In the upper third of the arm it passes through the interval between the pectoralis major and the deltoid muscle, lying in the same groove with the descending or humeral branch of the acromiothoracic artery. It pierces the costocoracoid membrane and crosses the axillary artery and terminates in the axillary vein just below the midportion of the clavicle. This vein is occasionally connected with the external jugular and subclavian veins by a branch which passes upward in front of the clavicle. The *basilic vein* is of considerable size and formed by the coalescence of the common ulnar vein with the median basilic vein at the elbow. It passes upward along the inner side of the biceps muscle and pierces the deep fascia a little below the middle of the arm. The vein ascends along the course of the brachial artery to the lower border of the tendons of latissimus dorsi and teres major muscles and continues upward as the axillary vein, being joined by the venae comitantes surrounding the brachial artery.

As the brachial artery passes through the antecubital fossa beneath the lacertus fibrosis is divides into the *radial* and *ulnar* arteries, most commonly at the level of the coranoid process of the ulna and the neck of the radius (Figure 4–2). The *ulnar artery* is the larger of the two terminal branches of the brachial artery and passes obliquely downward and medially before it passes straight down to the wrist. The ulnar artery passes through the deep fascia immediately above the flexor retinaculum and is accompanied by two venae comitantes throughout its entire course. It runs deep to the forearm muscles which arise from the medial epicondyle and the proximal portion of the artery is crossed by the heads of the pronator teres, flexor carpi radialis, the palmaris longus, and the flexor digitorum sublimis muscles and the median nerve. In its lower part, it is covered by the flexor carpi ulnaris, but near the wrist it comes close to the surface and lies under the deep fascia in the interval between the tendons of flexor carpi ulnaris and the tendons of the flexor sublimis. It is followed by the ulnar nerve through most of its course and is closely associated with the nerve at the wrist. The ulnar artery terminates as the superficial and deep palmar or volar arches. The superficial arch gives rise to the digital arteries, and the deep arch continues into an anastomosis with the deep arch termination of the radial artery. The anterior and posterior ulnar recurrent arteries arise near the elbow as the first branches of the ulnar artery and anastomose with the branches of the brachial artery in the front and back of the medial side of the arm. Approximately 2 cm below the origin of the ulnar artery, the interosseous

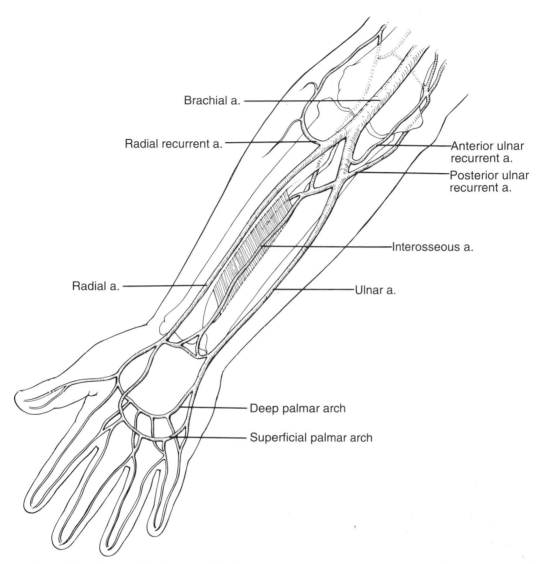

Brachial a.

Radial recurrent a.

Anterior ulnar recurrent a.

Posterior ulnar recurrent a.

Interosseous a.

Radial a.

Ulnar a.

Deep palmar arch

Superficial palmar arch

Figure 4–2.   Arteries of the forearm and hand.

artery originates and passes backwards to the upper margin of the interosseous membrane where it divides into the volar or anterior and dorsal or posterior interosseous arteries.

The *radial artery*, although the smaller of the two major branches of the brachial artery, is the direct continuation of the latter down the forearm. It originates opposite the neck of the radius and descends in the lateral part of the front of the forearm, to the wrist. It is unique in that no major muscles and no major motor nerves cross over it. It is covered by the brachioradialis in the upper forearm and throughout its entire course it is accompanied by venae comitantes. The radial nerve lies along its lateral side in the middle third of the arm, but distally above the wrist the nerve turns posteriorly away from the artery. The major branch of the radial is the radial recurrent artery which originates near the origin of the radial artery and contributes to the rich anastomosis about the elbow. Near its termination at the wrist, the radial artery gives rise to the superficial palmar artery. It then continues dorsally around the base of the first metacarpal into the hand to form the deep palmar arch, where it joins the deep branch of the ulnar artery.

ASSESSMENT

The manifestations of upper extremity arterial vascular injury differ depending upon whether the etiology is penetrating or blunt. Following penetrating injury, the manifestations may be the absence of distal pulses, a history of severe hemorrhage from the wound or ongoing hemorrhage from the wound, or more rarely, into the pleural cavity (Table 4–1). Where the injuries occur deep in the shoulder or arm, the manifestations may be an expanding or tense hematoma. When there is an associated venous injury, manifestations may be those of an arteriovenous fistula with a palpable thrill and audible bruit with or without changes in the distal pulses. Orcutt et al, in a study of 143 patients, found that a pulse defect was the most reliable sign of arterial injury and occurred in 75%, pulsatile bleeding occurred in 70%, pallor in 33%, parasthesias in 18%, and a bruit in 4%.[9] Of interest, in most series, 25% of major vascular injuries were thought to have normal pulses. The more proximal the injury the higher the incidence of palpable pulse so that with axillary injuries Orcutt found that 40% of the cases had a palpable wrist pulse.[9]

Following blunt trauma, particularly with open fractures, the manifestations may be those described for penetrating trauma. More commonly, blunt injuries are associated with stretch-type injury which usually results in thrombosis with a decrease in strength of pulses or absent distal pulses (Table 4–2). Because thrombosis tends to be more extensive in blunt injury, collateral flow may be compromised to a greater degree. Because of abundant collateral, both penetrating and blunt complete occlusions of the artery may still be associated with a distal pulse, though on careful palpation this is usually significantly less than that of the opposite extremity. For this reason, blood pressure should always be compared in the two arms when the location of the possible injury permits the application of a blood pressure cuff. Where possible, when injuries involve the forearm vessels, the Allen test may be useful to demonstrate radial or ulnar arterial injury. This is carried out utilizing alternate compression of the radial and ulnar arteries at the wrist with the fist closed. Then as the fist is opened refilling time is noted. Normally the ulnar artery is the dominant vessel and it is associated with the most rapid complete filling when the two vessels are compared.

In all penetrating injuries and major fractures of the arm, when there is any possibility

Table 4–1   Manifestations of Penetrating Trauma

Hypovolemic shock
Wound hemorrhage
Pleural hemorrhage
Wound hematoma—tense
Pulses ↓ or absent
Audible bruit
Palpable thrill

Table 4–2   Manifestations of Blunt Trauma

Pulses ↓ or absent
↓ blood pressure
Severe distal ischemia
Hemorrhage or hematoma

of vascular injury, careful auscultation along the course of the major vessels should be done. Partial occlusions may be manifest by a bruit, and arteriovenous fistula by a systolic-diastolic murmur and accompanying thrill. In many arteriovenous communications the initial examination may not be positive, but with the passage of time the flow between artery and vein progressively increases so that 24 hours later, a thrill or bruit not present initially may be manifest for the first time.

When vascular laboratory assessment is available, this may be of help in diagnosis where there are wounds of proximity or elbow injuries which put the blood vessels at risk. Vasli found that in supracondylar fractures in children, Doppler velocity wave form accurately identified the presence or absence of arterial injury.[11] Rutherford found that differential pressures in the two extremities was sufficient to justify arteriography.[12] A triphasic Doppler signal indicates no significant proximal lesion, an exaggerated reverse flow component at end systole—early diastole indicates increased peripheral flow resistance as may be encountered with vasospasm or compartmental compression. A low-pitched monophasic signal indicates proximal obstruction. High end-diastolic velocity and no end-systolic reversal is seen in postischemic hyperemia or a distal arteriovenous fistula.[12]

In the absence of any swelling or any significant evidence of bleeding, arteriography is probably not indicated in the upper extremity wounds of proximity.[13] This is because of the excellent collateral which, should thrombosis occur, still permits the adequate distal circulation without serious morbidity. However, if there are large hematomas, extensive soft tissue injury, or any evidence of pulse weakness or deficits, arteriography or direct exploration is indicated.

In penetrating trauma where there is evidence of arterial injury, the location of the lesion is usually obvious and immediate surgery rather than arteriography is warranted. The only exception would be in axillary injuries where the morbidity of negative exploration may be considerable due to the extensive dissection necessary about the shoulder, and the need to mobilize the brachial plexus to adequately expose the artery. In these circumstances, in the absence of ongoing hemorrhage or severe distal ischemia, which demand immediate attention, arteriographic assessment prior to surgery is usually indicated. One alternative always available to the surgeon is the use of operative arteriograms after proximal exposure of the vessel.

When major fractures are present, particularly comminuted or open fractures of the shaft of the humerus or elbow fractures or dislocations are present, a high index of suspicion for vascular injury should exist. If there is any evidence of pulse deficit when one extremity is compared to the opposite side, arteriography is indicated. Following blunt trauma, particularly where orthopaedic surgery is necessary or the extremity is going to be enclosed in a cast, a high index of suspicion for vascular injury is warranted and minimal findings usually justify arteriography.

Neurologic function should be assessed, for as noted previously, nerve injury will be found in approximately 50% of cases and this injury, more than any other, will determine late disability. Should motor or sensory changes be identified, the changes should be related to specific anatomy so that the location and nature of the neurologic lesion can be identified. If the wound is explored, the nerve lesion should be repaired at the time of operation or marked for repair at a later date. Orthopaedic consultation should be obtained pre-operatively if bony injury is present and a plan for stabilization of the extremity developed.

PREOPERATIVE MANAGEMENT

As with any trauma patient, it is imperative for the evaluating surgeon to be aware of priorities. Airway patency and respiratory function must be assessed and assured. Intra-venous access should be obtained with large bore catheters and hypovolemia treated. Bleeding from the upper extremity, should it be present, is best controlled by direct pressure, rather than tourniquet, if possible. A chest x-ray is required and should be done on all trauma patients regardless of the location of the injury. If there is evidence of intrathoracic bleeding and there is any possibility of axillary or subclavian artery injury, emergency anterior thoracotomy may be necessary to control bleeding into the chest. When vascular injury is suspected, particularly if shock has been present, a bladder catheter should be placed to monitor urinary output and monitor the response to resuscitation.

X-rays of the extremity are indicated to locate foreign bodies such as bone fragments, bullets or shards of glass. All wounds associated with a retained bullet must have the foreign body located to determine the path of the missile or, in rare circumstances, establish the probability of bullet embolism.

If the limb is severely ischemic, that is, paralyzed and anesthetic, immediate operation is mandatory as final results relate directly with revascularization time. When it takes longer than 6 to 8 hours from the time of injury to restore blood flow to an ischemic extremity, loss of some degree of limb function will occur. Fortunately collateral flow is usually adequate to maintain viability of the arm for most upper extremity injuries unless they are associated with extensive soft tissue injury.

Preoperative antibiotics directed against skin organisms should be given prior to taking the patient to surgery and continued for 24 hours postoperatively.

OPERATIVE EXPOSURE

The trauma surgeon needs to be familiar with the anatomy of the upper extremity (see previous section). As is true in all forms of surgery on the arterial system, proximal control is essential prior to exposing the area of probable injury. In presumed injuries of the proximal portion of the axillary artery, supraclavicular exposure of the artery may be necessary. For all other injuries, from the middle of the axillary artery downward, proximal control is usually possible in the extremity. With those injuries which are presumed to be distal to the lower half of the upper arm, proximal control is readily obtainable by a tourniquet on the upper arm. This permits the site of injury to be exposed directly with the assurance that should uncontrollable bleeding occur, the tourniquet can be inflated and complete hemostasis ensured. For vascular injuries of the forearm, digital compression above the site of bleeding is usually adequate for control.

Axillary Artery

For exposure of axillary artery injuries, the arm is extended at right angles to the side. The incision is made from approximately two finger breadths from the sternoclavicular joint, outward in the infraclavicular area, approximately 2 cm below the inferior margin of the clavicle (Figure 4–3). For injuries involving the proximal portion of the axillary artery, the incision can be curved upward over the clavicle at its junction with the medial and the middle third and carried further proximally supraclavicularly. At this point the dissection is carried out just superior to the vein down through the scalene fat pad to expose the scalenus anticus muscle. This muscle should be carefully divided taking care to preserve the phrenic nerve on its anterior surface. The artery can then be identified and encircled. If necessary, the proximal half of the clavicle can be resected out to the coracoid process with minimal associated morbidity. This may be necessary in subclavian-axillary artery injuries where exposure is compromised by the clavicle.

In exposing the axillary artery the subclavian vein should first be identified and a plane

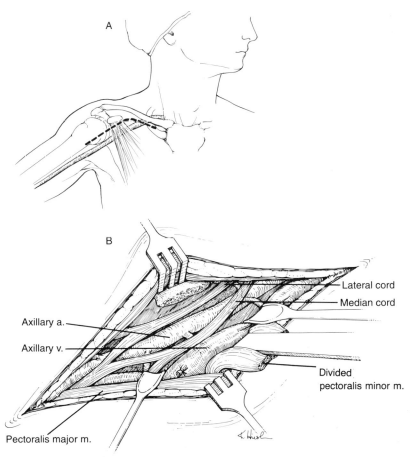

Figure 4–3. **A:** Incision for operative exposure of the axillary artery. **B:** Relationship of the axillary artery to the brachial plexus.

of dissection on the vein obtained so that it can be retracted downward to expose the artery. This will often require division of thoracoacromial branches as well as the cephalic vein. With the vein retracted downward, the axillary artery is usually palpable just posterior and slightly superior to the upper edge of the vein. Control of the artery is best obtained in the proximal third where only the highest thoracic artery, a diminutive branch, is present. Once the artery is encircled the dissection can be carried distally and the pectoralis minor detached from the coracoid process to expose the second portion of the axillary artery. An effort should be made to preserve major collateral branches when the injury exposure permits, since should thrombosis of the reconstruction occur, these collaterals will generally ensure viability of the arm. The third portion of the artery is exposed by dividing the attachment of the pectoralis major to the humerus, preserving approximately 1 cm of the tendon for reanastomosis (the pectoralis minor tendon does not require reanastomosis). Care should be taken to identify the cords of the brachial plexus and if possible the branches to the pectoral muscles preserved. Following thrombosis or proximal occlusion of the artery, the collapsed brachial artery can resemble cords of the brachial plexus and careful identification is best obtained by dissecting the artery from the proximal location of the occluding clamp distally and gently retracting the brachial plexus in the course of exposing the artery. Any severed portions of the brachial plexus should be carefully identified for possible reanastomosis. Because of the excellent collateral, back bleeding from the injury site is usually vigorous until distal control is obtained.

Brachial Artery

For injuries of the upper portion of the brachial artery, proximal control can usually be obtained by exposing the axillary artery in the axilla where it is very superficial (Figure 4–4). The pulse is usually palpable through the skin with the arm extended at right angles to the body. A longitudinal axillary incision will then expose this portion of the artery for proximal control. The brachial plexus must always be kept in mind since at this level it surrounds the artery and a junction of the lateral and medial cords constitute the median nerve which courses over the artery. Usually the brachial plexus can easily be parted sufficiently to encircle the artery for proximal control. In the upper third of the arm, the brachial artery can be exposed by an incision over the inner side of the coracobrachialis muscle with the subcutaneous tissue and the subadjacent fascia carefully divided so as to avoid injuring the medial cutaneous nerve or the basilic vein. The latter may run on the surface of the artery as high as the axillary. After the fascia is divided the ulnar and musculocutaneous nerve can be identified on the inner side of the artery, the median on the outer side. The latter occasionally is superficial to the artery in this location. The venae comitantes also surround the vessel on either side and these must be carefully separated and their communications divided as necessary. Care should be taken to preserve the profunda brachii arterial branch if at all possible for its collateral potential. Rather than dividing this collateral in order to approximate the injured vessel ends, a vein graft should be used.

From the middle of the arm downward, the brachial artery can be exposed by making an incision along the inner margin of the biceps muscle (Figure 4–4). If the forearm is bent so as to relax the muscle, it is more easily retracted. With the fascia divided, the median nerve can usually be seen lying on top of the artery, although sometimes it is beneath. It is possible also to misidentify the inferior profunda artery as the main trunk, particularly if it is providing the collateral circulation, and once again, this vessel should be preserved if

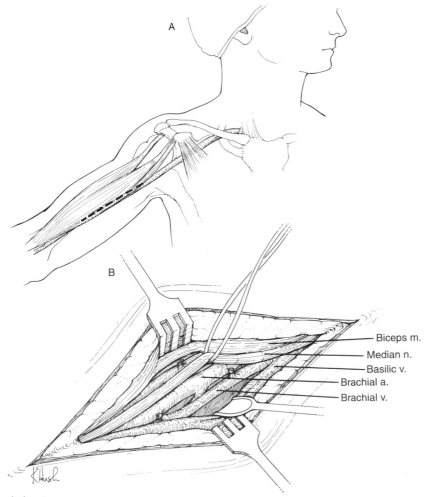

Figure 4–4. **A:** Incision for the exposure of the brachial artery. **B:** Deep exposure of the brachial artery.

at all possible. In the lower portion of the arm, the artery is exposed along the medial border of the biceps tendon; the median nerve must be identified and preserved. The bicipital fascia requires division, avoiding dividing brachial veins if possible (Figure 4–5).

Radial Artery

The radial artery is relatively superficial through its entire course (Figures 4–5 and 4–6). It is only overlapped in the upper part of its course by the fleshy belly of the brachioradialis muscle, the medial head of which can be retracted to expose the artery as far as the wrist. At the wrist it lies lateral to the tendon of the flexor carpi radialis which is readily palpated on the radial side of the wrist. In its entire course, there are no major anatomic structures which interfere with the exposure.

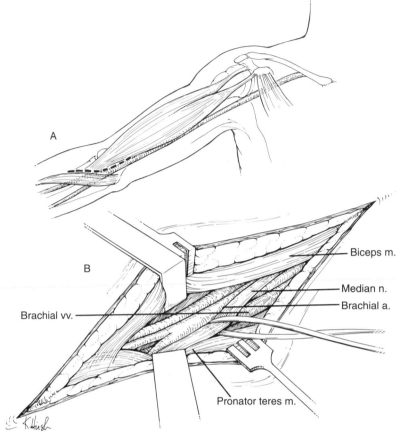

Biceps m.

Median n.

Brachial a.

Brachial vv.

Pronator teres m.

Figure 4–5. **A:** Incision for exposure of the brachial artery at the elbow. **B:** Deep exposure of the brachial artery.

Ulnar Artery

The proximal portion of the ulnar artery is buried beneath the muscles taking origin from the medial epicondyle. So for injuries of the upper third, these muscles must be divided (Figure 4–7). It is usually preferable to identify the origin of the ulnar artery at the brachial artery, retract the median nerve, and then carefully divide the muscles to permit definitive exposure of the artery. For lesions distal to the proximal fourth of the artery, the flexor muscles of the forearm and wrist can be retracted medially to expose the artery. For distal third lesions, it is appropriate to identify the artery at the wrist and dissect proximally, utilizing the tourniquet to ensure proximal control. The incision is best made just anterior to the ulna and the dissection carried over the top of the ulna to identify the artery in the lower third of the arm. The ulnar nerve is closely associated with the artery in the distal part of the forearm and must be protected.

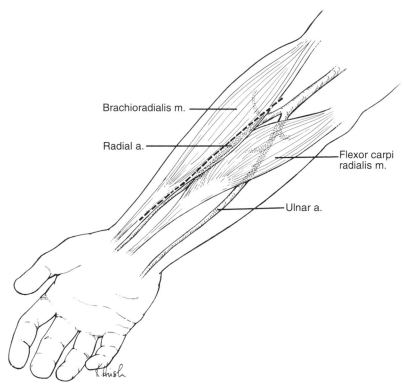

Figure 4–6. Incision for exposure of the radial artery.

VASCULAR REPAIR

Principles of vascular repair utilized on all other arteries are appropriate here. Generally, the arteries are muscular and relatively easily handled, and technical results are quite good.

Radial and Ulnar Arteries

In isolated injuries of the radial or ulnar artery where the opposite vessel is known to be intact, ligation of the injured vessel may well be the most appropriate treatment. In heavily contaminated injuries and injuries when there has been loss of soft tissue coverage, or in the presence of complex or comminuted open fractures, the risk of hemorrhage may outweigh any advantages gained by repair. Following simple lacerations, from stabs or cuts with glass, repair is usually appropriate. Whereas, with more complex injuries such as gunshot wounds where interposition grafting may be required, ligation is usually preferable to complex repairs. The exception being injuries to both arteries where usually it would be appropriate to repair both if the soft tissues permit, to ensure patency of one.

As regards simple longitudinal lacerations or partial divisions of the artery from sharp cuts, freshening of the margins of the cut may be appropriate. However, if the laceration is clean, simple approximation with fine interrupted monofilament 5-0 or 6-0 suture is

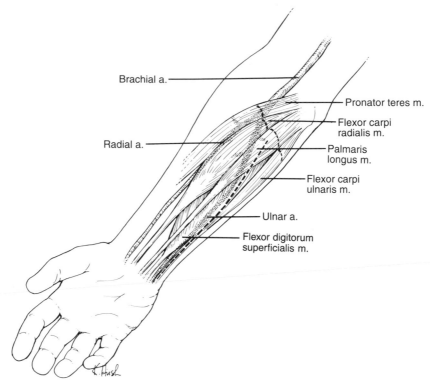

Figure 4–7. Incision for exposure of the ulnar artery.

appropriate (Figure 4–8). For optimum results, care should be taken, where possible, to obtain intima-to-intima approximation which is best obtained by an everting type of suture. For complete transections interrupted repair is almost always preferable to running repair. The reason for this is that when dealing with small vessels, it is very easy to purse-string the anastomosis, particularly when working with monofilament suture. Two small horizontal mattress sutures placed at opposite sides of the vessel will initiate eversion. This can be followed by a series of interrupted sutures. Loss of up to two centimeters of the radial or ulnar artery can usually be compensated for by mobilization of the artery, particularly if this does not involve the division of a large collateral such as the interosseous or an elbow collateral. When an artery must be approximated under tension, at least half the circumference of the vessel should be encompassed by sutures before the ends of the vessel are approximated and the sutures tied. The latter is facilitated by the assistant holding the two vascular clamps and approximating the ends under tension while the posterior row is tied. Following this the integrity is usually such that even if there is temporary relaxation of tension on the approximating clamps, the vessel will not tear.

Brachial Artery Injuries

For all practical purposes, all brachial artery injuries should be repaired, even when immediate soft tissue coverage is lacking. In the latter instance a vein graft can be placed

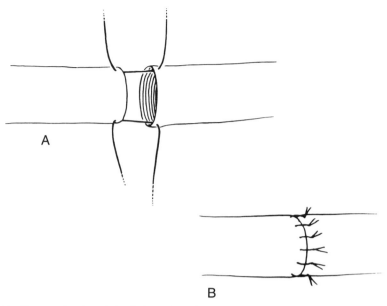

Figure 4–8. Reapproximation of simple laceration. **A:** Lining up vessel ends. **B:** Completion of repair with interrupted sutures.

extra-anatomically in such a fashion so as to preserve flow and maintain integrity of the circulation. Lacerations from sharp knives or glass can usually be approximated with simple interrupted sutures after vascular control is obtained. Complex lacerations or contused injuries associated with blunt trauma or gunshot wounds will usually require excision of the artery to the point of intact intima proximally and distally. The divided vessel end should be freshened and obliquely cut so that the circumference of the anastomoses will exceed the circumference of the vessel. Using olive-shaped dilators, the vessel can be gently dilated and spasm broken. Alternatively, Papaverine can be infused into the vessel to relax spasm and facilitate anastomosis of the larger lumen. Either interrupted or running closure of the brachial artery is appropriate depending upon the skill and experience of the surgeon (Figure 4–9). As many brachial arteries are quite small, interrupted closure is technically safer. As with smaller vessel injuries, horizontal everting sutures are placed 180° apart to initiate the closure, followed by interrupted sutures a millimeter or two apart. Approximately 2 cm of the brachial artery can be resected and the ends still reanastomosed. When large collaterals would require division to approximate the vessel ends, it is safer to utilize an interposition vein graft to restore continuity. The vein should be bevelled on both ends to match the bevelled artery. Care should be taken to identify the direction of the valves to ensure that the ends of the vein are reversed. If running suture is elected, two sutures should be used so that everting sutures can be initiated at 180° from one another with a running stitch carried between—care being taken not to purse-string the vessel. Prior to placement of the last few sutures, dilators can be passed proximally and distally to ensure the patency of the anastomosis.

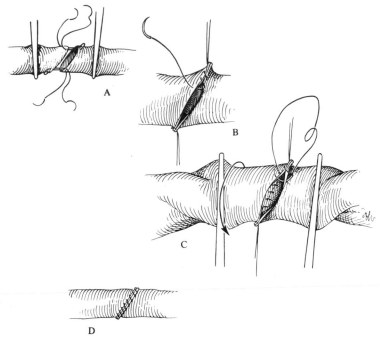

Figure 4–9.   Repair of brachial artery. **A:** Horizontal mattress sutures at 180 degree to each other to evert the edges. **B:** Running suture between two initial sutures. **C:** Running suture on back side of vessel. **D:** Completed repair.

Axillary Artery

Repair of axillary artery involves techniques which are similar to those used for the brachial artery. The larger caliber of this vessel provides more latitude for technical error. For lesions involving the distal third, particularly when exposure around the brachial plexus is difficult, a vein bypass around the area of injury may be more appropriate than attempting to carry out anastomosis within the three cords of the brachial plexus, particularly when one of the latter may require concomitant or subsequent repair. Either running or interrupted anastomoses can be carried out and several centimeters of the vessel can be resected as necessary. Care must always be taken to ensure that there is integrity of the intima at the site of anastomosis and that an everting anastomosis is utilized.

Venous Repairs

Simple lacerations of veins of the forearm and arm rarely require repair, but when exposed concomitantly with exposure of the artery, simple lacerations can be approximated with everting interrupted or continuous suture. Complex injuries are best treated by ligation. Axillary vein injuries, when identified, are appropriately treated by repair, though complex injuries are best treated by clean ligation rather than interposition vein grafts. Attempts to repair complex injuries will usually result in venous thrombosis. Extension of the thrombus, under this circumstance, threatens collateral more than clean ligation. The vein can be mobilized for approximately one centimeter but because of its fragile nature it lends itself less well to anastomosis under tension. It is absolutely essential in venous repairs to ensure eversion of the anastomosis and careful intima to intima approximation with fine sutures— either interrupted or continuous. Techniques required are similar to those for arterial repair but even a more meticulous technique is essential. Though some have advocated placement of a distal arteriovenous fistula to maintain early vein patency, this is introducing a second lesion to facilitate repair of the first. Except in rare instances, it is not warranted.

Associated Fractures

In all instances of vascular injury, save those with normal perfusion, vascular repair takes precedent over orthopaedic fixation. Even though subsequent orthopaedic manipulation could compromise the repair, this is most unusual and if necessary the repair can be redone. Limbs are lost from delays in vascular repair, rarely from delay in stabilization.[6]

POSTOPERATIVE CARE

The vessels of the upper extremity are smaller, and therefore more technically difficult to manage than those elsewhere. Therefore, failure of the reconstruction is more common. For this reason, we routinely carry out operative arteriograms following completion of the anastomosis and prior to wound closure. Twenty milliliters of contrast injected as rapidly as possible through a #20-21 needle will provide information about patency and flow. Alternatively, the hand can be inspected prior to contaminating the surgical table and reintervention or arteriography done immediately if the appearance of the circulation is less than optimal.

Postoperatively, the pulses and capillary reflow should be monitored closely for the first 24 hours. Any change for the worse should lead to operative or arteriographic assessment.

For injuries about the elbow, posterior splints should be utilized for 2 to 3 days to protect the anastomosis. The wound should be monitored for bleeding so that bulky dressings which obscure the wound should be avoided. The fascia should have been closed loosely so that bleeding, should it occur, can decompress and the fascia should be opened if the arm becomes tense or any numbness or weakness develops so as to avoid the compartment syndrome. Antibiotics started preoperatively should be continued postoperatively. Physical therapy should be initiated as soon as the wound and any fractures permit.

COMPLICATIONS

Although all series describe thromboses of the repairs, early recognition usually permits successful reoperation, and severe distal ischemia is usually not present. Reperfusion hypercoagulability is not a major problem as it is in the lower extremities.

Another complication is the compartment syndrome (see Chapter 20). Because preservation of function is essential in the upper extremity, it is rarely appropriate to close the fascia following arterial repair if there is any evidence of increase in tension. If muscle has been damaged, as is true in gunshot wounds, and especially with blunt trauma, it may be appropriate to open skin and fascia the entire length of the involved compartment to prevent perfusion compromise.[14] The results are best when swelling is due to hemorrhage or direct muscle contusion. When muscle swelling is due to ischemic damage, the results of fasciotomy are at best a tradeoff. Compartment perfusion may be improved but exposure of ischemic muscle may lead to infection and slough of the compartment.

RESULTS

In all series the results of upper extremity arterial or venous repair are excellent. This is probably because many technical failures go unrecognized because of the presence of good collateral.[15] This emphasizes the importance of preserving all collateral possible during operative treatment.

The primary cause of limb loss is associated injury, primarily that of massive soft tissue destruction infection, or major neurologic injury, particularly those involving the brachial plexus or its nerve roots.[10] The flail extremity is of little value and a prosthesis is more optimal from the point of view of function. When several roots or cords of the brachial plexus are functional, muscle and nerve transfers can often produce a useful extremity which is superior to a prosthesis.

The upper extremity is relatively clean, and infection is much less common than injuries to the lower extremity. An extra anatomical bypass can be used when lack of adequate soft tissue coverage results in thrombosis of the repair. Alternatively, muscle flaps can be mobilized to cover the repair.

In all series the incidence of overt thrombosis of repairs is less than 5% and loss of extremities from failure of vascular repair is rare, providing that preceding precautions are followed.[14] Hughes reported no amputations were necessary following brachial artery repairs.[1] Rich noted that in Vietnam, of 276 brachial artery injuries treated by reconstruction, only 13 extremities required amputation.[15] He did note on late follow-up of 91 patients that some of the patients had complete thrombosis but remained asymptomatic. Overall, the amputation rate following vascular injury approximates 5%.

As regards ultimate function in late follow-up, arterial and vein problems are rarely the cause of disability even when the repair has thrombosed. The primary cause of disability is nerve injury. Visser reported a series of 37 upper extremity nerve injuries associated with vascular injury. The injured nerve was completely transected in 23 cases. Twenty of these nerves were treated with primary or secondary repair. Seven patients failed to regain any function, motor or sensory, another eleven regained partial motor or protective sensory function. Only five patients with nerve transection regained complete return of neurologic function. Nichols, in his review of nerve injury, noted that they were associated with a 24% to 44% incidence of long-term disability. Hardin et al reported a similar experience. He noted, as did others, that the more proximal the injury, the worse the result.

REFERENCES

1. Hughes CW. Historical aspects of vascular trauma. In: Rich NM, Spencer FC, eds. *Vascular Trauma*. Philadelphia, Pa: WB Saunders; 1978:6–21.
2. Carrel A. Results of transplantation of blood vessels, organs and limbs. *JAMA*. 1908;51:1662.
3. DeBakey ME, Simeone FA. Battle injuries in World War II. An analysis of 2,471 cases. *Ann Surg*. 1946; 123:534.

4. Bunt TJ, Malone JM, Moody M, Davidson J, Karpman R. The frequency of vascular injury with blunt trauma induced extremity fracture/dislocation. *Am J Surg*. 1990;160:226.
5. Drapanas T. Etiology, incidence and clinical pathology. In: Rich NM, Spencer FC, eds. *Vascular Trauma*. Philadelphia, Pa: WB Saunders; 1978:22–43.
6. Perry MO, Shires GT. Vascular trauma in the extremities. In: Carter, Polk, eds. *Trauma*. London, Engl: Butterworth's; 1981:185–191.
7. Hardin WD, O'Connell RC, Adinolfe MF, Kerstein MD. Traumatic arterial injuries of the upper extremity: determinants of disability. *Am J Surg*. 1985;115:266–270.
8. Visser PA, Hermreck AS, Pierce GE, Thomas JH, Hardin CA. Prognosis of nerve injuries incurred during acute trauma to peripheral arteries. *Am J Surg*. 1980;140:596–599.
9. Orcutt MB, Levine BA, Gaskill HV, Sirinek KR. Civilian vascular trauma of the upper extremity. *J Trauma*. 1986;26:63–67.
10. Nichols JS, Lillehei KO. Nerve injury associated with acute vascular trauma. *Surg Clin North Am*. 1988; 68:837–852.
11. Vasli LR. Diagnosis of vascular injury in children with supracondylar fractures of the humerus. *Injury*. 1988; 19:11–13.
12. Rutherford RB. Diagnostic evaluation of extremity vascular injuries. *Surg Clin North Am*. 1988;68:683–691.
13. Hartling RP, McGahan JP, Blaisdell FW, Lindfors KK. Stab wounds of the extremities: indications for angiography. *Radiology*. 1987;162:465–467.
14. Fazi B, Raves JJ, Young JC, Diamond DL. Fasciotomy of the upper extremity in patients with trauma. *Surg Gynecol Obstet*. 1987;165:447–448.
15. Rich NM, Spencer FC. *Vascular Trauma*. Philadelphia, Pa: WB Saunders; 1978:362–365.

5

Lower Extremity Vascular Injury

F. WILLIAM BLAISDELL, M.D.

HISTORY: The management of vascular injuries of the extremities has historically constituted the most challenging problem of wound management. Tight pressure bandages have been used since antiquity to control hemorrhage but the development of the principle of the tourniquet was slow. In 1674, Morrel, a military surgeon, introduced a stick into the bandage and twisted it until arterial flow stopped.[1] This type of crude tourniquet became a temporary means of controlling hemorrhage and permitted the more frequent use of the ligature since control of bleeding permitted deliberate exposure of the injured vessel. Whether or not subsequent amputation was required there was a high rate of secondary hemorrhage after the ligation due to infection in the wound.[2] In the limbs which remained viable, back bleeding from the arterial wound was another cause of secondary hemorrhage as collateral flow was mobilized. This problem was solved by Bell in 1801, who performed both proximal and distal arterial ligation and obtained better results due to a decreased incidence of secondary hemorrhage.[3]

In 1896, J. B. Murphy of Chicago carried out the first successful end-to-end arterial anastomosis in man.[4] His patient was a 29-year-old male who was shot in the femoral triangle. Proximal and distal ligatures were temporarily placed around a common femoral aneurysm. The damaged portion of the artery was resected. After mobilization of the vessel, the proximal end was invaginated into the distal artery for a distance of 1 cm and the anastomosis maintained with adventitial sutures.

The next development came in 1906 when Goyanes excised a popliteal artery aneurysm and used the accompanying popliteal vein to restore continuity.[5] He used the suture technique developed by Carrel and Guthrie which consisted of first triangulating the arterial orifice with three sutures followed by continuous suture between.[6] Intermittent success was reported with arterial repair from that point on. The German surgeons in World War I attempted repair of acutely injured arteries[7]; however, ligation of injured vessels was considered the treatment of choice up through World War II.

As noted in the previous chapter, the Korean conflict was notable for a number of medical advances, one of the major of which was the introduction of techniques of arterial and, to a lesser degree, venous repair as the treatment of choice for vascular injuries.[7] The overall amputation rate was 13% in this conflict, compared to that of 49% in World War II.

The amputation rate for extremity vascular injuries dropped even further, to 8%, in the Vietnam War.[7]

INTRODUCTION

Lower extremity vascular injuries are arbitrarily classified as those involving the common femoral artery distally to the branches of the tibial arteries to the foot. Thus defined, the incidence of injury to vessels of the lower extremity represent the commonest of all vascular injuries. The principal method of treatment, through all major conflicts and in peacetime practice up to nearly the present time, has been ligature of the artery involved. Since the collateral circulation of the lower extremity is nowhere near as adequate as that of the upper extremity, amputation was usually the end result of arterial ligation.

INCIDENCE AND LOCATION OF INJURIES

The overall incidence of vascular injuries to the lower extremity approximates 60% of total arterial injuries.[8] The true incidence of venous injuries is not known since many venous injuries go unrecognized. Because of the relative larger size of the veins as opposed to the arteries, the incidence of venous injuries must be equal or higher than those of arterial injuries.

The incidence of the injuries to the individual arteries in the lower extremity parallels their relative length.[8] Thus the common femoral artery injuries are approximately 5% of lower extremity vascular injuries. That of the profunda is reported to approximate 2% to 3% although the incidence of injury to this vessel is not known since the more distal injuries are probably not identified nor require treatment in most instances. Injuries to the superficial femoral artery are the most commonly recognized of all arterial injuries, averaging 11% to 20% civilian injuries and 30% for military injuries.[7,9,10] The higher frequency of injuries to the upper extremity with household and industrial accidents accounts for the lower incidence of leg injuries in civilian casualties.

The incidence of popliteal artery injuries has been high in military experience, being 12% of all arterial injuries in World War I, 20% of all arterial injuries in World War II, 25% in the Korean conflict, and 22% reported by Rich for Vietnam.[11] In 1969, Brewer and his associates, in reviewing multiple series of civilian arterial injuries, found an overall incidence of approximately 12%.[12] Penetrating or blunt injuries of the popliteal artery in all series constitute the highest risk for amputation of any arterial injury with knee dislocation constituting the most frequent cause in civilian injuries.[13]

The true incidence of injuries to the anterior tibial, posterior tibial, and peroneal arteries is not known as many of these injuries are overlooked. However, in the series reported by DeBakey and Simeone during World War II, the injuries to these vessels constituted more than one fifth of all the arterial injuries.[15] In the majority of civilian reports the incidence of injury to these vessels has been approximately 2% to 3%.[16]

ANATOMY

The *common femoral artery* starts as the vessel emerges from under the inguinal ligament midway between the anterior superior iliac spine and the pubic tubercle. In this area, the femoral triangle is covered only by fascia making the femoral artery the most clinically accessible large artery in the body (Figure 5–1). Three to five centimeters from its origin, the common femoral artery branches into the superficial femoral and the profunda femoral arteries. The *common femoral vein* lies medial to the artery, being composed of the superficial and profunda femoral vein; in addition, it is joined midway between its origin and the inguinal ligament by the greater saphenous vein. Both the artery and the vein in the femoral triangle are contained within a common fibrous sheath. The femoral nerve lies on the lateral side of the artery in a relatively protected position covered by fibers of the iliopsoas muscle and its fascia. The common femoral artery can be mobilized with

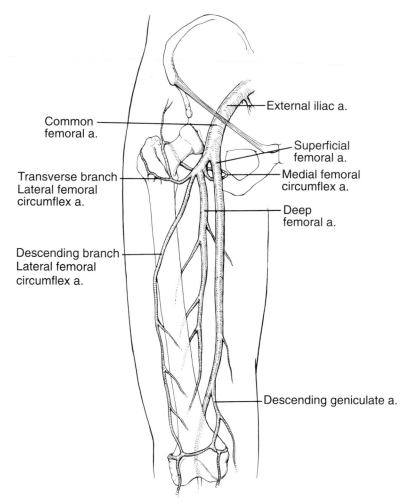

Figure 5–1. Anatomy of the femoral artery.

impunity as it gives rise to only several small branches. These are the superficial circumflex iliac, laterally, and the superficial epigastric artery, anteriorly, both of which arise just below the inguinal ligament. The smaller pudendal vessels arise more distally and pass in front of and behind the femoral vein.

The *profunda femoral artery* arises posteriorly at the common femoral bifurcation, and immediately gives rise to medial and lateral circumflex branches. As it leaves the femoral triangle, it passes behind the adductor longus muscle continuing down the thigh on the adductor magnus muscle, giving off four perforating arteries which pass posteriorly to supply the thigh musculature. All of these branches have rich communications with collateral vessels about the hip and with the obturator artery, a branch of the hypogastric artery which passes medially through the obturator foramen down the thigh. The distal branches of the profunda femoral anastomose with the geniculate branches taking origin from the proximal popliteal artery.

The *profunda femoral vein* parallels that of the artery, progressing upward, somewhat posterior and lateral to the artery. Approximately 1 cm distal to the origin of the profunda artery, the vein passes anterior to the artery to join the superficial femoral vein forming the common femoral vein.

The second major branch of the common femoral, the *superficial femoral artery*, passes down the medial aspect of the thigh to penetrate the adductor magnus muscle approximately two finger breadths above the medial condyle of the femur to become the popliteal artery. The course of the superficial femoral artery is a relatively straight one, changing from a relatively anterior location proximally to a posterior medial location distally. Along most of its course it is covered by the sartorius muscle which is referred to as the adductor or Hunter's canal. Several small branches in the thigh occasionally provide collateral circulation. However, the only major branch is the superior geniculate artery which originates from the distal superficial femoral artery in the lower part of the adductor canal just before it penetrates the adductor magnus muscle. This branch descends to join a rich anastomosis about the knee joint. Near its origin, the superficial femoral artery in the femoral triangle lies near the medial surface of the shaft of the femur, separated from it only by the vastus medialis muscle. Distally, the artery lies slightly posterior to the femur and in close proximity to it.

The *superficial femoral vein* courses upward from the popliteal vein and lies medial and anterior to the artery. Occasionally, however, it is a bifid vein surrounding the artery with numerous communicating channels between the two. The remaining important vein in the thigh is the saphenous vein which runs in a subcutaneous course from just behind the medial condyle of the femur up the midmedial portion of the thigh to curve from its medial position to join the common femoral vein.

The *popliteal artery* is the continuation of the superficial femoral artery and becomes such as the former emerges posteriorly from the adductor magnus muscle (Figure 5–2). It extends in the popliteal space distally to its terminal branches, the anterior and posterior tibial arteries. The anterior tibial frequently takes its origin as high as at the level of the knee joint. On occasion, the popliteal artery may terminate in a true trifurcation of the anterior tibial, posterior tibial, and the peroneal arteries. The proximal portion of the popliteal artery lies behind the distal third of the femur and lies nearly in the midline of the posterior aspect of the knee behind the capsule of the knee joint. It terminates variably but usually at the distal border of the popliteus muscle. Throughout its entire course the popliteal artery lies deep in the popliteal fossa. Proximally the artery is covered by the semimembranosus

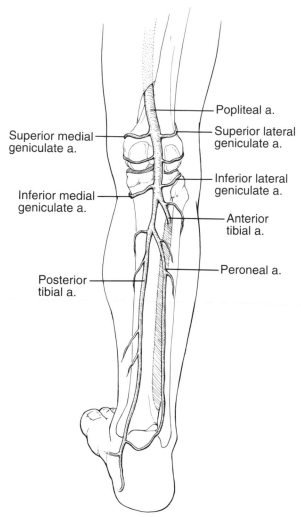

Superior medial geniculate a.

Inferior medial geniculate a.

Posterior tibial a.

Popliteal a.

Superior lateral geniculate a.

Inferior lateral geniculate a.

Anterior tibial a.

Peroneal a.

Figure 5–2.   Anatomy of popliteal, posterior tibial, and peroneal arteries.

muscle. At the level of the condyles of the femur it is covered mostly by subcutaneous tissue and fat. Distally, the plantaris muscle and nerves to the lateral head of the gastrocnemius muscle cross over the artery. At its termination it is covered by the triceps surae composed of the two heads of the gastrocnemius muscle and the soleus muscle. The sciatic nerve lies lateral to the upper portion of the artery, but after division into the peroneal and tibial nerves, the tibial nerve lies posterior and overlies the popliteal artery in the lower third of the popliteal fossa. The popliteal artery gives off multiple geniculate branches medially and laterally as it courses down the popliteal fossa. The proximal branches anastomose with the profunda femoral artery and the distal branches with the anterior recurrent tibial artery and lateral collaterals from the peroneal and posterior tibial artery.

The *popliteal vein* is deep and slightly medial to the popliteal artery. It receives numerous geniculate collaterals, paralleling the branches at the artery, and also receives a major vessel, the lesser saphenous vein, which joins it in the midportion of the popliteal space.

The *anterior tibial artery*, after leaving the popliteal, passes forward through the proximal interosseous membrane between the tibia and fibula to the anterior compartment of the leg (Figure 5–3). In its upper portion it lies deep in the anterior compartment close to the medial side of the neck of the fibula. It descends on the anterior surface of the interosseous membrane, passing over onto the anterior surface of the tibia in the region of the ankle. It terminates in front of the ankle joint where it becomes quite superficial

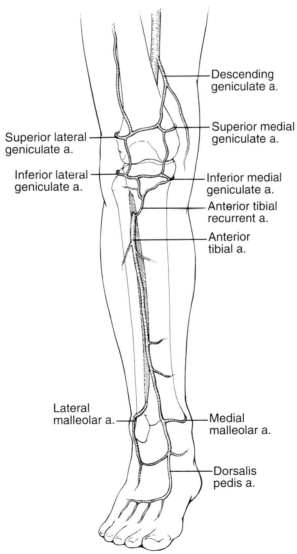

Figure 5–3.   Anatomy of the anterior tibial artery.

and continues as the dorsalis pedis artery which passes down over the second metatarsal to terminate in the dorsal plantar arch. In the upper third of the leg, the anterior tibial artery courses between the tibialis anterior medially and the extensor longus digitorum laterally. In the middle third of the leg it lies between the tibialis anterior and the extensor hallucis. Just above the ankle it is crossed by the tendon of the extensor hallucis longus and lies between it and the innermost tendon of the extensor longus. The anterior tibial artery gives rise to numerous muscular branches as it passes down the leg. Two venae comitantes carry blood upward on each side of the artery. The peroneal nerve courses around the outer side of the neck of the fibula and comes in close relationship with the lateral side of the artery shortly after the artery passes through the opening in the interosseous membrane. In about the middle of the leg, the nerve is superficial to the artery. In the lower part of the leg, the nerve is generally on the lateral side of the artery.

The *posterior tibial artery* is usually the direct continuation of the popliteal beyond the origin of the anterior tibial at the lower border of the popliteus muscle (Figure 5–2). It extends downward in an oblique fashion, lying behind the tibia. At the ankle it courses midway between the medial malleolus and the tuberosity of the calcaneus terminating by dividing into medial and lateral plantar arches on the sole of the foot. It is covered throughout most of its course by the transverse fascia of the leg, separating it from the gastrocnemius and soleus muscles. It is accompanied by the posterior tibial nerve which passes downward on the lateral posterior side of the artery and is accompanied by two venae comitantes which surround the artery. The posterior tibial artery gives off numerous muscular branches as it passes down the leg. As it descends the posterior tibial artery lies successively upon the tibialis posterior, flexor digitorum longus and finally the posterior aspect of the tibia above the ankle joint. At its termination, it is covered by the adductor hallucis muscle. In the lower third of the leg, where it is more superficial, it is covered only by the integument and the fascia and runs parallel with the inner border of the Achilles tendon.

The *peroneal artery* originates from the posterior tibial artery at a variable distance below the origin of the anterior tibial (Figure 5–2). In some instances, its origin is at the same site as the anterior tibial. In most instances its origin is 2 to 3 cm distal to the origin of that vessel. It is the largest branch of the posterior tibial and runs downward in an oblique lateral direction under the soleus muscle to the fibula. Descending parallel to the fibula it emerges just above the ankle joint from beneath the flexor hallucis longus muscle. It terminates in lateral calcaneal branches at the level of the heel. It is accompanied by the venae comitantes. The peroneal artery has numerous collateral branches between it and the posterior tibial and anterior tibial arteries as it courses down the leg. In the upper portion of its course it is contained in a fibrous canal between the tibialis posterior and the flexor hallucis longus. It is covered in the upper part of its course by the soleus and below by the flexor hallucis longus.

Two superficial veins which are of importance in the lower leg, if for no other reason than they make excellent arterial substitutes, are the *greater and lesser saphenous vein*. The former can be identified in the grove anterior to the medial malleolus. It passes upward in a medial and posterior course lying on the fascia. It passes just posterior to the medial femoral condyle at the level of the knee. The lesser saphenous vein can be found posterior to the lateral malleolus at the ankle. It then passes medially and posteriorly and in midleg comes to lie in the midline. In the upper third of the leg it passes deep to the fascia where it joins the popliteal vein just before the knee joint.

ASSESSMENT

The assessment of penetrating injuries is relatively easy. The absence of distal pulses, weak distal pulses, the presence of bruits, thrills, expanding hematomas, or overt external hemorrhage provides a clue, not only that arterial injury is present, but also its location (Table 5–1). Under these circumstances, direct intervention is indicated. In instances where there is a pulse deficit, particularly when the limb is profoundly ischemic with loss of sensation and motor function, a major emergency exists and immediate operation is indicated.

The greater problem, with penetrating trauma, involves wounds of proximity where there is no direct evidence of vascular injury. For knife wounds, the absence of a history of hemorrhage or any of the above findings usually dictates management by observation and follow-up.[17] If there is a bruit present or any question of pulse deficit, then arteriograms or direct operative intervention is indicated.

Gunshot wounds which occur in proximity to the artery can injure the vessel without touching it. The decision whether or not to carry out arteriography must be weighed carefully and if there is major associated soft tissue injury in proximity to the artery, arteriograms are indicated. For low velocity missile injury with no evidence of hematoma, loss of arterial pulses, or hemorrhage, limbs can be safely observed.[18,19]

Blunt trauma is a more difficult problem. Extensive soft tissue injury may be associated with "spasm" which may be nothing more than a slight stretch of the vessel or hemorrhage in proximity. Although shards of bone can result in penetrating injuries to blood vessels, the most common injury from blunt trauma is a stretch-type injury.[20] The classic injury is that associated with knee dislocation. Here the pulses may be present initially and the injury, if exposed at this point, consists of nothing more than a slight disruption of the intima. However, with passage of time the intima may have a tendency to roll up like a window shade which it does naturally in a completely divided vessel. This results ultimately in occlusion of the vessel. The progressive exposure of the basement membrane with intimal injury also results in the gradual buildup of thrombus.

Because of the high incidence of popliteal artery injury associated with both anterior and posterior dislocation, these injuries should have arteriographic assessment. This can be done in the operating room in conjunction with an orthopaedic procedure or it can be done prior to orthopaedic operative intervention by the radiologist in the x-ray department. Injuries at the condylar area and tibial plateau level also are associated with the risk of popliteal artery injury, but to a lesser degree. Femoral shaft fractures, because of proximity to the superficial femoral artery, may result in injury to this vessel. When there is any asymmetry of pulses between the injured and the normal extremity, even though the limb is viable, the injury is best assessed by arteriography. Many of these limbs when badly injured

Table 5–1 Signs of Arterial Injury

- Severe ischemia
- Weak or absent pulse
- Bleeding
- Tense hematoma
- Bruit

are hidden away in splints and casts. Thus ischemic complications may not be evident when they develop, and the ischemic pain may be ascribed to the orthopaedic problem.

PREOPERATIVE MANAGEMENT

Once recognized, every attempt should be made to repair arterial injuries of the lower extremity promptly. In those patients with ischemic manifestations, blood flow should be restored within 6 to 8 hours, since occlusion of muscular arterial branches and death of muscle are universal in severe ischemia beyond this period. This is the reason why the results are poorest for delayed repairs and there is a high incidence of amputation. Moreover, there is significant systemic morbidity from reperfusion of severely ischemic extremities (this is not necessarily true of the upper extremity where the relative volume of ischemic tissue is low). The large masses of skeletal muscle which are reperfused in the lower extremity release thromboplastins and inflammatory components. These tear up the vascular system, result in increased vascular permeability, third spacing, and result in diffuse organ failure as manifest by the respiratory distress syndrome, myocardial infarction, and renal failure. For this reason, when pulses are absent, and the limb is ischemic, particularly if paralyzed and anesthetic, a major emergency exists. Immediate operative treatment is indicated. If arteriograms are necessary to locate the lesion, these are best obtained in the operating room utilizing percutaneous femoral arteriography or direct needle puncture following proximal exposure of the artery. In this manner, the operation can proceed concomitantly with the obtaining of x-rays.

For those patients in whom the presence of injury is questionable, but in which hemorrhage or hematomas are present, arteriography may be indicated if there is question of major arterial involvement and operative treatment of the wound or fracture is not otherwise indicated.

Preoperative administration of a gram of a second-generation cephalosporin is indicated in the emergency room. Blood should have been sent to the laboratory for typing and cross-match. Plain x-rays of the involved extremity are indicated if there is any question of retained foreign body or bony injury.

If other injuries are present, the extremity injury management may have to await its priority for treatment since other potentially life-threatening injuries may take precedent.

EXPOSURE

All of the vessels of the lower leg are best exposed by generous longitudinal incisions. The *common femoral artery* is best demonstrated by a longitudinal incision which overlaps the inguinal ligament at the point of the femoral artery pulse, and extends slightly medially, obliquely downward (Figure 5–4). The incision is best placed slightly lateral rather than slightly medial to the artery since the medial exposure risks injury to the adjacent saphenous vein and common femoral vein and their collaterals. In instances where the injury involves the proximal common femoral artery, proximal control can be assured by extending the incision obliquely upward as a suprainguinal incision. An oblique opening is made parallel to the fibers of the external oblique and carried down through the transversalis fascia to identify the external iliac artery just above the inguinal ligament. The iliac artery

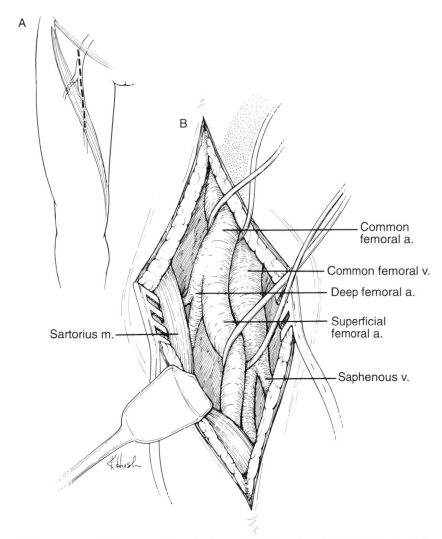

A

B

Common femoral a.

Common femoral v.

Deep femoral a.

Superficial femoral a.

Sartorius m.

Saphenous v.

Figure 5–4. Exposure of the common femoral artery and its bifurcation. **A:** Skin incision in relation to the femoral artery and sartorius muscle. **B:** Isolation of the vessels.

can be encircled and controlled and then further dissection carried out below the inguinal ligament to expose the femoral artery. Because it only gives off small branches, the entire femoral artery can be mobilized and freed if necessary to repair both anterior and posterior lacerations. If there is presumed concomitant injury to the common femoral vein an incision is better placed on the medial side of the artery so that the common femoral vein can be exposed easily in parallel. However, a simple extension of the incision proximally and distally, regardless of its location, usually permits adequate exposure of both vessels.

The *profunda femoral artery* can be identified by exposing the bifurcation of the common femoral artery, encircling the larger vessel first, followed by the superficial femoral artery. Then retraction of that vessel medially or laterally permits the dissection and exposure of the profunda. Caution must be exercised in dissecting the profunda femoral artery to avoid division of abundant collaterals and also to avoid hemorrhage from inadvertent transection of the profunda femoral vein. However, when exposure of the first 3 or 4 cm of the profunda femoral artery is necessary, the profunda vein can be transected with minimal morbidity. The ends should be secured with running suture since secondary hemorrhage from the vein is an embarrassing event which happens all too frequently unless running closure of the divided vein is carried out.

In injuries to the proximal *superficial femoral artery*, the common femoral artery is usually best exposed initially and dissection carried distally to its bifurcation where the origin of the superficial femoral artery can be exposed. If the medial edge of the sartorius starts to overlap the superficial femoral artery this muscle can be readily retracted laterally.

The portion of the superficial femoral artery in Hunter's canal is readily exposed by identifying the medial edge of the sartorius muscle and making the incision along the edge of this muscle (Figure 5–5). Its edge is mobilized, then the muscle retracted laterally, and the dissection carried under the muscle to expose the superficial femoral artery. The distal third of the femoral artery is best exposed by placing the incision along the anterior or lateral edge of the sartorius muscle and retracting the muscle posteriorly. At this level the artery is quite deep, lying between the vastus medialis and the adductor muscles. It can usually be located by following any of the venous or arterial collaterals which occur in the region. In this region the vein is usually intimately related to the artery and one or more of the venae comitantes must be dissected from the artery to permit adequate mobilization for exposure. For injuries to the distal superficial femoral artery, a proximally placed tourniquet will suffice for proximal arterial control. This should not be inflated unless necessary and should be deflated as soon as vascular control is obtained. This ensures a continued collateral flow which is an important preventative of distal thrombosis in both artery and vein.

The *popliteal artery* can be exposed from either the medial or posterior approach. In blunt trauma there is a considerable advantage in the posterior approach since no major muscles need to be taken down. This avoids adding to the instability of an already unstable knee. If the medial approach is considered appropriate, the knee should be flexed. The incision is made longitudinally just behind the tibial plateau and the femoral condyle. For adequate proximal exposure of the artery, the medial head of the gastrocnemius muscle can be divided. A short segment of tendon should be left to permit reapproximation of the muscle. The knee joint should be avoided by keeping the dissection posterior to the joint capsule and anterior to the nerve which, in the upper portion of the popliteal artery, usually lies lateral to the artery. The vein is usually encountered first and must be mobilized to facilitate exposure of the artery. For exposure of the distal portion of the popliteal artery, the knee should be kept sharply flexed and, if necessary, the soleus muscle can be separated from its attachment to the tibia permitting the fossa to be opened widely to the bifurcation or trifurcation. The tibial nerve is usually immediately posterior and may be misidentified as the artery. Care should be taken to preserve all the branches of the nerve if possible. When a segment of artery must be removed, the artery can be mobilized throughout its length to facilitate primary end-to-end anastomosis. The decision to do this must be weighed against the disadvantages of interrupting important collateral. If the leg has been clearly viable prior to operation, interposition vein graft may be more appropriate than mobilizing the artery so as to avoid risk to critical collaterals.

The posterior approach to the popliteal artery requires positioning the patient in a prone position (Figure 5–6). Although curvilinear incisions are advocated by some, we have found no problem with a straight linear incision carried the length of the popliteal

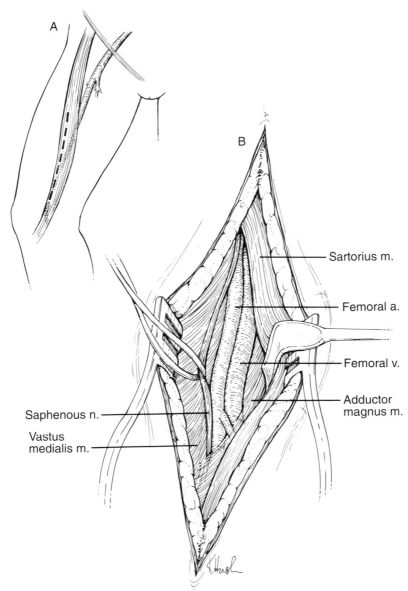

Figure 5–5. Exposure of the superficial femoral artery. **A:** Skin incision along the sartorius. **B:** Distal portion of the vessel between the vastus medialis and adductors.

space. The artery lies in a slightly medial position in the upper portion of the popliteal space but is in the midline in the lower two thirds. The dissection is carried down through the fascia. The artery can be seen located deep in the popliteal space just on top of the joint capsule. The tibial nerve must be identified as it crosses over the artery and vein and gently retracted. If the distal portion of the artery or trifurcation requires exposure, the gastroc-nemius muscle can be split between its two heads and the soleus mobilized from its posterior

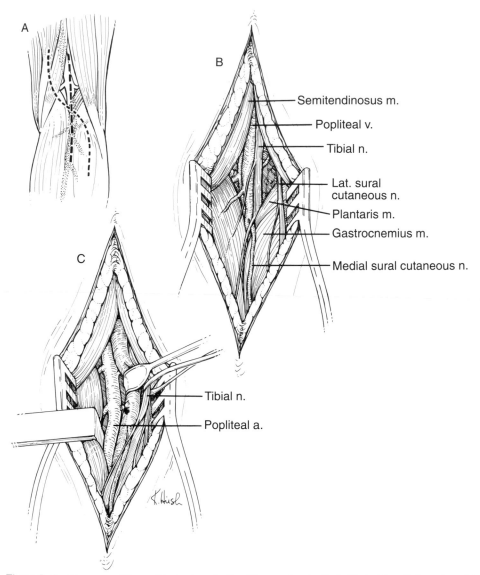

Figure 5–6.   Exposure of the popliteal artery. **A:** Curvilinear or longitudinal skin incision. **B:** Location of the neurovascular structures of the popliteal space. **C:** Retraction of the tibial nerve for exposure of the popliteal artery.

tibial attachment. The plantaris muscle can be divided as necessary for exposure and does not require reattachment.

Exposure of the first portion of *anterior tibial artery* can be quite difficult because it lies deep in the popliteal space and passes through the interosseous membrane and courses downward deep in the anterior compartment. The origin of the vessel can be exposed from either of the popliteal artery approaches just described and the interosseous membrane slit so as to facilitate an additional 1 cm or more exposure. For many injuries near the origin which require treatment, the lateral approach may be superior (Figure 5–7). In this

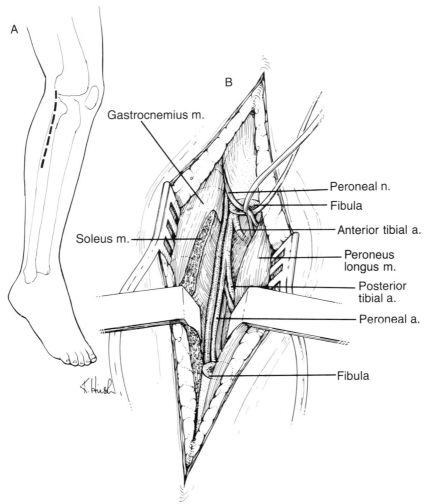

A

B

Gastrocnemius m.

Soleus m.

Peroneal n.

Fibula

Anterior tibial a.

Peroneus
longus m.

Posterior
tibial a.

Peroneal a.

Fibula

Figure 5–7. **A:** Skin incision. **B:** Lateral exposure of the anterior tibial artery via resection of the proximal fibula.

instance, the incision is made directly over the head and neck of the fibula with careful identification of the common peroneal nerve. As much as the proximal third of the fibula can be resected. This will give immediate and excellent exposure of the artery from its origin well down the leg. If complex fractures are present about the knee, however, this may add to the instability of the leg and decisions whether to repair or ligate must be considered, since exposure for ligation of the proximal portion of the artery is relatively simple compared to the exposure required for repair. For injuries distal to the first 3 to 4 centimeters, the vessel can be exposed on the interosseous membrane by dissecting down along the lateral aspect of the tibialis anterior, retracting the anterior compartment musculature medially and laterally. The distal third of the artery is easily exposed by dissection carried down along the lateral edge of the tibia. The vessel is best identified as it passes onto the tibia, and the dissection carried proximal from there as necessary. Distally it is superficial in its course down to the region of the second metatarsal and is readily exposed with preservation and retraction of any associated overlying tendons. The tibial nerve should be identified and carefully avoided.

The *posterior tibial artery*, the continuation of the popliteal, is exposed medially. Its upper third is best exposed by extending the incision used for the medial approach to the distal popliteal artery (Figure 5–8). The soleus is detached from the posterior aspect of the tibia and the artery and its accompanying veins identified. The lower portion of the artery can be exposed posterior to the medial malleolus and its course followed backward, or by dissecting in a plane just posterior to the tibia between the soleus and the plantar flexors of the foot (Figure 5–9). The posterior tibial nerve which accompanies the artery must be identified and preserved.

The *peroneal artery* can be exposed in its proximal portion by the medial approach used for the distal popliteal artery by taking down the insertion of the soleus muscle from its attachment to the tibia. However, unless the exposure needed is within the first 2 or 3 cm of the vessel origin, the best approach to the peroneal artery is laterally (Figure 5–7). The incision is made over the posterior edge of the fibula and carried down deep into the leg to expose the vessel. Generally, repair of the distal third of the artery is not indicated and ligation is appropriate. This can be done through quite a small incision.

PRINCIPLES OF VASCULAR REPAIR

In almost all instances where vascular injury of the lower extremity is assumed, the opposite leg should be prepped for potential removal of the saphenous vein for use as a patch or for arterial replacement as an interposition graft.

The *common femoral artery*, being a large vessel, lends itself to many different modes of repair. However, gunshot wounds or direct blunt trauma may require resection of the vessel. If the wound is relatively clean, a prosthetic graft of PTFE or Dacron can be successfully utilized. Even though the saphenous vein is much smaller in caliber it can be used as an interposition graft. If the size discrepancy is quite large, some type of patch or plasty technique may be more appropriate to repair the artery. In heavily contaminated wounds, it is possible to borrow a section of the external iliac artery and replace the artery with autogenous tissue. The vascular graft is then used to replace the external iliac artery. Simple lacerations are best debrided and approximated with interrupted or running monofilament suture (Figure 5–10). Injuries to the associated vein, if complex, are best treated by ligation since this provides less risk of thromboembolism. Simple vein lacerations can be closed with fine everting monofilament suture. While the saphenous vein is available as a patch it should ordinarily be left intact as a potential collateral.

Profunda femoral artery injuries can be treated with simple ligation, repair, a vein patch, or with resection and reanastomosis. However, this artery does not mobilize well because of its abundant branches and can be ligated with minimal disability since its collateral connections are excellent.

Superficial femoral artery is easily exposed and because of minimal branches it can be mobilized for 2 to 3 cm if necessary for end-to-end anastomosis. When anastomosis must be done under tension, at least half of the circumference of sutures should be placed prior to reapproximating the artery since an extremely steady assistant is required to maintain approximation of the vessel ends otherwise. Everting sutures are optimal, particularly

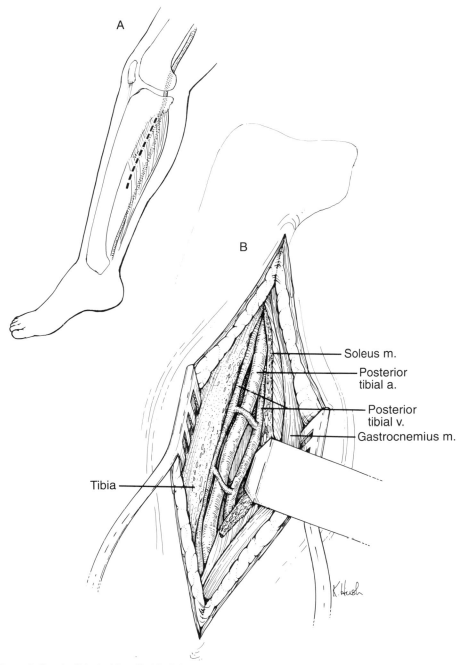

Figure 5–8. **A:** Skin incision. **B:** Medial exposure of the posterior tibial artery.

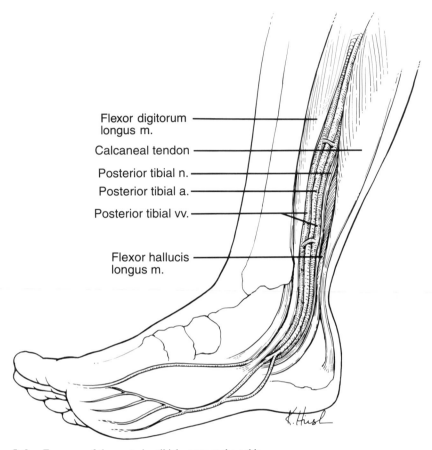

Flexor digitorum
longus m.

Calcaneal tendon

Posterior tibial n.

Posterior tibial a.

Posterior tibial vv.

Flexor hallucis
longus m.

Figure 5–9.   Exposure of the posterior tibial artery at the ankle.

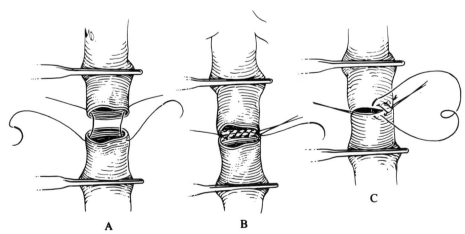

A

B

C

Figure 5–10.   Technique utilized for large vessel repair. **A:** Initial sutures 180° to each other to line edges up.
B: Running monofilament suture on back side of artery. **C:** Completion of repair.

in the smaller arteries found in females or children, to avoid thrombogenesis. An optimal way of performing the anastomosis is to place two horizontal everting mattress sutures at 180° of each other on the vessel wall, with running sutures placed between (see Figure 5–11). The vessel ends should be obliquely cut to ensure a larger diameter anastomosis and the vessel should be gently dilated with an olive dilator or treated with papaverine so it is not in spasm at the time of the anastomosis. Injuries to the associated veins are best ligated unless there has been extensive soft tissue injury and presumed damage to collateral. Under these circumstances interposition vein graft may be appropriate even though it functions only temporarily, as arterial inflow may be compromised if there is major venous outflow obstruction. If there is any question about the need to carry out simultaneous vein anastomosis, whether it is at the superficial femoral or popliteal level, pressure measurement should be obtained in the distal vein with the vein clamped or ligated. If the manometer pressure in the vein measures 40 cm of water or more, significant venous obstruction exists and repair of the vein is probably indicated. With pressures under this level, the decision whether to repair the vein is arbitrary. Usually, venous ligation will be associated with minimal morbidity unless extensive associated venous thrombosis occurs. However, this type of thrombosis is more likely to occur following complex repair than with clean ligation.

Popliteal artery injuries are most difficult to treat of all the common vascular injuries. The reasons are twofold. The collateral potential about the knee joint is the least of any arterial location because of the lack of bulk of tissues at this level. When there has been extensive injury, any existing collateral is easily damaged. The lack of collateral contributes to the problem by inducing severe distal stasis and when delay between injury and treatment is more than 6 to 8 hours, thrombosis of the side branches of the major arteries is likely, as is associated thrombosis of the draining veins. The latter may well interfere with flow through even the best arterial anastomosis and lead to both thrombosis of the repair and limb loss.

Popliteal artery repair must be particularly meticulous. All damaged or devitalized intima must be removed and anastomosis conducted with eversion to ensure intima-to-intima approximation even if this requires an interposition graft (Figure 5–11). For small arteries, interrupted everting sutures may be more optimal than a running suture which is more apt to purse-string the artery. Once arterial flow has been restored obstructed pressure in any adjoining vein injury can be assessed either by palpation or by direct measurement. If the vein is distended and tense, or pressure is above 40 cm of water, venous repair is indicated, even if a saphenous vein interposition graft is required. Because repairs of the popliteal artery are associated with a thrombosis rate varying from 0% to 25% and probably averaging about 10% to 15%, postoperative arteriograms are indicated to assess flow in the vessel and the status of the anastomosis.

Routine instrumentation of arteries to remove clot should be avoided if possible. Vigorous massage of the leg distal to the anastomosis should be done prior to completion of anastomosis to ensure presence of back bleeding or to force out any jelly-like clot. If there is a possibility of residual clot this is best detected with an arteriogram which can be done through a catheter inserted in the vessel prior to completion of the anastomosis. If clot is present, concomitant systemic administration of heparin should be considered and the risk of rethrombosis weighed against the risk of bleeding. Usually, however, the bleeding complication is more readily treated than the thrombotic complication. Should thrombosis develop on the operating table or immediately postoperatively, prompt return to the

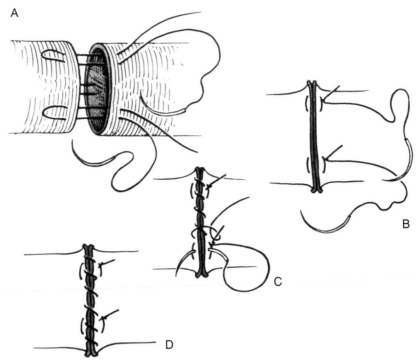

Figure 5–11.   Technique for closure of a moderate-sized artery. **A:** Everting initial sutures—there, three are used 120° to each other. **B:** Eversion of the vessel ends. **C:** Continuation of each mattress suture as a running suture. **D:** The completed repair.

operating room is indicated. Under these circumstances gentle instrumentation of the distal artery using a Fogarty catheter is appropriate. Several catheters can be placed simultaneously so that at least two out of three branches of the popliteal artery are cleared of clot. Once again, consideration should be given to the status of the associated vein and should there be evidence of low flow and much arterial spasm, concomitant venous repair should be considered.

Anterior tibial, posterior tibial, and peroneal arteries can be repaired using the exposure indicated in the previous section. In most instances, an isolated injury to any one of these three arteries does not necessarily require repair. In most instances, even if only one artery is patent, adequate peripheral circulation will be present. However, in complex injuries where there is evidence of poor distal perfusion, repair of one or two of these vessels may well be indicated.[20] Meticulous technique utilizing magnification is indicated and intima-to-intima approximation must be exact. Very fine interrupted suture technique should be utilized and vein patches and interposition grafts used liberally. If there has been extensive soft tissue injury, particularly when there has been major nerve injury, as is often the case when multiple lower leg vessels are injured, and severe distal ischemia exists, consideration should be given to amputation as an alternative to attempted vascular repair. Unless there is good soft tissue coverage and a clean wound, secondary hemorrhage from repaired vessels is a threat to the life of the patient.

COMPLICATIONS AND POSTOPERATIVE MANAGEMENT

The most acute complications following treatment of vascular injuries are those of thrombosis and hemorrhage. The true incidence of these complications is not available in most reports. In the Vietnam vascular registry, Rich found 63 complications in 290 patients undergoing vascular repair—or 20% of the group.[21] Two thirds of the complications were thrombosis and one third related to hemorrhage. The hemorrhage usually resulted from loss of covering soft tissues from either direct damage or, more commonly, from infection in badly damaged, contaminated tissue. In civilian casualties, the incidence of contaminated wounds is far less as is the incidence of secondary hemorrhage. Good judgment must be exercised and attempts to repair a vessel in a field where there is no adequate soft tissue coverage should be avoided. Under most circumstances, hemorrhage should be rare in civilian practice. Bypass grafts can always be placed extra-anatomically where there is anticipation of infection or soft tissue loss, or following secondary hemorrhage. If the limb had been viable prior to the vascular repair, or viable following thrombosis of a reconstruction, then further attempts at repair should be avoided and secondary repair carried out later if there is evidence of significant residual disability.

Most major hemorrhages from arterial suture lines are initially manifest by small initial hemorrhage and any hemorrhage which occurs from the wound 24 hours or more following repair should lead to consideration of an anastomotic leak. Bleeding is painless and patients can hemorrhage to death in bed without any overt warning. If wound bleeding occurs 24 or more hours following repair (Sentinel hemorrhage) then the burden of proof that hemorrhage does not come from anastomosis lies with the surgeon and operative exposure of the questionable vessel is usually indicated.

Thrombosis is the commonest complication. Most thromboses occur within 24 hours of surgery and most start on the operating table and are manifest within a few hours of surgery. For this reason, when there is ever any doubt about the adequacy of the vascular repair, operative arteriograms are indicated while the patient is still in the operating room. Alternatively, the extremity can be exposed by removing the drapes and the limb assessed for pulses. If pulses are decreased and arteriograms have not been done, the choice is either to reoperate or carry out arteriography. The best time to redo the operation is immediately following the first while the patient is still in the operating room.

Another complication related to vascular injury is the compartment syndrome. This can occur as a result of venous obstruction, compartment hemorrhage, muscle contusion or edema, or from muscle ischemia and swelling (see Chapter 20). In the latter instance, the decision for or against fasciotomy is controversial. Muscle does not swell significantly when it is perfectly viable. When the vascular injury is remote from the site of potential swelling, ie, common femoral artery injury, restoration of flow to the calf in less than six hours will not be associated with appreciable muscle damage or significant swelling. When fasciotomy is carried out when the limb has been ischemic longer than this, fasciotomy will expose ischemic and dead muscle with attendant risk of hemorrhage and poor wound healing and with little benefit in reversing muscle damage. Fasciotomy in these circumstances is at best a tradeoff. Whatever is gained in improving perfusion of marginally viable muscle is lost relative to the creation of an open wound. In the remaining circumstances, fasciotomy may be beneficial if skin and fascia are opened widely over the involved compartment or compartments.

The final major complication following revascularization of ischemic extremities is the "reperfusion syndrome."[24] As is true of the compartment syndrome, this complication relates directly to the duration and severity of the limb ischemia and to the mass of skeletal muscle involved. Blood loss with systemic hypovolemia also aggravates and escalates the problem. Reperfusion of ischemic and dead muscle results in the washout of breakdown products which enter the systemic circulation. These act as procoagulants which activate intravascular coagulation, produce a systemic inflammatory response, alterations in vascular permeability, and/or disseminated intravascular coagulation and the bleeding syndrome. Vascular permeability is associated with extravasation of fluid and colloid from the vascular system, resulting in the respiratory distress syndrome, refractory hypovolemia, and diffuse organ damage. This accounts for severe morbidity and the mortality associated with delayed revascularization. This syndrome comprises what was once referred to as the "fat embolism syndrome." It is associated with the high mortality noted following revascularization of limbs following acute arterial embolism. This is the primary reason why anticoagulation and/or amputation may be more appropriate treatment than ill advised attempts to restore blood flow to extremities which have been severely ischemic for more than 6 to 8 hours.

RESULTS

The results of lower extremity vascular repair correlate directly with two factors: the extent of associated soft tissue injury and the duration and severity of the ischemia associated with the vascular injury.[21,23,24] If there is major associated nerve injury such as transection of the sciatic nerve where there will be most certainly an insensate foot, amputation is usually superior to vascular repair. In this circumstance, vascular repair should be considered primarily to be able to ensure below-knee amputation. This involves making certain that profunda femoral flow is adequate since the superficial femoral artery patency is not required for successful BK amputation. Also the presence of associated injuries must be weighed in making therapeutic decisions. If the injury is confined to the extremity, an attempt to save a badly injured limb with comminuted fractures and soft tissue injury may be indicated. If there are other life-threatening injuries, however, amputation usually offers the best potential for salvage of life and no attempt to save a limb should be made if this involves potential compromise of survival (see Chapter 21). Modern prosthetics play a very significant role in successful rehabilitation of those patients who require amputation and who are usually young patients.

When the injury has been the result of profound ischemia with paralysis and anesthesia of the limb, particularly when the limb is blue and mottled and the ischemia has been longer than 6 or 8 hours, attempts to restore circulation will usually be unsuccessful due to the inability to reperfuse dead muscle. Moreover, should reperfusion be successful, systemic hypercoagulability or DIC may threaten the life of the patient or may result in prompt rethrombosis of the vascular repair. Since very few series provide data on the extent of soft tissue and bony injury which occur in parallel with vascular injuries and provide next to no information regarding the duration and severity of the ischemia, it is difficult to compare results. McLean demonstrated in World War II that clean ligation of the external iliac common femoral artery is associated with a 25% limb loss rate. Ligation of the superficial femoral artery is associated with a 50% limb loss rate and ligation of the popliteal artery,

75% limb loss rate. The results of successful vascular surgery in the Korean and Vietnam wars were markedly superior to these. Rich reported that the amputation rate for injuries of the common femoral artery was 15%, for the superficial femoral artery, 12.1%, and for the popliteal artery, 29%. Reports of civilian vascular injuries indicate that the success of popliteal artery repairs varied between 8% and 44%. No accurate data are available for treatment of isolated injuries of the lower leg vessels, but the amputation rate for individual injuries should be negligible.

REFERENCES

1. Schwartz AM. Historical development of methods of hemostasis. *Surgery*. 1958;44:604.
2. Blaisdell FW. Medical advances during the Civil War. *Arch Surg*. 1988;123:1045–1050.
3. Bell J. *Principles of Surgery, I*. DIS Course 9. 1801:404.
4. Murphy JB. Resection of arteries and veins in continuity end-end suture: experimental and clinical research. *Med Rec*. 1897;51:73.
5. Goyanes J. Neuvos trabajos de chirurgia vascular: substitution plastica de las arterias por las venas. *El Siglo Med*. 1906;53:561.
6. Carrel A. Results of transplantation of organs, vessels and limbs. *JAMA*. 1908;51:1602.
7. Hughes CW. Historical aspects of vascular trauma. In: Rich NM, Spencer FC, eds. *Vascular Trauma*. Philadelphia, Pa: WB Saunders; 1978:3–4.
8. Drapanas T. Etiology, incidence and clinical pathology. In: Rich NM, Spencer FC, eds. *Vascular Trauma*. Philadelphia, Pa: WB Saunders; 1978:22–43.
9. Makins GH. *Gunshot Injuries to Blood Vessels*. Bristol Engl: John Wright and Sons; 1919.
10. Rich NM, Spencer, FC. Chapter 23. *Superficial Femoral Artery Injuries*. Philadelphia, Pa: WB Saunders; 1978:510–525.
11. Rich NM, Spencer FC. Popliteal artery injuries. In: Rich NM, Spencer FC, eds. *Vascular Trauma*. Philadelphia, Pa: WB Saunders; 1978:526–548.
12. Brewer PI, Schramel RJ, Menendez CV, Creech O Jr. Injuries of the popliteal artery: a report of 16 cases. *Am J Surg*. 1969;118:36.
13. Wagner WH, Calkins ER, Wearer FA, Goodwin JA, Myles RA, Yellin AE. Blunt popliteal trauma: one hundred consecutive injuries. *J Vasc Surg*. 1988;7:736–748.
14. Bunt TJ, Malone JM, Moody M, Davidson J, Karpman R. The frequency of vascular injury with blunt trauma induced extremity fracture/dislocation. Presented at the Society of Clinical Vascular Surgery; January 1990. In press.
15. DeBakey ME, Simeone FA. Battle injuries of arteries in World War II: an analysis of 2,471 cases. *Ann Surg*. 1946;123:534.
16. Rich NM, Spencer FC. Anterior tibial, posterior tibial and peroneal artery injuries. In: Rich NM, Spencer FC, eds. *Vascular Trauma*. Philadelphia, Pa: WB Saunders; 1978:549–562.
17. Hartling RP, McGahan JP, Blaisdell FW, Lindfors KK. Stab wounds of the extremity: indications for angiography. *Cardiovasc Radiology*. 1987;162:465–567.
18. Rose SC, Moore EE. Trauma angiography: the use of clinical findings to improve patient selection and case preparation. *J Trauma*. 1988;28:240–245.
19. Reid JDS, Weigelt JA, Thal EA, Francis H III. Assessment of proximity of a wound to major vascular structures as an indication for arteriography. *Arch Surg*. 1988;123:942–946.
20. Drost TF, Rosemurgy AS, Proctor D, Kearney RE. Outcome of combined orthopedic and arterial trauma to the lower extremity. *J Trauma*. 1989;29:1331–1334.
21. Rich NM, Spencer FC. Sequelae of acute arterial trauma. In: Rich NM, Spencer FC, eds. *Vascular Trauma*. Philadelphia, Pa: WB Saunders; 1978:106–124.
22. Vitale GC, Richardson JD, George SM Jr, Miller FB. Fasciotomy for severe blunt and penetrating trauma of the extremity. *Surg Gynecol Obstet*. 1988;166:397–401.
23. Shah DM, Corsen JD, Karmode AM, Fortune JB, Leather RP. Optimal management of tibial arterial trauma. *J Trauma*. 1988;28:228–234.
24. Klausner JM, Paterson IS, Mannick JA, Valeri R, Shepro D, Hechtman HB. Reperfusion pulmonary edema. *JAMA*. 1989;261:1030–1035.

6

Extremity Nerve Injury

LAWRENCE H. PITTS, M.D.
F. WILLIAM BLAISDELL, M.D.

HISTORY[1,2]: The loss of irritability and fragmentation of fibers following nerve section were first recorded by Guenther and Schoen in 1840. It was with this background that August Waller, working in London in 1850, followed the sequence of axonal degeneration in the severed glossopharyngeal and hypoglossal nerves of the frog. He noted that cutting the nerves on both sides resulted in the animal's death but that when one side was cut, he noticed decreased power and sensation on the affected side of the tongue. During the subsequent 12 to 15 days he observed the breakdown of the medullary (myelin) sheath. In 1852, Waller made some additional fundamental discoveries. He observed the regeneration of glossopharyngeal nerve fibers into the tongue three to four months after section. In addition, he showed that when a spinal sensory nerve is cut below the ganglion, the degeneration is not carried back to the ganglion. If, however, the ganglion itself is removed the nerve degenerates. These observations supported Remak's thesis that axonal processes arose from the neuroganglion cells.

Ranvier (1878) noted the distance between each node (internodal length) was proportional to the diameter of the myelinated fiber. He believed that the myelin might protect the axon or that it might act as an insulator in a similar way to the insulating cover on a submarine cable. He proposed that nodal constriction might stop the semiliquid myelin from flowing along the nerve to its lower end or that breaks in the sheath might allow the diffusion of nutrients into the axon. In 1913 Cajal studied axon degeneration and regeneration in greater detail. He demonstrated that the proximal stump of the injured axon will usually degenerate back to the preceding node of Ranvier or the one before. After a few hours the tip of the proximal axon stump swells to form an end bulb from which axons will sprout on or about the second day. Distally, the axons and myelins start to fragment and the debris lies mainly in the Schwann cells.

INTRODUCTION

The most challenging aspect of extremity injury has been and remains injury to nerves. Far and away nerve injury has constituted the principal factor which accounts for limb loss and permanent disability. Major advances which laid the background for successful nerve repair were those in nerve physiology and these resulted from the introduction of techniques for measuring nerve conduction in intact animals.[3] In 1949, Dawson and Scott measured conduction velocities in sensory nerves with electrodes placed on the skin.[4] They found that the conduction velocities were reduced in regenerating nerves following injury.

As regards nerve repair itself, very little was done prior to World War II. Nerves were considered simple structures and their repair consisted of gross reapproximation by suture of the epineurium. The incidence of failure of the repair and of infection during and immediately after repair was high. As the documentation of the microanatomy became available it became clear that the poor results were predominantly the result of the consequence of failed axonal regeneration at the site of repair.[5–7] This stimulated more sophisticated techniques of nerve repair which included the identification of specific fascicles and repair of these fascicles by suture of the perineurium rather than the epineurium. The importance of not carrying out nerve repair under tension was emphasized and the use of nerve grafts, rather than extensive mobilization of nerves, resulted in marked improvement in results in the treatment of complex injuries of nerves.[8,9]

INCIDENCE AND MECHANISM OF INJURY

The exact incidence of peripheral nerve injury is difficult to ascertain because most large series are reported from referral centers and many peripheral and sensory nerve injuries are untreated and may even be unrecognized. Because of its smaller mass and greater concentration of neurologic structures, injuries to the upper extremities are approximately twice as likely to produce nerve injuries as are injuries to the lower extremity.[10] Very commonly the nerve injuries occur in association with other injuries. With penetrating trauma, associated vascular injuries are common.[10,11] The incidence of nerve injury is higher in patients with vascular trauma to the arm (75%) than in the leg (25%). As regards orthopaedic injuries, approximately 12% of humeral shaft fractures are accompanied by paralysis of the radial nerve and 15% to 20% of knee dislocations have accompanying injury to major nerves.

The three primary causes of nerve injury are, in order of frequency, penetrating trauma such as that from missiles, knife wounds, or sharp objects; traction injuries such as occur in association with fractures and dislocations, high velocity missile injuries, or surgery; least common, nerves may be compressed by tight-fitting casts, by tourniquets, or by compartment syndromes.

Sharp lacerations of nerves from cuts or stab wounds that result in a clean laceration of the nerve lend themselves to early intervention and repair. Common injuries following blunt trauma occur as a result of fractures, dislocations, traction, and gunshot wounds. In the majority of these instances, the nerve is not completely divided and it is difficult to accurately identify the extent of damage and determine whether it is functional or anatomic on the initial examination of the patient. Complete functional loss at the time of injury does not preclude complete recovery without intervention. Moreover, even should there be complete division as determined by exploration, it is difficult to determine how much resection of the nerve may be required for anastomosis of healthy tissue.

As previously noted, most of the peripheral nerve injuries associated with fractures occur in the upper extremity. Radial nerve injury associated with humeral fracture is the most common injury. The ulnar nerve is especially vulnerable at the elbow. The median nerve is least frequently injured in association with fractures.[9]

Neural injury is relatively common in association with major dislocations of the lower extremities and these result in stretch injuries. These are found most commonly in association with knee dislocations or posterior hip dislocations. Neural injuries associated with fractures have greater than an 80% incidence of spontaneous resolution, whereas recovery is much less common with neural injury secondary to dislocations.[9] Compression type injuries such as occur in compartment syndromes have a variable prognosis depending upon whether immediate decompression is done for the former or whether there is associated muscle or compartmental damage that may result in total infarction of the compartment and all the structures in it. Compartment syndrome secondary to direct contusion and hemorrhage, when recognized, should be treated promptly by decompression, and if done, the prognosis for nerve recovery is quite good.[12]

ANATOMY AND PHYSIOLOGY

Peripheral nerves contain variably numbered and sized nerve fibers (axons) individually enclosed within an endoneurial sheath (Figure 6–1). These axons are in turn bound together into bundles or fascicles by adjacent connective tissue—the perineurium. The bundles are

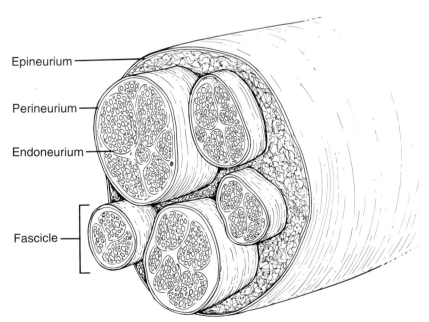

Figure 6–1.   Cross section of a divided nerve showing multiple fasciculi.

held together by a loose areolar connective tissue framework and the epineurium which provide most of the nerve's tensile strength and which separates the nerve from surrounding tissues. These sheaths, ie, the endoneurium, perineurium, and epineurium, are the connective tissue framework of the peripheral nerve which provide support, isolation, and insulation of its various components (Figure 6–2). Each of these have specific characteristics which should be understood.

The *endoneurium* is made up of Schwann cells and surrounds each individual axon. The *perineurium* invests each fascicle with a relatively thin but dense and distinctive sheath of fibrous tissue. When the fascicles at the end of a freshly cut nerve are carefully examined, it can be seen that they have the ability to move back and forth independently. The fascicular blood supply is contained between these septae. The *epineurium*, the outer sleeve which surrounds the entire peripheral nerve, also moves somewhat independently of its contents.

Injection studies demonstrate that the microcirculation of each funiculus runs in the perineurium. The internal circulation of the nerve is supplied to it segmentally through the mesoneurium in a relationship similar to that of the intestine and its mesentery. The nutrient vessels enter the nerve along the line where the mesoneurium attaches to the nerve and not the remaining portion of its circumference. A rupture of endoneurial tubes formed by Schwann cells leads to denuding of axons. The Schwann cells proliferate to reinvest the exposed or injured nerve and, if successful, will contain the regenerating axon. Otherwise uncontained axons will become entangled with proliferating fibroblasts arising from the connective tissue of the nerve. Thus, neuromas can occur even when there is continuity of the nerve if the endoneurium is ruptured.

The cell bodies of the motor nerve fibers (anterior horn cells) lie in the anterolateral aspect of the spinal cord gray matter. The axons of the anterior horn cells pass laterally out of the spinal cord forming the anterior or ventral spinal nerve roots (Figure 6–3). In contrast, the cell bodies of the sensory neurons lie outside the spinal cord in the dorsal root ganglion, which is in continuity with the spinal cord via the posterior or dorsal nerve roots. The ganglia lie within the foramina of the spinal canal where the ventral and dorsal nerve roots join to form the peripheral nerve. The preganglionic fibers make up the dorsal nerve root itself and travel between the ganglion and the spinal cord, whereas sensory fibers distal to the ganglion in the peripheral nerve represent postganglionic fibers.

The distinction between preganglionic and postganglionic fibers is important in the prognosis for long-term recovery from injury. Proximal nerve injuries involving the preganglionic fibers or dorsal root ganglion electrically and physiologically disconnect sensory nerve cells from the spinal cord and sensory recovery is virtually impossible. Motor

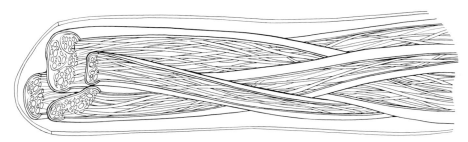

Figure 6–2. Longitudinal section of a nerve showing how fasciculi change in relationship to one another.

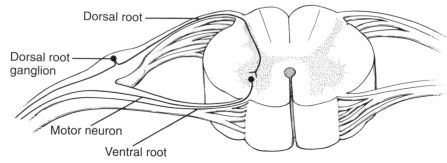

Figure 6–3. Cross section of spinal cord. Dorsal root ganglion containing sensory nerve cell lies inside vertebral body whereas motor nerve cell is in the anterior horn of the spinal cord.

recovery remains possible because the motor nerve cell body lies within the spinal cord itself. However, these proximal injuries are often associated with direct avulsion of nerve fibers from the spinal cord and motor recovery is rare. Preganglionic injuries by definition occur within or proximal to the neural foramina and therefore are not amenable to surgical repair. Postganglionic injuries distal to the neural foramina may be amenable to surgical exploration and repair and have a somewhat better prognosis.

Seddon used only three terms to classify injury.[6] These were neurapraxia, axonotmesis, and neurotmesis. *Neurapraxia* means simple shock to the nerve which could result from concussion or compression but with no loss of integrity of the axon. *Axonotmesis* indicates interruption and degeneration of the axon with no loss of integrity of the nerve sheath; *neurotmesis* is actual disruption of the nerve from interruption of isolated nerve fasciculi to complete interruption of the nerve itself.

A more practical classification is that of Sunderland in which there are five degrees of nerve injury (Table 6–1).[7] *First-degree injury* corresponds to Seddon's neurapraxia and usually results from concussion or compression of the nerve. Electrical conductivity of the nerve distal to the lesion is preserved. Surgical repair is not necessary and recovery is spontaneous and rapid within days or weeks. Recovery does not depend on regeneration of any neural element and should be complete.

Second-degree injury, equivalent to axonotmesis, occurs when anatomical continuity of the nerve and Schwann sheath is preserved but the axons are interrupted and must recover by axonal regeneration. There is complete motor, sensory, and autonomic paralysis and progressive muscle atrophy. Surgical repair is not necessary. Recovery from second-degree

Table 6–1 Classification of Injuries to Nerves

DEGREE OF INJURY	ANATOMIC DISRUPTION
First	Conduction loss only, without anatomic disruption
Second	Axonal disruption without loss of the neurilemmal sheath
Third	Loss of axons and nerve sheaths
Fourth	Fascicular disruption
Fifth	Nerve transection

From Sunderland S. *Nerves and Nerve Injuries*. Edinburgh, UK: Churchill Livingstone; 1978:127. Reprinted with permission injuries should be complete unless the injury is so proximal that atrophy of the motor end plate or sensory receptor occurs before the axon can grow back to these organs. Thus, recovery is faster and more complete after distal injuries in which regeneration distances are not excessive than after more proximal injuries in which substantially fewer nerve fibers may reach the appropriate end-organs before they atrophy. Recovery occurs at the rate of approximately one millimeter per day (1 inch per month).

Third-degree injuries involve disruption of the endoneurial sheaths along with the axons. Thus when axons regenerate they may enter the nerve sheaths of other axons, resulting in aberrant regeneration. With loss of the sheath there is increased intraneural fibrosis making it more difficult for axon regrowth to penetrate through the site of injury. Time for functional improvement depends upon the distance between the injury site and the end-organ. The axon grows at the same rate as those involved with second-degree injuries. Second- and third-degree injuries are equivalent to Seddon's neurotmesis.

In *fourth-degree injuries* nerve fasciculi are disrupted with a commensurately greater degree of intraneural scarring. To become functional, axons must grow through the intraneural scarring and re-enter endoneurial sheaths. When these injuries are minimal in extent, partial resection with anastomosis of the fascicles, utilizing meticulous technique, improves outcome.

Fifth-degree injuries consist of those in which the entire peripheral nerve is transected. Invariably there is considerable epi- and perineurial hemorrhage with subsequent scarring; neural function cannot recover without surgical intervention. Fifth-degree injuries can be limited to a very short section of nerve such as those associated with sharp transection or a very long segment as seen with gunshot injury or associated with stretch injury or compartment syndrome.

Following interruption of the continuity of the nerve, axonal sprouting begins at 10 to 20 days. If scar tissue blocks their entrance to the peripheral portion of the nerve, the sprouts will coil into a disorganized neuroma. In contrast, if the nerve has been repaired, axonal regrowth can proceed at the rate of about one millimeter per day, after an initial lag of 10 to 20 days. Recovery is always imperfect.

The rate and success of nerve regeneration is influenced by several factors. The younger the patient, the faster and more complete the recovery. The nerve involved is also important as pure motor or sensory nerves recover better than do mixed nerves. The radial and musculocutaneous nerves, which are primarily motor nerves, recover better than the mixed median nerve and the tibial division of the sciatic nerves fares better than the peroneal division.[9] An important factor is the level of the nerve injury and the duration of deinnervation. If more than 12 months is required for regenerating axons to reach a denervated muscle, a significant degree of muscle atrophy will have occurred and the muscle may not function despite some reinnervation. In contrast, sensory restitution may still be possible under these circumstances. Repair of a divided ulnar nerve near the axilla or the peroneal nerve above midthigh is unlikely to provide motor improvement. However, repair of the median nerve near the axilla or the tibial nerve about midthigh may allow return of at least some protective sensation.

Factors which influence the success of recovery are the length of the injury along the nerve, and whether or not primary approximation is possible, or nerve grafting is required. Associated injuries to adjacent tissues such as bones, blood vessels, muscles, and tendons also affect prognosis. Regeneration occurs more rapidly in the proximal portion of the extremity.

ASSESSMENT

Every injured extremity should have a careful assessment of sensory and motor function. If other life-threatening cranial or truncal injuries are present, this can be deferred until immediate life-threatening injuries are dealt with, but it is essential that prior to any orthopaedic manipulation, or any treatment of vascular injury of the extremity, examination be conducted to verify the presence or absence of nerve integrity.

The examination should consist of testing sensation which should be possible even in a severely injured hand, and for motor function which may not be feasible when there are major associated injuries. A gross examination should consist of asking the patient whether he notices any loss of sensation. Possible defects can then be assessed using sharp discrimination. A paper clip may be used to test two-point discrimination. Only light pressure should be applied and the area being examined held immobile so that the patient cannot press against the examining instrument. Normal value of two-point discrimination to fingertips is about 4 mm. It will be less acute or completely absent depending on the severity of the nerve damage. The motor examination should be tested by motor strength and graded by standard methods (Table 6–2).

Specific nerve evaluation of the upper extremity involves the brachial plexus (Figure 6–4), median nerve, and radial and ulnar nerves (Table 6–3). Proximal median nerve injuries can be assessed by determining the presence or absence of thumb joint flexion and distal interphalangeal joint function of the index finger. The distal median nerve can be assessed by the ability to oppose the thumb or carry out palmar abduction. The ulnar nerve can be tested by testing thumb adduction and by the ability to radially abduct the index finger or to flex the MP joint of the small finger. Proximal or upper arm radial injuries can be assessed by the ability to extend the wrist joint. Distal radial nerve injuries are assessed by presence or absence of metatarsophalangeal joint extension of the fingers and the ability to carry out forceful thumb interphalangeal joint extension (see table). A brief examination of the major peripheral nerves in the upper and lower extremities is outlined in Tables 6–3 and 6–4.

INITIAL MANAGEMENT

While management of nerve injuries must be individualized for a particular patient, certain general principles can be applied. Acute injuries may either be opened or closed. Since lacerating injuries often will interrupt part or all of the nerve, these injuries often will

Table 6–2   Grading of Motor Strength

GRADE	FUNCTION
0	Absent
1	Trace motion
2	Movement of a joint not against gravity
3	Movement of a joint against gravity
4	Movement against resistance
5	Normal strength

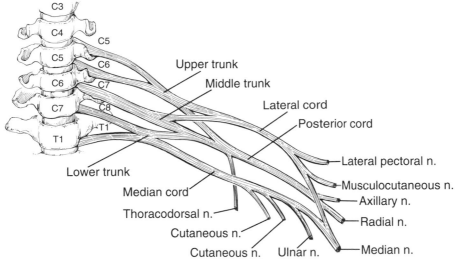

Figure 6–4. Anatomy of the brachial plexus.

Table 6–3 Findings of Peripheral Nerve Injury (Upper Extremity)

	SENSORY	MOTOR
Brachial plexus	Spotty and mixed loss.	Mixed weakness arm, forearm, and hand.
Median	Palmar hand, thumb, index, long, and radial fingers. Dorsal thumb, index, long, and radial fingertips only.	Below elbow: Loss of opposition of thumb with fingers, thenar muscle palsy. Above elbow: Inability to flex distal thumb and index fingers, inability to pronate forearm, flex wrist.
Radial	Dorsal hand to midfingers, thumb, index, long, and radial half of ring finger.	Below elbow: Wrist drop, inability to extend fingers at MP joint. High arm: Inability to extend elbow.
Ulnar	Ulnar wrist, hand, and fingers, ulnar ring, and all of 5th finger.	Inability to spread fingers or flex MP joints without phalangeal flexion. Clawing of 4th and 5th fingers.

Table 6–4 Findings of Peripheral Nerve Injury (Lower Extremity)

	SENSORY	MOTOR
Femoral	Medial leg, ankle, and feet (saphenous nerve).	Inability to extend knee.
Peroneal	Loss of sensation dorsum foot.	Foot drop, inability to extend toes.
Tibial	Anesthesia lateral foot.	Loss plantar flexion ankle and toes.
Sciatic	All of findings for peroneal and tibial (partial loss—any combination of the above).	

require surgical exploration. Generally, if the wound is clean or minimally contaminated, and after more immediate problems such as vascular injuries are corrected, the possibility for nerve repair can be assessed. If the nerve ends appear sharply divided with minimal hemorrhage or contusion, immediate repair is appropriate. Immediate repair can allow better identification and approximation of nerve fascicles, and is more easily done than after extraneural scarring obscures nerve anatomy. Nerve repair should be delayed if the penetrating object is blunt such as a missile, if the injury is dirty, if there is much associated soft tissue damage, if there are associated fractures, or if a vascular repair is particularly tenuous. In such circumstances it is best to clean and debride the wound, identify the nerve ends if it is divided, and fix these in proximity so they do not retract, reducing the need for subsequent mobilization at the time of repair. After the wound has healed, re-exploration is indicated for definitive repair about 3 to 4 weeks after injury.

One indication for acute surgical exploration is a progressing neurological deficit. This can occur with an enlarging false aneurysm from a vascular injury or from a compartment syndrome due to hemorrhage and swelling in a myofascial compartment with compression and ischemia of the nerve. With a worsening neurological deficit, emergency nerve decompression requires opening skin, fascia, and muscle constricting the nerve. The decompressed nerve should be covered with some soft tissue, although delayed skin closure may be necessary; the fascia should not be closed.

In all other instances of blunt trauma, delayed repair is recommended,[8,9] usually 2 to 3 months after injury, to allow recovery of neuropraxic lesions and to allow any possible axonal regrowth through the area of injury in axonotmetic lesions. With delayed exploration, intraoperative nerve action potentials (NAP) should be recorded to determine whether or not axonal regeneration has crossed the lesion in continuity. Intraoperative recording of nerve action potentials is much superior to waiting for electromyographic (EMG) evidence of motor recovery in proximally innervated muscles since EMG evidence of nerve regeneration requires an average waiting period of six months. To record NAPs, the lesion is surgically exposed and the nerve stimulated proximal to the injury site. Any contraction of distal muscles is a highly favorable prognostic sign and no further dissection is indicated. If no contraction is noted, the nerve is stimulated proximal to the lesion and NAP recorded from electrodes placed around the nerve distal to the lesion. The presence of an NAP suggests a very favorable prognosis and a continued conservative course is appropriate. Kline and Gudice reported 63 lesions that showed intact intraoperative nerve action potentials despite no clinical evidence of conduction. Ninety percent recovered function with only external neurolysis.[12]

If no NAPs are recorded, the nerve is resected proximal and distal to the injury site until a normal fascicular pattern is obtained. If possible, the nerve is then primarily reapproximated and the epineurium sutured or cable nerve grafts employed.

Decision whether to proceed with delayed exploration of a *brachial plexus lesion* must be guided by a combination of clinical, electrophysiological, and radiographic information. Useful recovery of motor function can be expected only if the period of muscle denervation does not exceed about 18 months. For a muscle located 12 inches below the plexus injury, useful recovery will occur after suture repair only if repair is done within six months. Even if suture repair is performed early, useful reinnervation can be expected only in the proximal muscles such as the deltoid, the biceps, and the triceps, the brachioradialis, and possibly some proximal forearm muscles. For this reason the areas of brachial plexus that the surgeon should be most concerned with at the time of re-exploration are those that carry with them the potential for reinnervation, primarily the superior trunk, the middle trunk, the lateral cord, musculocutaneous nerve, the posterior cord, and the axillary nerve. Electromyography may be useful during observation since motor unit potentials will be evident well in advance of clinical motor function. If nerve root avulsion is suspected, computerized tomographic (CT) scanning with intrathecal contrast may be of value in demonstrating a traumatic pseudomeningocele at the appropriate level. Root avulsion from the spinal cord cannot be repaired, and some other form of reinnervation such as the use of intercostal nerves can be considered.

Once preganglionic avulsion injury has been ruled out and no clinical or electromyographic evidence for recovery is seen, plexus exploration may be undertaken 3 to 6 months after injury. Intraoperative nerve action potential recordings should be used during surgery to prevent resection and suture of an electrically recoverable lesion. Surgical management of brachial plexus injuries should be done at centers specializing in repair of complex nerve injuries.

TECHNIQUE OF REPAIR

Nerve repair should be carried out using at least 2 to 4 power loupes or with an operating microscope using 12 to 20 power magnification.[13,14] It may be difficult to use a microscope when joints have to be flexed to bring nerve ends together. The two factors responsible for optimal nerve regeneration are accurate approximations of corresponding fascicles and the reduction of intraneural scar formation. The latter is very important as fibrous tissue obstructs and delays the sprouting of axons.

The techniques of repair are epineurial or perineurial. Epineurial repair should be utilized only when one is dealing with a small peripheral, preferably pure nerve, such as a digital nerve. With larger nerves with many fascicles successful epineurial repair depends in part on perfect alignment of the ends. The reason for this is that even though the repair may appear neat externally, only some fascicles will maintain their anatomical alignment within the epineurium. Others will be without a partner, and so sprouting axons will not be immediately opposite an appropriate endoneurial tube. Thus, the greater the number of fascicles in a nerve, the more important it is to suture the nerve ends without rotational distortion.

Epineurial Repair

If the repair is a secondary repair, proper alignment of the nerve can be assured by placing 5-0 or 6-0 monofilament nylon sutures at the lateral edges of the nerve above and below the portion to be resected. After the lateral loops are placed, the nerve is transected using a scalpel or razor blade against a moistened tongue blade. It is important to assure that the cut cross section of the nerve shows fascicular pattern without marked intraneural scarring. The cut end of the normal nerve will show some pouting of the fasciculi and the epineurium will gently slip back and forth over the fasciculi at the cut end. Hemostasis should be carefully assured, preferably with temporary packing and pressure.

Small nerves such as digital nerves should be repaired with 10-0 atraumatic nylon sutures placed through the epineurial cuff at points 180° apart (Figure 6–5). When fasciculi

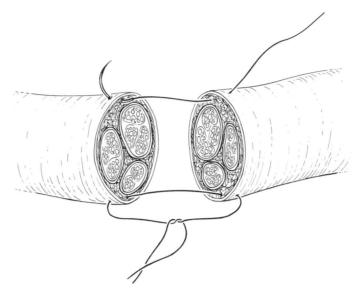

Figure 6–5.   Technique of epineurial repair of a small nerve.

are easily identifiable, they should be specifically secured with one perineurial suture. In practice, funicular suture is usually limited to situations where a primary repair is being done on a cleanly severed nerve. For primary epineurial repair, usually only minimal resection of the edges of the nerves is required. Perineurial and epineurial blood vessels can be identified for accurate alignment. In secondary epineurial repair, if more than 10 or 15 mm of gap is apparent, the issue is whether to use a nerve graft or nerve mobilization, with or without joint flexion, to approximate the divided ends. Nerve suture under tension must be avoided. The ulnar nerve in the upper arm has minimal branches and therefore can be mobilized extensively and can in addition be transposed anterior to the epicondyle. Length can be gained for the median nerve by liberating it from a deep position in the distal arm and the antecubital area and forearm so that it can come to rest subcutaneously. More arm flexion is necessary to approximate gaps in the median nerve than the ulnar nerve. The radial nerve can be mobilized from its spiral groove in a tunneling fashion and brought out on the medial aspect of the arm through a counterincision and rerouted straight across the antecubital fossa.

Interfascicular Repair

For interfascicular repair three to four millimeters of epineurium should be excised and the fascicles cut back to undamaged nerve tissue under the microscope. It is then necessary to identify common fasciculi in the proximal and distal portion of the resected nerve so that they can be matched and sutured directly (Figure 6–6). Fasciculi or fascicular groups are transected at slightly different distances from the neural stump in such a way that not all sutures are placed at the same level, thereby allowing for a slight staggering of individual anastomoses. Correct rotational alignment is identified by matching epineurial blood vessels and an epineurial stay suture is inserted to maintain the correct alignment of the

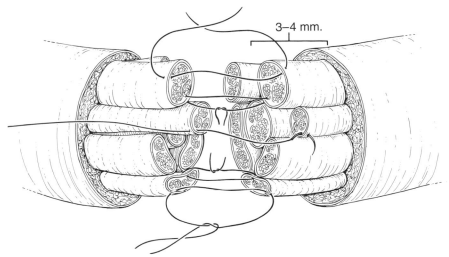

Figure 6–6.   Technique of interfascicular repair utilized for larger or mixed nerves.

nerve and facilitate perineurial repair with 10-0 nylon. A single 10-0 stitch is used to unite the perineurium of the fascicle with the perineurium of the opposing distal fascicle. A second suture may be used as necessary. All nerve repairs must be free of tension, as for epineurial repairs.

When the nerve cannot be approximated without tension, a nerve graft should be used. One of the most commonly used donor nerves is the sural nerve, which can be mobilized for a distance of 35 cm; a superficial radial nerve graft of 20 cm, and a medial ante-brachiocutaneous nerve graft of 12 cm also can be obtained. In placing the graft, the various sizes of funiculi of the proximal and distal stumps must once again be carefully mapped and matched by an appropriately sized graft (Figure 6–7). To reduce the amount of scar at the juncture of the graft and stump, the levels of repair of the various funiculi should be staggered by shortening some of them. Surgeons differ as to whether to use interfascicular grafting in preference to epineurial suture with extensive proximal and distal mobilization or extreme joint flexion to approximate the nerve ends. The amount of postoperative joint flexion needed to avoid tension at the completed nerve juncture must be determined before closing the skin. If there is no tension, postoperative immobilization is necessary only until the skin heals. When splinting is needed to prevent tension on the nerve juncture, it must be maintained for 3 to 4 weeks. If a sizable gap has been overcome by positioning, the flexed joints should gradually extend over 4 to 8 weeks after this period.

When there is total anesthesia the patient will lack any awareness of discomfort from a congested portion of the extremity. Accordingly, great care must be taken in applying dressings and casts in these circumstances.

POSTOPERATIVE CARE AND FOLLOW-UP

Splinting is usually advisable after repair of peripheral nerves to prevent stress on the suture line and avoid potential nerve repair disruption. This should be continued for 2 to 4 weeks by which time some regeneration of the axon should have started at the suture line and the

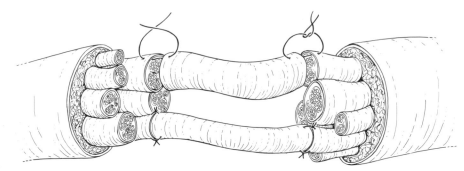

Figure 6–7.   Technique utilizing nerve graft repair.

suture line will have acquired some mechanical strength to withstand some distraction and stress. If there has been some tension on the repair, the application of a splint that allows some voluntary movement but prevents excessive extension of the joint may be appropriate. After nerve healing has begun but before innervation has occurred, the joints, tendons, and soft tissues should be passively exercised every day to prevent contractures from developing. Muscle wasting cannot be prevented but contractions of paralyzed muscles can be prevented by stretching with static or dynamic splints. These include cock-up splints for wrist drop, opponens splints for medial nerve lesions, and the anticlaw splint to prevent MP joint hyperextension.

Inactive limbs can become edematous although limb elevation and careful use of elastic bandages may prevent or reverse the problem. Patients must be instructed to avoid injury to their insensate limb and must learn to inspect the insensible areas on a daily basis. Inadequate return of muscle function may necessitate later tendon transfers or arthrodesis for optimal function of the extremity. The surgeon can monitor axonal regeneration across the repair site or distal anastomosis of the graft at regular intervals using Tinel's sign. The nerve is tapped from distal to proximal to the most distal point at which paresthesia is found. Utilizing this test, the rate of growth can be assessed which should approximate 1 mm per day after the initial 3-week delay for axon recovery. If at six months after surgery, no sign of nerve recovery has developed and Tinel's sign cannot be elicited distal to the repair site, reoperation may be required. The nerve should be re-explored and after nerve testing as previously described, the repair should be revised if there is no evidence of regeneration. Final results cannot be determined until two years or more after repair. At this point, final clinical testing can be done to determine the result and the need for tendon transfer. The order of appearance of sensory modalities during regeneration is Tinel's sign, deep pain, tingling, light touch and temperature, position sense, and epicritic sensibility.

Electromyographic testing may demonstrate early muscle reinnervation prior to objective clinical findings. The first changes are the decrease of muscle fibrillation and the appearance of slow polyphasic discharges produced by attempts at voluntary movement. Motor function is finally and definitively assessed by the appearance of active contraction and by the strength regained. Thorough examination necessitates the evaluation of independence of action of individual muscles, their excursion, speed, and power of action, and overall coordination and control of the extremity. Once motor functions begin to appear, progression may be very rapid.

COMPLICATIONS

A variety of pain syndromes often accompany injury to nerves. Inflammation such as arthritis, myositis, or tendinitis may develop after trauma. Avulsion of the brachial plexus or a nerve root may produce burning dysesthesias and paraesthesias as a type of central pain after de-afferentation. Painful neuromas and entrapment syndromes can arise at the site of injury causing exquisite local tenderness and pain. Partial nerve injuries which serve both motor and sensory function can lead to causalgia with severe hyperaesthesia and hypersensitivity to cold or muscle activity and increased pain in stressful situations.[14] Hyperpathia, trophic changes, and vasomotor hyperactivity are characteristic. Minor stimuli may produce severe pain. Although spontaneous remissions may occur, treatment should be instituted early. Sympathetic blocks and sympathectomy are specific diagnostic and therapeutic procedures. Aggressive physical therapy may be combined with peripheral blocks with guanethidine and reserpine. If pain remains severe, repeat neurolysis, creation of dorsal route entry zone lesions, dorsal column stimulation, or central pain procedures may be required.

Management of the problems of chronic pain are complicated and may not be successful. Initial management includes narcotic and nonnarcotic analgesics to which may be added tricyclic antidepressants such as amitriptyline or mild tranquilizers such as diazepam. Anticonvulsives, particularly carbamazepine, and less often phenytoin also can reduce pain after injury to nerves. Recent experience with surgical destruction of the spinal cord dorsal root entry zone (DREZ) has shown that dramatic improvement can be obtained in some patients with injuries to the brachial plexus, avulsion of nerve roots, and the pain of deafferentation. Finally, stimulation of the brain by electrodes in the thalamic or periaqueductal gray regions may be used for selected patients who fail to respond to more conservative measures.

RESULTS

Results of nerve repair are directly related to the location of the injury and the nature of the nerve involved.[15–18] The more distal the injury, the better the results. For pure sensory nerves such as those in the palm or in the digit, the results are usually excellent. One study, which compared the results of fascicular repairs with those of epineurial repairs of digital nerves in humans, showed no difference between the two as regards return of light touch, pin prick, and two-point discrimination.[19]

Haase et al reported relatively good results in more than 60 patients treated with interfascicular grafting in transected median and ulnar nerves.[20] Fifty percent to 63% of these patients had return of two-point discrimination and 70% to 90% had return of pain and tactile sensation throughout an anesthetic area. Millesi, who used interfascicular grafting, reported a 96% to 100% return of sensation throughout an anesthetic area in lesions of the median and ulnar nerves but only a 32% to 39% return of two-point discrimination.[21] The earlier series in which epineurial suturing was used, often without grafting, documented only a 46% to 82% return of sensation in previously anesthetic areas with only a 4% to 25% return of two-point discrimination.[9] Seddon reviewed the results of injury to specific nerves. He reported fairly good results with the primary or secondary suture in 78% of radial nerves, 98% of median nerves, 83% of ulnar nerves, and 35% peroneal nerves.[6] Kline reported improvement in 73% of sutured sciatic nerves.[22]

Nichols carried out an extensive review of outcome of brachial plexus injury.[12] He noted that the most common injury to the brachial plexus was stretch or blunt injury. He found that isolated stretch injuries to the upper trunk had the best prognosis for recovery, presumably because these nerves had the shortest distance to regenerate between the point of entry and the motor end plate. Another 19 patients had C-5, C-6, and C-7 root damage with 11 patients recovering some wrist and finger extension as well as biceps and shoulder abduction. In 50 patients with complete C-5, C-6, and C-7 lesions, one third recovered some elbow flexion and shoulder abduction. When the stretch injuries involved C-5 through T-1, there was poor prognosis for recovery. Follow-up at two years showed that recovery was limited to shoulder muscles. In 1982, Sedel reported on the outcome of 63 patients operated on for 32 complete and 31 incomplete lesions.[19] Repairs were done in 48 cases; 3 had direct anastomoses, 30 required nerve grafts, and 15 had either nerve transfers or neurolysis. Of the 32 patients with complete palsies clinically, 27 were found surgically to have complete lesions. They would never have recovered spontaneously. Twenty-six of these underwent repair and 11 recovered some use of elbow and wrist function but there was no further functional improvement. Of the 23 with partial palsies undergoing major repair, 20 were improved in at least one area.

Nichols in his assessment of lower extremity injuries[12] noted that proximally transected sciatic, peroneal, and femoral nerves tend to have a worse prognosis for recovery than more distal injuries, secondary to the length of the nerve needed to regenerate before reaching its appropriate musculature. In injuries involving the sciatic nerve the peroneal division is almost always the most severely involved—perhaps because of its oblique course through the thigh along with relative tethering at the head of the fibula. The peroneal nerve injured at or above the midthigh carried a particularly poor prognosis. Even though the injury was mostly axonotmetic, the axons usually did not arrive at the distal musculature in sufficient time to reverse the effects of long-term deinnervation because of the greater length of the nerve. In contrast to a proximal peroneal nerve injury, injury of the tibial nerve in the popliteal fossa or below generally carries a relatively good prognosis for recovery.

REFERENCES

1. Krücke W. Introduction to Dyck, Thomas & Lawbert. In: *Peripheral Neuropathy*. Philadelphia, Pa: WB Saunders; 1975.
2. Weller RO, Navarro JC. *Pathology of Peripheral Nerves*. London, Engl: Butterworths; 1977.
3. Hodes R, Larrabee MC, German W. The human electromyogram in response to nerve stimulation and the conduction velocity of motor nerves. *Arch Neur Psych*. 1948;60:340.
4. Dawson GD, Scott JW. The recording of nerve action potentials through skin in man. *J Neurol Neurosurg Psychiatry*. 1949;12:259.
5. Haymatter W, Woodhall B. *Peripheral Nerve Injuries: Principles and Diagnoses*. 2nd ed. Philadelphia, Pa: WB Saunders; 1953.
6. Seddon H. *Surgical Disorders of the Peripheral Nerves*. 2nd ed. Baltimore, Md: Williams & Wilkins; 1975.
7. Sunderland S. *Nerves and Nerve Injuries*. 2nd ed. New York, NY: Churchill Livingstone; 1978.
8. Graham, W. Nerves. In: Kilgore, Graham, eds. *The Hand*. Philadelphia, Pa: Lea & Febiger; 1977: chap 15.
9. Pitts LH, Rosegay H. In: Mattox KL, Moore EE, Feliciano DV, eds. *Trauma*. San Mateo, Calif: Appleton & Lange; 1988: chap 43.
10. Rich NM, Spencer FC. *Vascular Trauma*. Philadelphia, Pa: WB Saunders; 1978.
11. Visser PA, Hermreck AS, Pierce GE, Thomas JH, Hardin CA. Prognosis of nerve injuries incurred during acute trauma to peripheral arteries. *Am J Surg*. 1980;140:596.
12. Nichols JS, Lillehes KO. Nerve injury associated with acute vascular trauma. *Surg Clin North Am*. 1988; 68:837.

13. Dolenc VV. Contemporary treatment of peripheral nerve and brachial plexus lesions. *Neurosurg Rev*. 1986; 9:149.

14. Edwards MS, Brown BA. Traumatic peripheral nerve lesions. In: Way, LW, ed. *Surgical Diagnosis and Treatment*. 8th ed. San Mateo, Calif: Appleton & Lange; 1985: chap 39.

15. Harden WD, O'Connell RC, Adinolf MF, Kerstein MO. Traumatic arterial injuries of the upper extremity: determinants of disability. *Am J Surg*. 1985;150:266.

16. Orcutt MB, Levine BA, Gaskill HV, Sirinek KR. Civilian trauma of the upper extremity. *J Trauma*. 1986; 26:63.

17. Wilkins RH. Peripheral nerve injuries. In: Sabiston DC, ed. *Textbook of Surgery*. 13th ed. Philadelphia, Pa: WB Saunders; 1986: chap. 11.

18. Wolf YG, Reyna T, Schropp KP, Harmel RP. Arterial trauma of the upper extremity in children. *J Trauma*. 1990;30:903.

19. Sedel L. The results of surgical repair of brachial plexus lesions. *J Bone Joint Surg*. 1982;64:54.

20. Haase J, Bjerre P, Simesen K. Median and ulnar nerve transections treated with microsurgical interfascicular cable grafting with autologenous sural nerve. *J Neurosurg*. 1980;53:73.

21. Milesi H, Meissl G, Berger A. The interfascicular nerve grafting of the median and ulnar nerves. *J Bone Joint Surg*. 1972;54A:727.

7

Open Fractures and Dislocations

JAMES P. KENNEDY, M.D.

HISTORY: The treatment of open fractures has plagued physicians through-out history. The Edwin Smith Papyrus (circa 3000 to 2800 BC) described an open humerus fracture as "an ailment not to be treated." [34]

Hippocrates treated open fractures by cleansing the wound, sealing it with pitch or balsam, and then wrapping the limb in wine soaked bandages. He gave these patients a poor prognosis. [1] *During the age of "laudable pus," Galen advocated frequent manipulations of wounds with application of potions and poultices to induce purulence, feeling this necessary for proper wound healing.*

The renaissance of wound and open fracture treatment began with the cultural Renaissance. Brunschwig in the 15th century introduced the concept of removing nonvital tissue from wounds, although the Hippocratic and Galenist methods were still standard protocol in the Middle Ages.

In the 1700s Pierre-Joseph Desault began using his technique of incising and exploring wounds to remove devitalized tissue and provide drainage which he called "debridement." Surgical debridement then be-came the standard, but in spite of these advances, infection continued unabated. During the US Civil War the Surgeon General noted that out of 6576 cases of open femur fractures, the mortality rates for debridement and amputation were equal at about 50% each. [26]

With Lister's introduction of aseptic technique, the patient with an open fracture finally had a good chance of survival with an intact limb. Lister first used his aseptic techniques in March of 1865 on a patient with an open fracture. [34] *Lister sterilized the surgical instruments, surgeon's hands, and air about the wound with carbolic acid. The wounds were then dressed with occlusive dressings of carbolic acid. Using these techniques, he reported a mortality rate of only 9%.* [23]

During World War I, aggressive and thorough debridement was com-bined with occlusive dressings to protect the wounds from the outside contaminants and rigid fracture immobilization, a technique perfected by H. Winnett Orr during the evacuation of soldiers back to the United States. [29] *Using these techniques, but adding open packing of the wound to allow drainage, during the Spanish Civil War José Trueta noted infection in 8 patients and gas gangrene in 1 out of a total of 1073 with open fractures.* [45]

Due to the simplicity of Orr and Trueta's technique, it was widely used during World War II which also saw the use of sulfanilamide introduced directly into wounds for local antibiotic action. Although penicillin saw only limited use (due to its availability) for open fractures at the end of World War II,[20] by the time of the Korean War systemic antibiotics were widely available and routinely used.

INTRODUCTION

The prognosis following an open fracture is very different from that of the same closed fracture, and therefore the approach to and philosophy of their treatment is much more complex than just treating a fracture and a traumatic wound.

The fact that an open fracture is present means that a greater deal of energy was delivered to the bone in order to produce the soft tissue disruption. Given this, it can also be inferred that there is more soft tissue stripping (muscle, periosteum, and ligament) from the bone resulting in its relative devascularization.[10,15] Accompanying this, there is a variable degree of contusion, crush, and devascularization of the soft tissues as well. All of these factors significantly influence the rate of healing, incidence of nonunion, and risk of infection. Extraordinary measures are sometimes required to improve the chances of obtaining a good end result.

The principles used today for the treatment of open fractures—aggressive debridement, open wound treatment, soft tissue and bone stabilization, and systemic antibiotics—have reduced the high fatality rate due to open fractures in ancient times to essentially zero. Amputations, which were inevitable during the Civil War, are necessary today for only the severest of open fractures.

CLASSIFICATION

A multitude of classification systems have been developed to predict the outcome and assist in planning the treatment of open fractures. Anderson and Gustilo[4,16,17] have developed a simple, well-accepted classification for open fractures (Table 7–1). A Grade I fracture is a

Table 7–1   Classification of Open Fractures

	WOUND SIZE	SOFT TISSUE
Grade I	< 1 cm	No or minimal tissue damage
Grade II	> 1 cm	Moderate tissue damage
Grade III	Any size	Major tissue damage
		Soft tissue loss
		Bone loss
		Gross contamination
Grade IIIa		Bone can be covered
Grade IIIb		Bone cannot be covered
Grade IIIc		Vascular injury

relatively low-energy injury associated with a small (less than 1 cm) often "pinprick" wound without significant injury or stripping of the soft tissues.

Grade II fractures demonstrate a moderate amount of soft tissue damage with open wounds larger than 1 cm, but without major loss of soft tissue (Figure 7–1).

Grade III fractures are associated with a severe degree of soft tissue damage and exhibit soft tissue loss. Grade IIIa fractures, although presenting with soft tissue loss, still have sufficient soft tissue to allow coverage of bone. Grade IIIb fractures do not have adequate soft tissue available for bone coverage and usually require plastic surgery reconstruction with flaps (Figure 7–2). Grade IIIc fractures are the most severe form of injury and represent a near-amputation. These fractures are characterized by major arterial injury causing ischemia and necessitating vascular repair to revascularize the limb.

High velocity gunshot wounds are open fractures that must be approached somewhat differently. Due to the high forces usually imparted into the soft tissue, a fracture that behaves as a Grade III injury due to soft tissue injury may look like a Grade I injury based on the small skin wound. These injuries are covered in more detail later.

Fractures which exhibit bone loss are also classified as Grade III, as are fractures with smaller Grade I- or II-sized soft tissue wounds, but with severe soft tissue contusion and periosteal stripping. A final caveat is that any fracture, regardless of the size of the wound or amount of soft tissue injury, that is associated with gross contamination such as farmyard injuries, or that has significant vegetable matter or soil within the wound, is treated as a Grade III injury due to the risk of clostridial infection or clostridial myonecrosis.

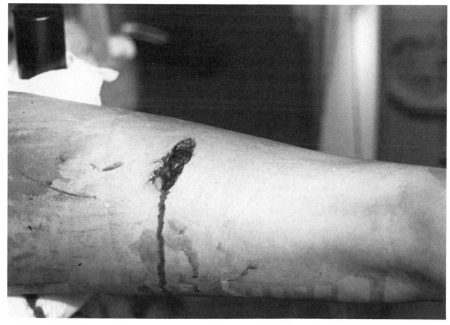

Figure 7–1.   Grade II Open Fracture. Six-cm wound associated with open femur fracture. No significant tissue loss.

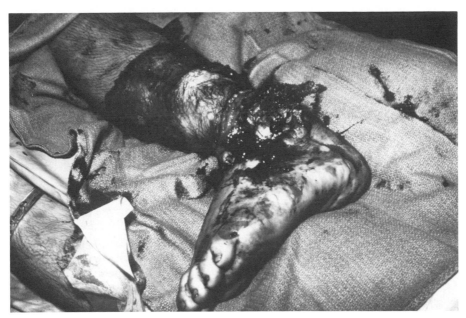

Figure 7–2. Grade IIIb Open Fracture. Significant soft tissue damage and loss associated with distal tibia fracture. Insufficient tissue remained following debridement for coverage of bone. Delayed free-flap was required for wound closure.

EVALUATION

Following the initial resuscitation in the Emergency Department, the usual orthopaedic exam is directed toward the injured extremity with particular attention to evaluation of the neurovascular status. Compartment syndrome should be carefully ruled out in those fractures at risk (see Chapter 20). A common fallacy is that an open fracture automatically decompresses its compartments and therefore cannot develop a compartment syndrome. Up to 10% of open tibia fractures will have a compartment syndrome due to the severe associated soft tissue injury.[7]

Historical factors such as mechanism of injury, time elapsed since the injury, other associated injuries, and preinjury medical condition of the patient are determined. The grade of the open injury is then assessed. Gross foreign material that is easily accessible is removed from the wound[10] followed by a quick "saline dump." Pouring a quick liter or two of saline in the Emergency Department will help wash gross contamination from the wound and prevent tissue dessication. If the limb is malaligned, a gentle gross reduction will align the limb and can help relieve any vascular compromise.

A sterile, moist saline or betadine dressing is then applied to the wound. It is appropriate to spend a few moments making this protective dressing secure. Merely taping a gauze dressing on the wound is not adequate as it will invariably become dislodged during transportation and positioning of the patient. Ideally, once the wound is assessed and the dressing applied, the dressing should not be removed until the surgical prep in the operating room, as the incidence of infection is directly related to the number of times the dressing is removed to allow inspection of the wound. Keeping a sterile dressing in place can reduce infection rates from 18.2% down to 4.3%.[46]

Following the application of a secure dressing, apply a temporary splint to the limb so the patient can be transported for the necessary x-rays. Cardboard splints are convenient for this as they are inexpensive, disposable, and do not interfere with the x-rays.

DECISION MAKING

The initial decision to make is whether the limb with an open fracture can be salvaged or whether a primary amputation is required. With proper aggressive early treatment, there is a high rate of functional healing of Grades I and II fractures. Some of the more severe injuries with vascular and neurologic injury may be unsalvageable—essentially traumatic amputations still connected by a bridge of skin. Although technically in some cases such a limb may be salvaged, the high incidence of infection after such injuries requires multiple operations and often results in the late amputation of a functionless, painful, or infected limb. In one series,[9] Grade IIIc injuries of the tibia had a late amputation rate of 78%. For this reason, it is often preferable to perform a primary amputation in Grade IIIc injuries of the lower extremity.[21]

As will be discussed further in Chapter 18, Grade IIIc fractures with associated posterior tibial nerve disruption or Grade IIIc fractures which due to severe tissue damage will not be functional if salvaged are absolute indications for primary amputation.[18] A primary amputation will often save the patient years of painful treatment for costly complications[8] and is psychologically easier to accept than a delayed amputation.[18] Delayed amputation is two to three times more expensive than amputation performed primarily, and often a higher level of amputation will be required.[8] A lengthy salvage attempt will remove the patient from productive society, often never to return.

Every open fracture requires emergent surgical treatment. The occurrence of infection is related to the delay in initiating surgical treatment. An anoxic Grade IIIc limb needs to be revascularized with all possible haste if salvage is to be successful. Surgical treatment should ideally be initiated within six hours of injury.[2,10,33,36] The surgical treatment depends upon the type and grade of the fracture, and its priority relative to the patient's other injuries as well as any corresponding delay in treatment. The factors that are most helpful in reducing infection are antibiotic treatment, timely aggressive surgical debridement, fracture stabilization, and proper treatment of wounds.[2,32,33,46] Often, other life-threatening injuries require intervention before the open fracture can be appropriately treated. This necessary delay will ultimately determine the type of treatment possible for the open fracture.

OPEN FRACTURE PROTOCOL

A convenient protocol[12] for open fracture treatment is as follows (Table 7–2). Prophylaxis for tetanus is given as needed (see Table 2–1). The single most important factor in reducing the rate of infection is the early administration of broad spectrum antibiotics,[33] so an intravenous antibiotic regimen (Table 7–3) is started as soon as possible in the Emergency Department.

Table 7–2   Protocol for Open Fracture Treatment (Grade I, II, and III)

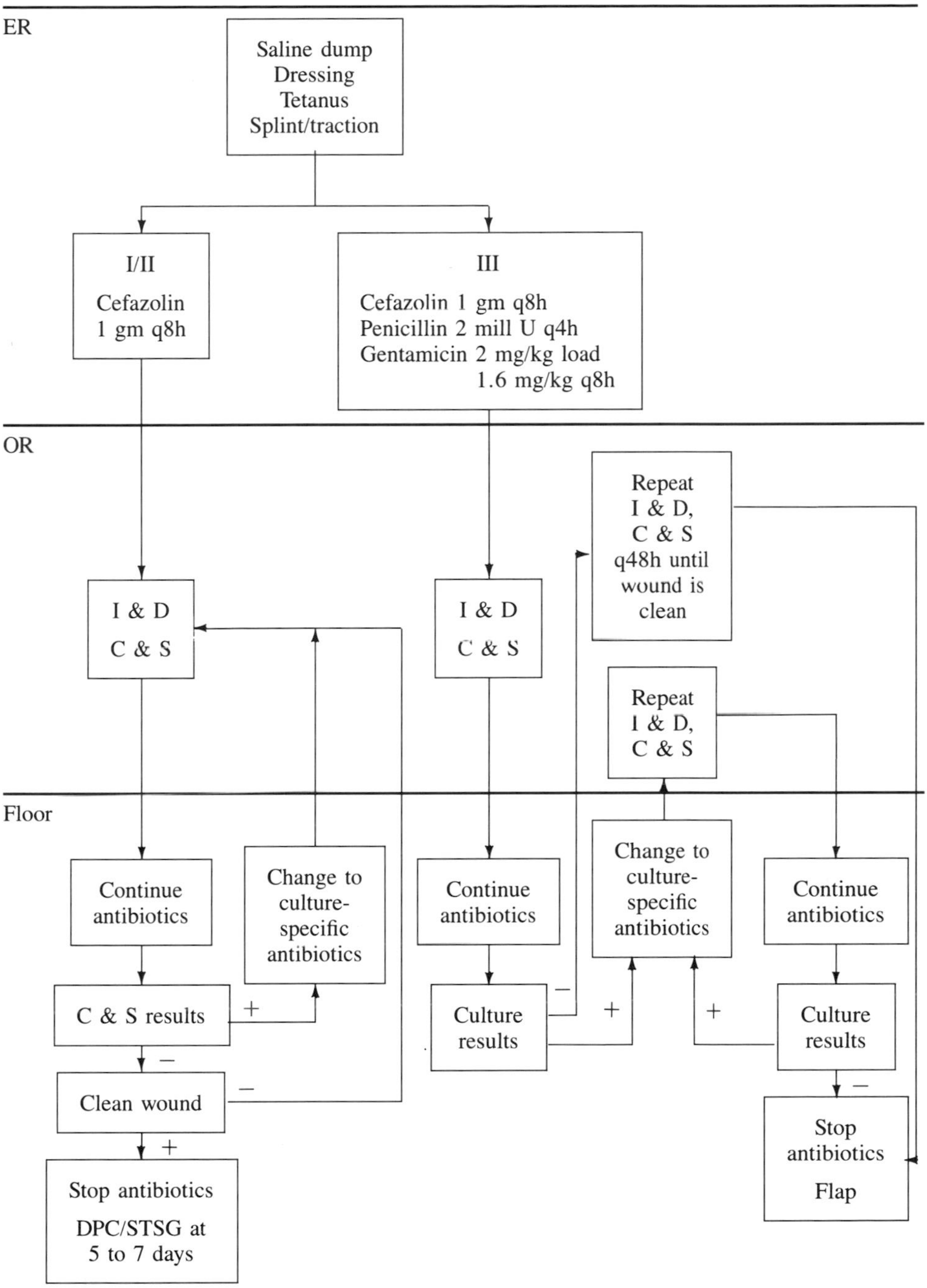

ER

```
                    ┌─────────────────┐
                    │  Saline dump    │
                    │  Dressing       │
                    │  Tetanus        │
                    │  Splint/traction│
                    └─────────────────┘
```

I/II	III
Cefazolin 1 gm q8h	Cefazolin 1 gm q8h Penicillin 2 mill U q4h Gentamicin 2 mg/kg load 1.6 mg/kg q8h

OR

Repeat I & D, C & S q48h until wound is clean

I & D C & S

I & D C & S

Repeat I & D, C & S

Floor

Continue antibiotics — Change to culture-specific antibiotics

Continue antibiotics — Change to culture-specific antibiotics — Continue antibiotics

C & S results   +

Culture results   −   +   +   Culture results

Clean wound   −

Stop antibiotics   −

Stop antibiotics DPC/STSG at 5 to 7 days   +

Stop antibiotics Flap

I&D: Irrigation and debridement; C&S: Culture and sensitivity; DPC: Delayed primary closure; STSG: Split thickness skin graft.

Table 7–3   Antibiotic Regimen

Grade I	Cefazolin 1 gm q4h while in OR, q8h thereafter
Grade II	Cefazolin as for Grade I Fractures
Grade III	Cefazolin as for Grade I Fractures
	PCN-G 2 million Units q4h
	Gentamicin 2.0 mg/kg load for young & healthy
	1.6 mg/kg load q8h maintenance

Cultures of the wound should be performed at some point, as it has been shown that if an infection ensues, in three fourths of the cases, the causative organism will be present on initial cultures.[31] A deep culture is more accurate,[3,35] and this is best obtained in the operating room. As well, samples can be harvested at this time for tissue or quantitative cultures. Results from postdebridement cultures obtained in the operating room are available just as quickly as those from the Emergency Department, are more accurate, and are probably all that are necessary.

DEFINITIVE OPERATIVE TREATMENT

Open fractures are irrigated and debrided in the sterile, controlled environment of the operating suite.[2] Although it may be possible to "get away" with "washing out" Grade I open fractures in the Emergency Department, a significant number of these fractures will be found to contain dirt or grass on the bone ends once they are adequately examined in the operating room.

The traumatic wound is surgically extended in an extensile fashion. This extension must be compatible with any fracture fixation that might be necessary.[10] All devitalized, crushed, or contused soft tissue is aggressively debrided[2,11,39,41] back to normal, clean bleeding tissue. "When in doubt, cut it out."

The tourniquet, which is sometimes used for surgical debridement, should not be inflated unless absolutely necessary as this will lead to further tissue ischemia,[32] and will eliminate muscle contractility which is the best indication of muscle viability. If uncontrollable bleeding is encountered, the tourniquet may be inflated for the few minutes required to maintain hemostasis, and then deflated. Deliver the fracture ends into the wound to allow their inspection and adequate irrigation. Any devitalized and stripped loose bone fragments that are not crucial to attaining a reduction or maintaining its stability must be removed.[2] Devascularized bone is debrided if at all possible until punctate bleeding is seen, being careful to maintain soft tissue attachments to the bone to preserve vascularity.[10] Avascular bone fragments are retained only if they are structurally crucial to obtain an acceptable reduction.[41]

Eight to ten liters of physiologic solution are used with a pulsatile lavage system to irrigate the wound and bone ends (Figure 7–3). (A smaller volume such as 4 liters may be used for small Grade I wounds.) At this point, specimens of tissue are taken for tissue culture. The irrigation is then completed by 2 more liters of fluid with 100,000 Units of bacitracin added.[5]

Wound extensions that have been surgically created may be closed being certain that

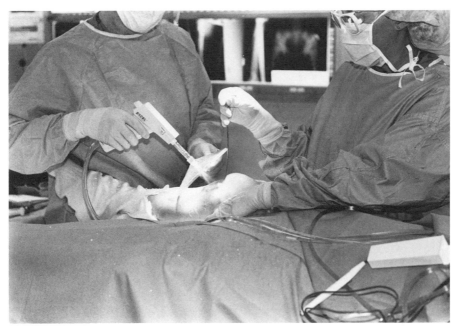

Figure 7–3. Pulsatile surgical lavage irrigating an open fracture. Note protective eyewear to prevent splashing of body fluids.

the traumatic wound is left widely open (Figure 7–4A,B). For small wounds, part of these surgical extensions must be left open to allow adequate drainage and prevent the traumatic wound from sealing off prematurely.[2] Every attempt is to be made to cover bone, joint surfaces, and implants as well as sensitive structures such as tendons, nerves, and vessels with available local soft tissues, but this must be done without tension.[2,10] The type of suture used may have some influence on the incidence of infection, as discussed in Chapter 2. Generally, synthetic monofilament sutures are preferred,[12] and of these, polydioxanone shows the lowest affinity of bacterial adherence.[13]

Following the initial debridement, the patient is continued on the antibiotic regimen for 24 to 48 hours. At this point if the postdebridement culture results are positive, the antibiotics are changed to those appropriate for the infecting organism. If cultures are negative, antibiotics may be stopped if the wound is clean.

Any Grade I or II wound with positive cultures and all Grade III wounds are returned to the operating room every 48 hours for repeat irrigation and debridement until they are healthy and clean. In addition to punctate bleeding, tetracycline labelling and a Wood's lamp, and laser doppler flowmetry can be helpful in determining whether bone is vascularized or should be debrided.[43] Similarly, intravenous fluoroscein used with a Wood's lamp[10] or transcutaneous oxygen measurements can help assess the viability of skin and soft tissue. Each time the patient is returned to the operating room, antibiotics are restarted until the wound is closed. New operative tissue cultures are obtained at each debridement session, and the antibiotics are adjusted accordingly.

Quantitative cultures are often helpful.[28] Bacterial counts greater than 10,000 organ-

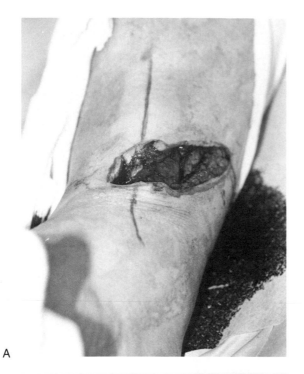

A

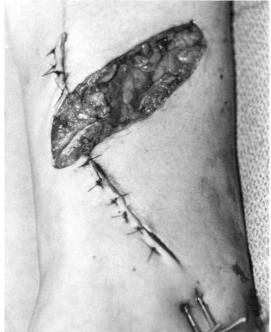

B

Figure 7–4. Technique of debridement of open fracture wounds. **A:** Grade II open wound with the extensile incision and edges of wound to be debrided marked. **B:** Following debridement of all internal devitalized soft tissue and bone, irrigation, and fracture fixation, the surgical wound is closed; the traumatic wound is left open for later skin grafting or delayed primary closure.

isms per gram of tissue are associated with the development of infection; counts less than this tend to be colonizations and do not usually lead to infection.[37,38]

Grade I and II wounds in which the initial cultures are negative can be allowed to close by granulation and secondary intention or may be returned to the operating room at 5 to 7 days for delayed primary closure. Larger wounds will often require a split-thickness skin graft. Grade III wounds with negative cultures are returned every 48 hours to the operating room for further irrigation and debridement until all devitalized tissue has been removed and the wound is healthy.

For wounds in which the cultures were positive, closure can be accomplished after further irrigation and debridement when tissue cultures become negative and there is no clinical sign of infection. Grade III wounds often require some type of flap for soft tissue coverage. This is best done early, at 5 to 10 days postinjury.

OPERATIVE FIXATION

It is beyond the scope of this monograph to discuss the specific details of operative fixation for open fractures. An entire treatise can be written on this topic alone, and it is much more complicated than the seemingly straightforward question of whether or not to fix. Bérenger-Féraud first advocated internal fixation of open fractures in 1870,[6] and orthopaedists have been debating its use ever since. Some of the issues include not only open vs closed treatment, but also acute vs delayed surgery, open reduction and internal fixation vs external fixation, plates vs rods, reamed vs unreamed nails, etc. Suffice it to say that severe open fractures are being treated more and more aggressively, and the frontier of treatment for these injuries is gradually advancing. It has been proven that for many types of fractures, proper operative fixation will yield better functional results with no higher rates of infection than the closed treatment of open fractures.[2,10,11,36,41]

Internal fixation of open fractures is indicated for intra-articular fractures[2,10,41] so that better cartilage healing is obtained. This is accomplished through anatomic reduction and lag-screw fixation so that early range of motion can be achieved.[40] Also, open fractures associated with massively traumatized limbs, patients involved with multisystem poly-trauma, and fractures associated with vascular injuries should be primarily internally fixed if at all possible.[10,46]

Generally, it is desirable to stabilize the open fracture (as it is for any fracture) at the initial operative procedure. Restoring the anatomy through a reduction and stabilization improves circulation; promotes healing of the bone and soft tissues; decreases inflammation, bleeding and dead space; and increases revascularization of devitalized tissue.[12] It will also result in the early mobilization and improvement of the overall status of the multiple trauma patient,[2,36] as discussed in the introduction.

Despite a lack of general agreement among orthopaedic trauma centers on many issues in the treatment of open fractures, some accepted techniques do exist. Isolated Grade I open fractures treated promptly can usually be handled by the same techniques as their closed counterparts, with the exception of the tibia (see Chapter 18). Grade II injuries in ideal situations in favorable areas such as metaphyseal bone, the forearm, hand, foot, humerus, and femur[10] can also be treated with the internal fixation techniques used for closed fractures. Acute internal fixation of intra-articular fractures in all areas is also desirable.

Fractures in other situations such as open tibias and Grade III fractures are more safely

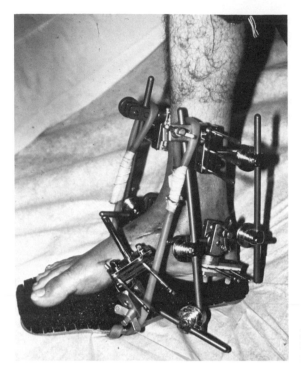

Figure 7–5. External fixator on right ankle for open hindfoot fracture. (Wounds not visible.)

treated conservatively with either modified internal fixation techniques, or immobilization through external fixators (Figure 7–5). Traction followed by delayed internal fixation once the wound declares itself is possible for isolated injuries. Certainly, there will rarely be criticism for not treating an open fracture with acute, internal fixation, but the surgeon may be condemned for fixation so in the wrong circumstances. If the treating surgeon is not very familiar and experienced with these types of injuries, it is best to err on the side of non-operative treatment.

Items of importance regarding specific open fractures will be addressed in the chapters addressing each anatomic area.

GUNSHOT WOUNDS

Gunshot wounds are a special subclassification of open fractures that merit some mention. Gunshot wounds are not sterile wounds due to the heat of the entering projectile as many contend.[44] The velocity of the projectile and whether or not it has passed through other materials before entering the body affect its potential for inoculation of the wound.

The amount of damage imparted by a missile is heavily dependent upon its velocity, as this is the prime factor in determining both the power (v^3) and kinetic energy ($\frac{1}{2} mv^2$) of the bullet (Figure 7–6). Today, guns are available that provide a wide range of muzzle velocities (Table 7–4).

Most handguns have muzzle velocities in the range of 1000 ft/sec, with very few having the capacity to fire up to 2000 ft/sec.[48] At ranges of 1000 ft/sec, damage is mostly

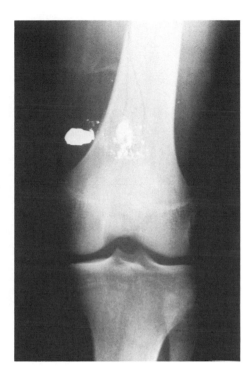

Figure 7–6. Rifle bullet injury. The patient was struck from a large distance, therefore the bullet's velocity (and kinetic energy) had significantly diminished so that only a small crack occurred when it struck the femur. Note mushrooming of soft lead slug.

confined to the bullet tract itself due to the low velocity[25] (Figure 7–7). As velocities in the realm of 2000 ft/sec are reached, cavitation occurs. Liquids, unlike gases, are noncompressible. When a high velocity missile enters soft tissues, the liquid component cannot be compressed and therefore must be displaced—creating a momentary cavitation in the tissue. The resulting expansion of the cavity which exceeds the elastic capacity of the soft tissues causes additional tissue damage due to the explosive characteristics of the energy released. The vacuum produced behind the bullet and by cavitation can suck outside debris and bacteria into the wound.[48] Also, bullet fragments can carry pieces of contaminated clothing into the body.

Gunshot wounds are rarely as grossly contaminated as the wounds produced by automobile or industrial accidents. The major risk with infection appears to be related more to the amount of soft tissue damage—which may not be obvious to the unsuspecting surgeon.

With the advent of military-style assault rifles and specialized ammunition that

Table 7–4   Missile Velocity

Low velocity	1000 ft/sec
High velocity	2000 ft/sec
Military/assault weapons	3000 ft/sec
Handguns	1000 ft/sec
0.38	900 ft/sec
0.38 Special	1200 ft/sec

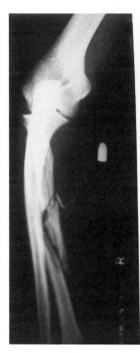 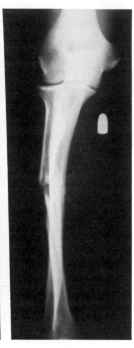

Figure 7–7. War injury from an officer's handgun resulting in a low-energy fracture. Note trail of bone dust behind the intact copper clad bullet marking the bullet tract.

explodes or mushrooms on impact to deliver greater wounds, the civilian surgeon is now seeing injuries which previously were only experienced during times of war. Military weaponry have muzzle velocities in excess of 3000 ft/sec. Not only is the degree of suction of outside material into the wound increased at these velocities, but also the degree of cavitation and soft tissue damage. The wound tract produced by these types of weapons has a cross sectional area far exceeding 30 to 40 times that of the bullet.[14] Bullets which mushroom and thereby increase their surface area dramatically on impact will correspondingly increase the soft tissue damage from the wound tract.

Although there may not be a large wound with military weaponry, it is possible to have soft tissue injury comparable to a Grade III open fracture hidden beneath the intact skin as a result of the cavitation and shock wave. It is not uncommon to find a bone completely shattered into dust due to the extreme energy imparted into it (Figure 7–8). These fractures with their benign appearing wounds, but with the sleeping specter of a Grade III soft tissue injury hidden below, are best treated through closed means by the prudent surgeon. Opening these fractures to fix them, beyond what is necessary for irrigation and debridement of the wound, is only asking for trouble. Surgical devascularization of fragments can precipitate nonunion or infection. Often the bone fragments are so small as to be irreparable surgically. These fragments will then serve as a vascularized bone graft for the fracture if their soft tissue attachments are not surgically disrupted.

Thorough neurovascular exams are mandatory with gunshot wounds. One cannot predict sparing of vital structures based upon the location of wounds. Once a projectile enters the body its path is entirely unpredictable. As it encounters variable resistance, it begins to tumble and take an erratic path "bouncing" off the structures it hits. More than

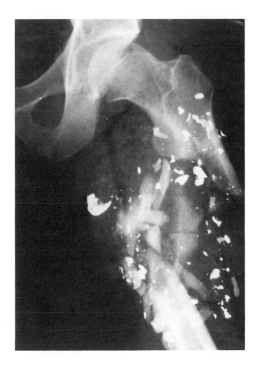

Figure 7–8. High-velocity explosive-type injury from high-powered rifle. Both bone and bullet are extensively fragmented.

one person has been saved from a fatal chest wound when a bullet strikes a rib and tracks around the thorax to exit without even entering the chest cavity.

Low velocity civilian handgun wounds may be treated with local cleansing and skin debridement as necessary in the emergency department, followed by a course of oral antibiotics.[48] Hospitalization is dictated purely by the nature of any orthopaedic or vascular injury. High velocity military-style missile wounds, due to their significant soft tissue injury components, require surgical debridement.

Shotgun wounds require a few special considerations. Shotguns are not precision instruments. They are designed to hit anything and everything within a short distance. Due to the expanding spray of pellets, depending on the distance of the victim from the gun muzzle, there may be either a devastating wound or simple peppering of the skin by low velocity pellets (Figure 7–9). At close range the tissues absorb the full complement of pellets with release of explosive energy into the flesh causing a great deal of soft tissue injury and fracture. The surgeon must also be aware that the wadding or other shell packing material is often driven into close-quarter wounds as well, serving as an excellent nidus for infection if not removed.

Generally, any metallic shrapnel fragments can be left as is. It is obviously impossible to satisfactorily debride the hundreds of pellets from a shotgun wound. Fragments encountered during the debridement are excised. Also, major fragments near vital structures may warrant removal to prevent late migration and damage.[19]

The other type of bullet fragment that demands removal is the intra-articular foreign body. A thorough evaluation is required to determine whether a fragment in the proximity

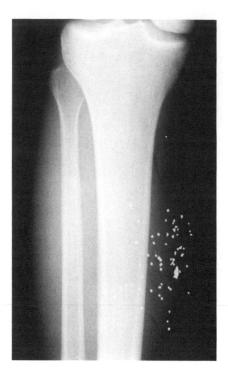

Figure 7–9.   Peppering of soft tissues from shotgun pellets. Injury occurred from some distance resulting in low-velocity soft tissue injury.

of a joint is indeed intra-articular. Plain radiographs are often confusing and a CT, although accurate, is time consuming and the patient may not always be stable enough to allow this. An arthrogram will quickly demonstrate any intra-articular metallic object by coating it with contrast material. Visualization can be improved through double contrast arthrography. Once a fragment is identified in the joint it should be removed. It can cause mechanical symptoms of joint locking or crepitation. Eventual joint destruction from mechanical wear is also possible. Of a more serious nature is lead arthropathy. If the fragment contains lead, the lead will gradually leach out into the synovial fluid where it is toxic and cause complete joint destruction. If the fragment is large enough, systemic levels of lead can become high enough to cause lead poisoning.

OPEN DISLOCATIONS

The same protocol for open fractures is followed for open dislocations—antibiotics, irrigation, and debridement. A few special details unique to joints must be addressed however. The articular surface must be kept moist. The cartilage has already suffered the blow dealt it by the force of impact and may not be able to tolerate any further insult. In rabbit knees, full thickness articular necrosis occurs after sixty minutes of exposure to room air without being moistened, and partial injury can occur as early as thirty minutes.[27]

Other than the treatment for the open nature of these dislocations, they are generally treated similarly to their closed counterparts. This consists of gentle reduction under anesthesia. Following thorough irrigation of the joint and debridement as required, the capsule of the reduced joint is closed[47] over a suction drain, and the remaining traumatic wound is left open.

There is probably no indication for in-and-out drainage systems where a through-and-through drain continuously flushes the joint. These tend to be messy and can introduce pathogens into the joint. Large Grade III injuries with soft tissue loss may not permit coverage of the articular surface, and warrant immediate reconstruction with local or distant flaps to maintain articular cartilage viability. In these instances, only the joint cartilage should be covered. The remaining portion of the wound must be left open.

Following the surgical treatment, the joint is immobilized to maintain reduction the same as for closed dislocations, and the subsequent treatment of the traumatic wound is identical to that for open fracture wounds.

REFERENCES

1. Adams F, trans. *The Genuine Works of Hippocrates*. Baltimore, Md: Williams & Wilkins; 1939.
2. Allgöwer M, Border J. Management of open fractures in the multiple trauma patient. *World J Surg*. 1983; 7:88–95.
3. Altemeier WA, Gibbs EW. Bacterial flora of fresh accidental wounds. *Surg Gynecol Obstet*. 1944;78:164.
4. Anderson JT, Gustilo RB. Immediate internal fixation in open fractures. *Orthop Clin North Am*. 1980; 11:569–578.
5. Benjamin JB, et al. Efficacy of a topical antibiotic irrigant in decreasing or eliminating bacterial contamination in surgical wounds. *Clin Orthop*. 1984;184:114–116.
6. Bérenger-Féraud, LJB. Traité de l'immobilisation directe des fragments osseux dans les fractures. Paris, Fr: Adrien Delahaye; 1870.
7. Blick, SS, et al. Compartment syndrome in open tibial fractures. *J Bone Joint Surg*. 1986;68–A:1348–1353.
8. Bondurant FJ et al. The medical and economic impact of severely injured lower extremities. *J Trauma*. 1988; 28:1270–1273.
9. Caudle RJ, Stern, PJ. Severe open fractures of the tibia. *J Bone Joint Surg*. 1987;69–A:801–807.
10. Chapman MW. The use of immediate internal fixation in open fractures. *Orthop Clin*. 1980;11:579–591.
11. Chapman MW. The role of intramedullary fixation in open fractures. *Clin Orthop*. 1986;212:26–34.
12. Chapman MW, ed. *Operative Orthopaedics*. Philadelphia, Pa: JB Lippincott; 1988.
13. Chu CC, et al. Effects of physical configuration and chemical structure of suture materials on bacterial adhesion. A possible link to wound infection. *Am J Surg*. 1984;147:197–204.
14. Dugas R, D'Ambrosia R. Civilian gunshot wounds. *Orthopedics*. 1985;8:1121.
15. Edwards CC, et al. Severe open tibial fractures. *Clin. Orthop*. 1988;230:98–115.
16. Gustilo RB, Anderson JT. Prevention of infection in the treatment of one thousand and twenty-five open fractures of long bones. Retrospective and prospective analyses. *J Bone Joint Surg*. 1976;58–A:453–458.
17. Gustilo RB, et al. Problems in the management of type III (severe) open fractures. A new classification of type III open fractures. *J Trauma*. 1984;24:742–746.
18. Gustilo RB, et al. The management of open fractures. *J Bone Joint Surg*. 1990;72–A:299–303.
19. Hopkins DAW, Marshall TK. Firearm injuries. *Br J Surg*. 1967;54:344.
20. Innes A, Ellis VH. Battle casualties treated with penicillin. *Lancet*. 1945;1:524.
21. Lange RH, et al. Open tibial fractures with associated vascular injuries: prognosis for limb salvage. *J Trauma*. 1985;25:204–208.
22. Larrey DJ, Richard Willmott Hall, trans. *Memoirs of Military Surgery and Campaigns of the French Armies*. Baltimore, Md: Joseph Cushing; 1814.
23. Lister J. On a new method of treating compound fractures, abscess, etc., with observation on the condition of suppuration. *Lancet*. 1867;1:326, 357, 387, 507.
24. Macleod GHB. *Notes on the Surgery of the War in the Crimea with Notes on the Treatment of Gunshot Wounds*. London, Engl: John Churchill; 1858.
25. Marcus NA, et al. Low velocity gunshot wounds to the extremities. *J Trauma*. 1980;20:1061.
26. *Medical and Surgical History of the War of the Rebellion, II*. Part III. Washington, DC: Government Printing Office; 1883.
27. Mitchel N, Shepard N. The deleterious effects of drying on articular cartilage. *J Bone Joint Surg*.1989;71-A: 89–95.
28. Moore TJ, et al. The use of quantitative bacterial counts in open fractures. *Clin Orthop*. 1989;248:227–230.

29. Orr HW. *Osteomyelitis and Compound Fractures and Other Infected Wounds: Treatment by the Method of Drainage and Rest.* St. Louis, Mo: CV Mosby; 1929.
30. Paré A. *The Case Reports and Autopsy Records of Ambroise Paré.* Hamby WB, ed. Springfield, Ill: Charles C Thomas; 1960.
31. Patzakis MJ, et al. The role of antibiotics in the management of open fractures. *J Bone Joint Surg.* 1974; 56–A:532.
32. Patzakis MJ, et al. Considerations in reducing the infection rate in open tibial fractures. *Clin Orthop.* 1983; 178:36–41.
33. Patzakis MJ, Wilkins J. Factors influencing infection rate in open fracture wounds. *Clin Orthop.* 1989; 243:36–40.
34. Peltier LF. *Fractures.* San Francisco, Calif: Norman Publishing; 1990.
35. Pulaski EJ, et al. Bacterial flora of acute traumatic wounds. *Surg Gynecol Obstet.* 1941;72:982.
36. Rittmann WW, et al. Open fractures. Long-term results in 200 consecutive cases. *Clin Orthop.* 1979; 138:132–140.
37. Robson MC, et al. Quantitative bacteriology and delayed wound closure. *Surg Forum.* 1968;19:501.
38. Robson MC, et al. Rapid bacterial screening in the treatment of civilian wounds. *J Surg Res.* 1973;14: 426–430.
39. Rockwood CA Jr, Green DP. *Fractures in Adults.* 2nd ed. Philadelphia, Pa: JB Lippincott; 1984.
40. Salter RB. The biologic concept of continuous passive motion of synovial joints. *Clin Orthop.* 1989;242: 12–25.
41. Schatzker J, Tile M. *The Rationale of Operative Fracture Care.* New York, NY: Springer–Verlag; 1987.
42. Sharp WV, et al. Suture resistance to infection. *Surgery.* 1982;91:61–63.
43. Swiontkowski MF, et al. Adjunctive use of laser doppler flowmetry for debridement of osteomyelitis. *J Orthop Trauma.* 1989;3:1–5.
44. Thoresby FP, Darlow HM. The mechanisms of primary infection of bullet wounds. *BJS.* 1967;54:359.
45. Trueta J. El tratamiento de las fracturas de guerra. Biblioteca Medica de Cataluña; 1938.
46. Tscherne H, et al. Osteosynthesis of major fractures in polytrauma. *World J Surg.* 1983;7:80.
47. Tscherne H, Brüggemann H. Die Wiechteilbehandlung bei Osteosynthesen, insbesondere bei offenen Frakturen. *Unfallheilkunde.* 1976;79:467.
48. Woloszyn JT, et al. Management of civilian gunshot fractures of the extremities. *Clin Orthop.* 1988; 226:247–251.

Fractures and Dislocations of the Shoulder; Scapula and Clavicle Injuries

JAMES P. KENNEDY, M.D.

HISTORY: Shoulder dislocations were known to and treated by the ancients. The first known orthopaedic case was a shoulder dislocation described in the Edwin Smith Papyrus, which dates as far back as 3000 BC.[42] Around 400 BC, Hippocrates described reduction techniques as well as a method for the treatment of recurrent dislocation[1] using much of the same rationale for treatment that we use today. However, unlike the anatomically based surgery of today directed toward reconstructing the lax soft tissues, the ancient Greeks applied a hot iron to the shoulder, then bound the arm to the body. The resultant scar formation would "tighten" the shoulder and prevent disloca- tion,[34] but also would result in a stiff joint.

INTRODUCTION

Fractures that occur about the shoulder, including those of the scapula, clavicle, and humeral head, result from direct violence to the region, or from indirect forces transmitted up the arm from the reflexive action of falling onto an outstretched hand. Ligamentous disruptions leading to subluxation or dislocation may occur at any of the three articulations in the shoulder girdle—the glenohumeral, acromioclavicular, and sternoclavicular joints.

SHOULDER DISLOCATION

The shoulder, particularly prone to dislocation, is the most commonly dislocated joint.[34] The stability of the shoulder joint is primarily a result of the ligamentous and soft tissue

115

structures about the shoulder, and only to a minor degree due to the bony architecture itself. The shoulder is a nonconstrained joint. Unlike the constrained hip joint with a large deep acetabulum, the ball and socket joint of the shoulder has evolved into the very shallow and small glenoid. This allows the high degree of mobility necessary at the shoulder in order to position the hand in space permitting highly technical and complex activities.

Mechanism

Shoulder dislocation usually occurs as an isolated injury, often as the result of a sporting accident in which a rotational or translational force occurs with the extremity in a vulnerable position. The anterior dislocation is caused by a force levering the humeral head out of its joint with the arm extended, externally rotated, and abducted—the position of the quarterback's arm who is starting a forward pass.

A posterior dislocation results from the production of the opposite forces of forward flexion, internal rotation, and adduction. This can be the result of a fall on an outstretched hand, but occurs more commonly from electrical shock or convulsion[21] during which the muscle forces generated by the strong internal rotators are sufficient enough to overpower the opposing weaker external rotators resulting in the dislocation. These cases are often bilateral.

Shoulder dislocations are occasionally seen in the multiple trauma patient. The shoulder is not as vulnerable as the lower extremities and pelvis in vehicular injuries. In vehicular trauma, force applied to the upper extremities is either a direct blow to the shoulder from the body striking against the interior of the auto resulting in a fracture, or an axial force transmitted through the hands holding onto the steering wheel. Direct blows only rarely will result in a dislocation.[34] In cases where axial force is directed up the arm, the elbow is usually in a flexed position so the force is not directly transmitted to the shoulder. Rather, the energy is absorbed causing wrist or forearm fractures, or dissipated by the "shock absorber" effect of the bent elbow. By the time the force reaches the shoulder, it is both insufficient to result in a dislocation, and applied in the wrong direction to do so.

Classification

Around 95% of shoulder dislocations are anterior. These are further subclassified into the subcoracoid, subglenoid, and subclavicular variants, with the subcoracoid being most commonly seen.[34] Posterior dislocations make up only 2% to 4% of dislocations,[24] and the remaining inferior, superior, and intrathoracic types are even more rare. It is important to be able to diagnose a posterior dislocation because this is the type most often missed due to the difficulty in diagnosis. Trauma is one of the most common causes of this form of dislocation.[13,24] Therefore, it is likely that the traumatologist will occasionally encounter cases of this nature.

The inferior dislocation, "luxatio erecta," is rare, but the characteristic "Statue of Liberty" position of the patient unable to lower his upraised arm is easily recognized. The superior and intrathoracic dislocations are the rarest forms.[34] The intrathoracic dislocation requires extremely severe trauma because high forces are needed to drive the humeral head between the ribs into the thorax.

Evaluation

The anterior dislocation is generally easily recognized. The shoulder looks abnormal with anterior fullness secondary to the abnormal position of the humeral head, squaring of the shoulder from the now prominent acromion, and absence of the humeral head beneath the deltoid. The arm is held in a position of abduction and external rotation. Radiologic exam easily confirms the diagnosis.

Posterior dislocations are difficult to diagnose unless there is a high index of suspicion. Sixty percent to 80% are missed at the time of presentation,[34] and they may go undetected for years.[13] On inspection, a subtle fullness is present posteriorly, which will be missed in the multiply injured trauma patients being examined in the supine position. As the two most common causes of posterior dislocation, electric shock and seizure, commonly result in bilateral dislocations, the deformity of bilateral dislocations will appear symmetric and is in danger of being assumed to be normal. The arm is held in a position of internal rotation and adduction,[13] and there is often limited supination of the forearm.[35]

Radiographs can be deceptive as well, as the routine anterior-posterior films of the shoulder are not sufficient to diagnose the posterior dislocation.[34] Therefore in these cases the only reliable clue available to the physician is the mechanism of injury. The history of a seizure or electrical shock alone should prompt specific investigation for a possible posterior dislocation.

Vascular injuries rarely occur with shoulder dislocations unless the patient is elderly or has atherosclerotic vessels.[4] Neurologic lesions, however, are commonly seen in up to 35%. Most are compression neuropraxias that will resolve with time following a prompt reduction. The axillary nerve is most commonly affected (10% to 20% incidence) followed by the musculocutaneous nerve. The radial and median nerve are less commonly involved.[34]

The older patient, especially, should be evaluated for integrity of the rotator cuff after relocation, as cuff tears are not uncommon.[12,28] It has been hypothesized[22] that in the younger patient, the dislocation is a result of failure of the glenohumeral ligament, but in the patient over 40 years of age is more commonly due to a rotator cuff rupture due to degeneration of the tendon with aging.

It is important to diagnose any cuff tear that may be present, because if surgical repair is needed, better functional results will be obtained through early rather than late repair. If the patient is cooperative, the cuff can be functionally tested through active range of motion[30] in the stable zone. Inability to actively abduct the shoulder is suggestive of a cuff tear. Acutely, the patient will not be able to do this because of pain. Intra-articular injection of local anesthetic is helpful, or the exam can be performed at ten to fourteen days[28] postinjury. If rotator cuff pathology is suspected, it may be confirmed through arthrography, a CT arthrogram, ultrasound, or MRI.

Radiology

A proper radiologic exam will clearly diagnose the type of dislocation and show any associated fractures. Tuberosity avulsions generally do not add to the morbidity of the injury and usually heal uneventfully. The humeral head impaction fracture, or Hill-Sachs lesion,[17] can add significantly to the injury. The Hill-Sachs lesion occurs when the humeral head impinges on the glenoid rim at the time of dislocation, causing a "V" shaped impaction fracture (Figure 8–1). These may be quite large and contribute to residual instability or posttraumatic arthritis.[5,34]

Films should include AP views in internal and external rotation taken in the plane of the chest, an AP in the plane of the scapula (true shoulder joint AP), a scapular "Y" lateral view, and an axillary lateral view[25,34] (Table 8–1). In many institutions, the anterior-posterior films of the shoulder in internal and external rotation are the only films obtained in the series. These are inadequate for the trauma patient,[25] as posterior dislocations will often be missed on these films. For the trauma patient, a complete trauma shoulder series is required (especially the axillary view) so that a posterior dislocation will not be missed. The rotation films should never be done until an initial film confirms that a fracture is not present. Rotating the shoulder in the presence of a fracture will cause pain and may displace the fracture.

The views which are often of poor quality due to improper technique are the axillary and scapular "Y" laterals. The scapular "Y" view is taken in the plane of the scapula, easily identified by the spine of the scapula. The technician directs the beam of the x-ray along the spine which can even be marked on the patient's skin if necessary (Figure 8–2).

The "Y" of the scapula in the lateral projection is formed by the body of the scapula inferiorly, the acromion posteriorly, and the coracoid anteriorly. The glenoid is located at the junction of these three arms and the humeral head should normally be located here (Figure 8–3). Displacement of the humeral head confirms a dislocation in either the anterior (in the direction of the coracoid) (Figure 8–4) or posterior (towards the acromion) (Figure 8–5)

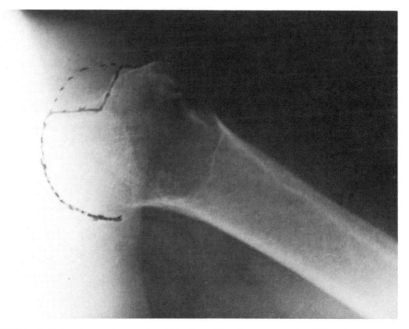

Figure 8–1. Hill-Sachs lesion in anterior portion of head resulting from a posterior dislocation.

Table 8–1   Radiographic Shoulder Trauma Series

AP in Plane of Chest	Internal Rotation*
	External Rotation*
True AP of Shoulder in Plane of Scapula	
Scapular "Y" Lateral	
Auxillary Lateral	

*Only if a fracture is not present.

direction. The anterior orientation is easily demonstrated by the presence of the ribs and chest wall.

The axillary view is the easiest on which to see a posterior dislocation (Figure 8–6), and will also easily document the presence of a Hill-Sachs lesion. Anterior and posterior orientation is easily determined by the location of the coracoid and acromion respectively. To obtain this view, the patient is placed supine and the injured arm gently abducted only far enough to allow the x-ray beam to pass between the arm and body (approximately 15° to 20°). The arm can relax on the table, or the patient may hold an IV pole in his hand to stabilize the arm. The head is rotated and laterally flexed away from the injured side, and the film is placed superior to the shoulder.

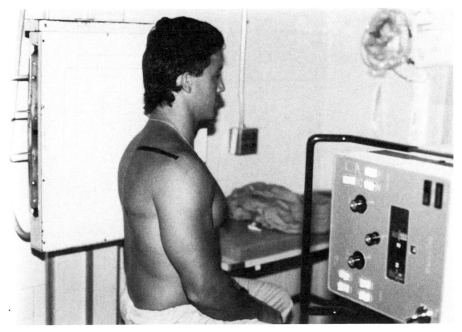

Figure 8–2. Technique for taking scapular "Y" x-ray by lining tube up with scapular spine marked by black line.

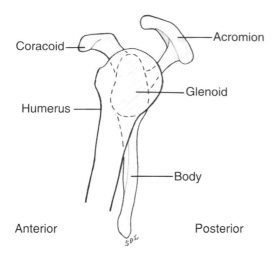

Anterior   Posterior

Figure 8–3. Configuration of scapula and shoulder as seen on the scapular "Y" x-ray.

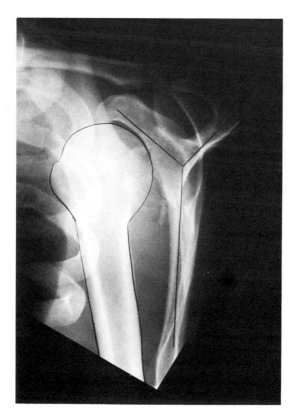

Figure 8–4. Scapular "Y" x-ray showing anterior dislocation with displacement of the humeral head in the direction of the thorax.

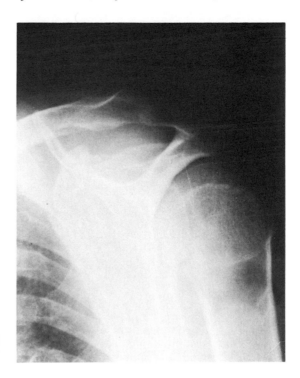

Figure 8–5. Scapular "Y" x-ray showing posterior dislocation. Humeral head is displaced away from the thorax.

TREATMENT

Relocation of any dislocated joint should be done on an urgent basis, certainly within six hours of injury. If there is any neurovascular compromise, this is a more emergent matter, and reduction should be done with all prudent haste. Included are those fracture dislocations where, due to the nature of the fracture, the vascular supply to the fracture fragments is impaired.

When the patient must be taken quickly to the operating room for other reasons, reduction may be done immediately following induction of anesthesia, without delaying other necessary surgical procedures. If the patient requires diagnostic workup prior to surgery such as angiography or CT scanning, reduction can be performed prior to these studies, or in the midst of them during a "lull in the action."

The shoulder should be gently reduced using one of the many techniques that have been described.[34] The various maneuvers can be divided into procedures using traction and those requiring leverage. Those methods requiring leverage should generally be avoided due to risk of fracturing the humerus and causing increased soft tissue damage. The incidence of recurrent dislocation after levering maneuvers such as the Kocher technique[34] has been found to be three times that using traction methods,[23] presumably due to increased capsular stretching and tearing.

All of the traction techniques employ steady longitudinal traction along the axis of the humerus with gentle rotation to coax the head back into the glenoid. The anterior dislocation usually requires accentuation of the external rotation to unlock the head from the glenoid followed by internal rotation to reduce the shoulder. This maneuver is reversed for

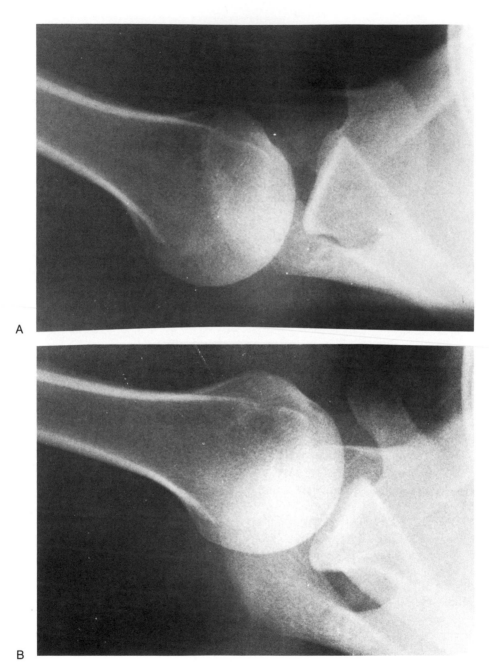

Figure 8–6. Axillary view of posterior dislocation. **A:** Humeral head displaced towards acromion. **B:** Reduced position of head in alignment with glenoid and between the coracoid and acromion.

the posterior dislocation. Acute dislocations can often be handled "at the scene" by one person with simple straight line traction. Many team physicians are familiar with this simple method of reducing dislocations on the playing field minutes after they occur. One of the earliest described techniques is the Hippocratic method which is useful when only one person is available to perform the reduction. The surgeon puts the plantar arch of his stocking foot in the patient's axilla, and uses his hands to manipulate the arm and apply traction.

The Eskimo technique,[33] a native treatment used in Greenland when no physician is available, can likewise be performed by one person. The patient lies on the floor in the decubitus position with the injured side up. The surgeon slowly lifts the body of the patient off the floor through the arm which is dislocated. The patient's body weight then supplies the traction to reduce the shoulder.

By the time most dislocations are seen at the hospital, muscle spasm is present requiring stronger force, muscle relaxation, analgesia, and countertraction to effect a reduction. A useful reduction technique is to employ a helper holding a bedsheet slung around the patient's chest through the axilla. The helper applies countertraction through this sheet. The surgeon takes a second sheet and ties it closely about his waist. The patient's arm is placed through this sheet. The surgeon may now use both his hands to manipulate the arm while applying steady traction through the sheet with his body weight (Figure 8–7).

Children (and some adults) may be apprehensive about or uncooperative with such maneuvers. In these instances, the modified Stimson[38] maneuver may be helpful. Originally described for the reduction of posterior hip dislocation, this technique has been adapted to

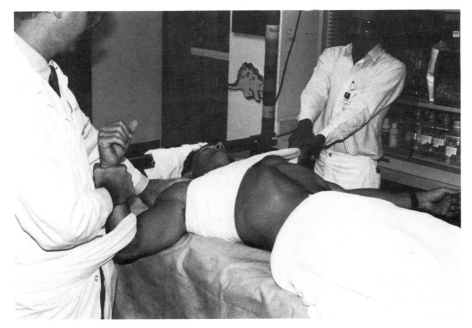

Figure 8–7. Traction/countertraction reduction technique using sheets.

shoulder dislocations as well. The patient is placed prone with the injured arm hanging over the edge of the bed. Traction is supplied by 5 to 10 pounds of weight attached to the wrist or held in the hand—although the weight of the arm alone may be sufficient. The joint will then reduce after 15 to 20 minutes, often without the need for narcotics or muscle relaxants. Alternatively, the wrist may be fastened with a cloth strap to a hook attached to the floor. The bed is then elevated an inch or so every few minutes to supply the traction.

An alternative method to use on the prone patient with the arm hanging dependently is scapular manipulation. The medial border of the scapula is gently elevated and protracted laterally. This method, in effect, reduces the glenoid to the dislocated humerus.

The surgeon should use the method he is most comfortable in performing, and the one most appropriate for the circumstances. If unsuccessful, a different approach using another technique should be attempted. The key with any of these techniques is not so much the maneuver, but assuring good analgesia and muscle relaxation so that a gentle reduction can be performed without risk of further damage. Occasionally a shoulder will require a general anesthetic to get adequate relaxation for reduction. Rarely, soft tissue or bony interposition, or buttonholing of the head through the capsule, will prevent a closed reduction and necessitate that an open reduction be performed.

Following reduction, the shoulder should be immobilized in a stable position appropriate for the type of dislocation. If the patient has a good anesthetic, the shoulder can be examined for the position of maximum stability, but generally this can be done without undue pain and risk only under the influence of a general anesthetic. For the majority of cases, therefore, the stable position will be determined by the type of dislocation and its mechanism.

The unstable position for an anterior dislocation is external rotation, abduction, and extension. The arm is therefore placed in internal rotation, adduction, and flexion. This position is easily maintained by a sling and swathe. A pad coated with zinc oxide and placed in the axilla will help prevent maceration.

The stable position for a posterior dislocation (external rotation, extension, and abduction) is more difficult to maintain. This can be done through casting the arm then connecting it with a bar to a band of cast material placed around the waist. Somewhat less cumbersome (for compliant patients) are "airplane splints" or "shoulder pillows."

The length of immobilization is related to the age of the patient, as younger patients almost always have recurrences and older patients almost never do.[16] Following three weeks of immobilization, 64% of patients less than 22 years old have been found to redislocate,[15] and the incidence is probably 90% or greater for adolescents. Older patients will develop severe restriction of motion following lengthy immobilization whereas young patients can tolerate a longer period of immobilization. Young patients are generally immobilized four to six weeks permitting early careful passive range of motion only in the stable position. Then immobilization is discontinued and a formal rehabilitation program instituted. With older patients, the passive motion is started much sooner—often within the first week.

There is no indication for acute surgical treatment of shoulder dislocations, except in the few instances where closed reduction is unsuccessful and an open reduction is required, cases of fracture dislocation in which the fracture component needs operative intervention, or cases of open dislocation where an irrigation and debridement is needed. Following the timely reduction of a fracture dislocation, the method of treatment (as described below) most appropriate for the reduced fracture pattern is recommended.[3,34,36]

PROXIMAL HUMERUS FRACTURE

Introduction

Fractures of the proximal humerus account for 4% to 5% of all fractures.[37] These fractures are more commonly seen in trauma patients than isolated dislocations as their mechanism of injury is that of a direct blow to the region. In the elderly patient these fractures are often caused by a fall. The goals of treatment are a healed, pain-free shoulder with functional motion.

These injuries can result in intra-articular avascular fragments in as many as 8% of all cases,[19] with an incidence of up to 100% in certain types.[26] Therefore, the surgeon should recognize how the blood supply to these fragments has been affected. Those cases with compromised vascularity are at risk for avascular necrosis, nonunion, and late pain.

Classification

The classification system for humeral head fractures has been described by Neer,[25] and is universally accepted. Treatment and prognosis are based on the type of fracture. The shoulder is divided into four anatomic areas—the greater tuberosity, the lesser tuberosity, the articular surface of the head (demarcated by the anatomic neck), and the shaft (demarcated by the surgical neck) (Figure 8–8). To classify the fracture and decide upon its treatment, the number of displaced "parts" is determined.

Fractures can occur as 2-, 3-, or 4-part patterns (Figure 8–9). Unacceptable position

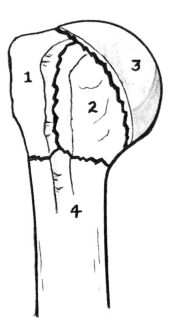

Figure 8–8. The four parts of the humeral head as used for fracture classification: 1, greater tuberosity; 2, lesser tuberosity; 3, articular head (anatomic neck fracture); and 4, shaft (surgical neck fracture).

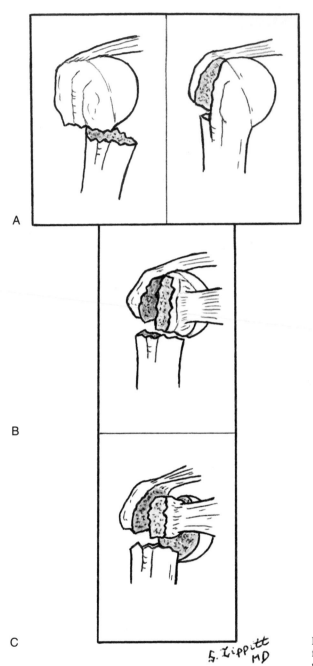

A

B

C

S. Lippitt
MD

Figure 8–9. Examples of humeral head fractures. **A:** Two-part fractures; **B:** Three-part fracture; **C:** Four-part fracture.

is considered to be greater than 45 degrees of angulation between parts or more than 1 cm of displacement of any part.

Dislocations may also occur with any of the types of fractures. Due to a common mechanism, the greater tuberosity fracture is associated with anterior dislocations, and lesser tuberosity fractures with the posterior dislocation. When isolated tuberosity fractures occur (especially if displaced), careful evaluation for concomitant dislocation should be performed. Fractures of the greater tuberosity are found in 10% of anterior dislocations.[41]

The final fracture variants are the intra-articular fractures. The impression fracture (Hill-Sachs lesion) has already been mentioned. Head splitting fractures usually occur in the presence of a dislocation. In this fracture pattern, extensive comminution of the articular surface is present due to impaction of the humeral head against the glenoid.

Evaluation

The evaluation for shoulder fractures is essentially the same as that for the shoulder dislocation. In addition to ruling out associated injuries in the region, the neurologic and vascular status must be carefully assessed. The trauma shoulder series of x-rays are indicated for these injuries (Table 8–1).

If there is doubt about the size or significance of a Hill-Sachs lesion or head splitting fracture, a CT scan can be helpful in treatment planning.

TREATMENT

Nondisplaced fractures (less than 45 degrees angulation, less than 1 cm displacement) can be treated by simple immobilization with a sling and swathe with the expectation of a good result (Figure 8–10). Range of motion through Codman's pendulum exercises can be started early.

Displaced 2- and 3-part fractures need to be reduced if a good functional result is to be expected (Figure 8–11). The rotator cuff cannot compensate for displacement greater than that noted above. Closed reduction will often restore the anatomic relationships of the fragments, although soft tissue interposition (especially the biceps tendon) can make these fractures irreducible through closed means.[27] If closed reduction fails to convert the fracture into a stable configuration that can be treated nonoperatively then the fragments must be openly reduced and internally fixed (Figure 8–12).

The difficulty with this plan of treatment arises with fixation technique. Even in younger individuals, the cortex of the humeral head can be "egg-shell" thin and does not lend itself well to screw fixation. There can also be compression defects, leaving voids in the cancellous humeral head, requiring bone grafting. In middle age or older individuals, screw fixation can be very tenuous. If screw fixation is not possible, the nonabsorbable suture[3] or tension-band wire[11,14] technique of Hawkins can work well.

Four-part fractures are rarely nondisplaced. In the unusual patient who does have a nondisplaced 4-part fracture, nonoperative treatment can be attempted.[36] For the vast majority of 4-part fractures which are displaced, this is not possible. The problem is that all soft tissue attachments (the capsule and the rotator cuff insertions onto the tuberosities)

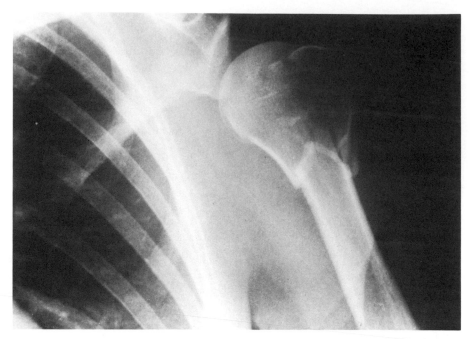

Figure 8–10.   Nondisplaced three-part (head, greater tuberosity, shaft) fracture that can be successfully treated with closed technique.

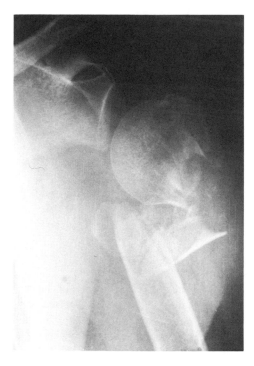

Figure 8–11.   Displaced comminuted two-part fracture at the surgical neck.

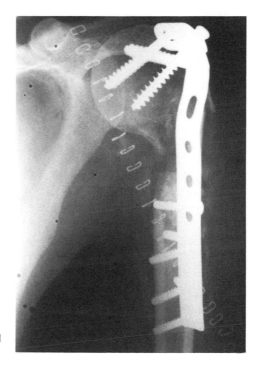

Figure 8–12. Internal fixation of humeral head fracture using plate and screws.

have been disrupted from the head of the humerus. The articular surface is likewise separated from the shaft. Therefore, no blood supply remains to the humeral head, and avascular necrosis is assured. The generally accepted proper treatment for these injuries is removal of the humeral head and insertion of a shoulder prosthesis.[3,26,34,36,39] A few authors feel that although avascular necrosis will occur in these cases, the fracture will nonetheless heal, rapidly revascularize, and give good results without collapse or degenerative change.[20]

Fracture-dislocations should be expeditiously reduced, new x-rays obtained, and treatment of the fracture based on the postdislocation reduction picture.[3] Often, displaced fracture fragments will correct themselves back to anatomic position following reduction of the dislocation. Fracture-dislocations involving the surgical neck will usually need open reduction as the arm cannot be used to manipulate the free-spinning humeral head into a reduced position.

Head splitting fractures need to be carefully assessed, and if the joint is incongruous or rendered unstable by the fracture, reduction and fixation is warranted. If these fractures are extensive, or involve poor bone stock, a prosthesis is required.[39]

Treatment of the Hill-Sachs impression fracture is directed toward its effect on the stability of the reduced shoulder. If 20% or less of the articular surface is involved, the shoulder generally is stable.[34] For those involving more than 50% of the head, a prosthesis is indicated before the incongruent surface induces glenoid changes as well.[34] For lesions of 20% to 40% of the head's surface, transfer of the lesser tuberosity and attached subscapularis tendon into the defect will render these unstable shoulders stable.[22]

CLAVICLE INJURIES

The clavicle is an S-shaped bone and serves as the sole bony connection of the upper extremity to the body. It articulates with the sternum through the sternoclavicular joint and with the scapula through the acromioclavicular joint. Subcutaneous in nature, it is therefore exposed to injury from direct trauma. Indirect forces from a fall onto the point of the shoulder can cause a shearing fracture in the midportion,[32] or an acromioclavicular injury.

Clavicle injuries can be divided into the ligamentous injuries of acromioclavicular and sternoclavicular joint dislocations, and the bony fractures. In the multiple trauma victim, clavicle injuries are often incidental to other problems. In fact, many probably go undiagnosed and therefore untreated in the badly traumatized victim without any sequelae. However, there are a few instances where these injuries must be recognized and treated, and one that is even potentially fatal.

ACROMIOCLAVICULAR JOINT DISLOCATION

Acromioclavicular joint dislocation was described by Hippocrates[1] who cautioned physicians against mistaking it for a shoulder dislocation and trying to reduce it. These injuries, known as the "AC separation" or "separated shoulder" in the athlete, are generally benign. Galen himself suffered this injury while wrestling.[1]

A result of a tear of the three ligaments about the acromioclavicular joint, namely the coracoclavicular, coracoacromial, and acromioclavicular ligaments, the clavicle is generally displaced superiorly and posteriorly by the pull of the trapezius. The rare inferiorly displaced dislocation can result in compression of the brachial plexus or subclavian vessels and therefore needs to be reduced in a timely fashion.

Diagnosis is usually straightforward. There is pain on palpation in the region of the joint. In more severe injuries, a deformity will be noted from the elevated distal end of the clavicle. This will also be noted on radiographic exam of the clavicle (Figure 8–13). In less severe injuries, films of both clavicles can be taken while the patient is holding 5 to 10 pounds of weight in each hand. The weight will cause depression of the humerus and scapula. If the acromioclavicular joint ligaments are torn, the clavicle will remain in its anatomic position resulting in distraction of the joint.

Using the three grades of severity common to the classification systems for sprains, a Grade I injury is a sprain without any joint disruption, Grade II shows partial subluxation due to partial ligament failure, and a Grade III injury is a complete tear with dislocation of the joint. These first three grades should be treated nonoperatively with symptomatic care.

Treatment of Grades I to III is generally that of benign neglect. Analgesics and a sling are helpful for pain control. The patient should be cautioned that a bony deformity will persist due to the displacement of the clavicle, but that this will not cause impairment. Hippocrates[1] noted this when he stated that a "tumefaction" would be present upon healing as the bone "cannot be properly restored to its natural situation."

Various types of slings, harnesses, and straps have been used to attempt to maintain the clavicle in a reduced position with varying rates of success. These are as trying for the patient as they are uncomfortable, must be worn continuously for six weeks, and have the risk of neurovascular compromise and skin necrosis from pressure.[34] Figure-of-eight bandages, commonly used for clavicular fractures, may afford some comfort, but cannot

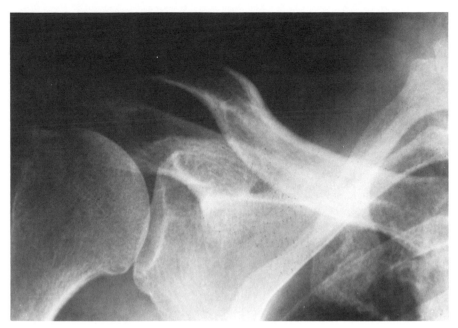

Figure 8–13.   Third-degree acromioclavicular joint dislocation. Note high-riding tip of clavicle in comparison to the acromion.

reduce the dislocation. Operative repair is successful in restoring joint anatomy, but function is generally not improved and the patient is "trading a bump for a scar." Excellent results that are equal to or better than those seen in shoulders which are operated upon for this injury can be expected with closed treatment.[8]

More severe degrees of acromioclavicular joint injury can occur. A Grade IV injury is characterized by posterior displacement of the clavicle which becomes impaled in the trapezius muscle, and a Grade V injury does so in the superior direction into the neck. Open reduction is required to free the clavicle in these instances due to its severe displacement in order to prevent disfunction of the joint and the trapezius muscle. Various types of stabilization can be performed.[5,34] One should be cautious if pins are chosen—because they notoriously migrate from the shoulder into such places as the great vessels, heart, trachea, or spinal cord.[34]

Sternoclavicular Joint Dislocation

Sternoclavicular joint dislocations may occur anteriorly or posteriorly. These are also difficult to diagnose in the multiply injured patient who is unable to complain about his injuries. Due to the subtle deformity this injury produces, the diagnosis is often missed initially. Lordotic or special sternoclavicular radiographic views are helpful, and the injury is clearly diagnosed on CT scans of the chest.

Anterior dislocations can be treated with benign neglect with expectation of good results. The posterior dislocation is a potentially dangerous injury. Due to the proximity of vital structures, these injuries can be fatal. Compression or laceration of the great vessels or trachea can occur. Posterior dislocations should be closed reduced by shoulder retraction. An interscapular roll and a towel clip to pull the clavicle anteriorly are often helpful. However, prior to reduction, the surrounding vital structures should be carefully evaluated and distal pulses and circulation noted. If the clavicle has punctured a vessel, it may be "plugging the hole in the dike,"[34] and removing it may lead to exsanguination.

CLAVICLE FRACTURE

Clavicle fractures make up 5% of all fractures[34] and occur most frequently in children as isolated injuries. Fractures of the clavicle are also a commonly ignored or missed injury in the presence of multiple trauma. In some cases, they will already be healed by the time the patient recovers and is ready to leave the hospital. There are few indications for the operative fixation of clavicle fractures per se. However, as discussed below, clavicle fractures sometimes need to be plated when there is an unstable scapular fracture present.

Other indications[3] for operative treatment of clavicle fractures include open fractures, widely displaced fractures impaled into the trapezius with resultant soft tissue interposition, and fractures which are explored due to neurovascular compromise. The latter are rare.[4]

If a fracture of the first or second rib is noted, it is indicative of high energy trauma applied to the region. The first two ribs are protected by the clavicle. If enough force remains following a clavicle fracture to fracture the underlying ribs, injury to the subclavian vessels or brachial plexus commonly occurs.

Treatment

Treatment of clavicular fractures is one of symptomatic relief until healing. Traditionally, a figure-of-eight bandage has been used with the additional theoretical benefit that the strap crossing the clavicle helps hold the fracture in a reduced position. In practice this seldom is true. In order for the bandage to hold a fracture in the reduced position, it must be applied very snugly to the point that it is too uncomfortable for most patients. For this method to be successful, it must be worn constantly and needs frequent adjustments as the straps tend to loosen and stretch. Due to all of these reasons, the bandage is often abandoned by the patient early in the course of treatment. A better form of treatment is the use of a simple arm sling. A sling is well tolerated, causes less discomfort than the figure-of-eight bandage, and gives equally good cosmetic and functional results.[2]

SCAPULAR INJURIES

Fracture

Scapular fractures are rare, accounting for approximately 1% of all fractures.[15,29] Until recently, all scapular fractures were treated by closed methods.[3,9,10] However, with the onset of modern fracture fixation techniques and the development of fracture fixation registries, the indications for the fixation of scapular fractures are now being determined. This is the last anatomic area for which clear indications for and techniques in the surgical management of fractures have yet to be proven and accepted.

Severe scapular injuries are the result of massive crushing injuries and are often associated with multiple rib fractures, pneumothoracies, hemothoracies, or flail chest segments.[40] Fortunately, these severe cases are rare as the scapula is a thin, low-profile bone which is protected from injury by a thick covering of muscle and its free mobility over the thorax.[15]

The usual scapular fracture is a simple, basically nondisplaced stellate fracture of the body, or consists of small fractures involving the prominences of the bone. These can be treated symptomatically with a sling or sling and swathe with the institution of early mobilization to maintain shoulder function.

Scapular fractures which require operative reduction and internal fixation are exceedingly rare, and are estimated to constitute approximately .03% of fracture fixations.[3] Fractures that will subsequently interfere with function of the upper extremity need to be reduced and stabilized. These include disruptions of the glenoid that are intra-articular or alter its position, fractures that render the shoulder joint unstable, or unstable fracture patterns through the glenoid neck with an associated acromioclavicular joint disruption or clavicle fracture. These last injuries sever the attachment of the arm to the body and should be stabilized through operative fixation of the affected clavicle or acromioclavicular joint.

Scapulothoracic Dislocation and Dissociation

The scapulothoracic "articulation" is not a true joint as articular cartilage surfaces are not present. However, motion does occur here. In scapulothoracic dislocations, the inferior angle of the scapula becomes caught beneath a rib. These injuries are easily treated by manipulation and reduction.

Scapulothoracic dissociation, however, is an entirely different matter. These are the most severe of shoulder girdle injuries. Luckily, they are also exceedingly rare, with only fifteen cases having been reported in the literature.[6,7] These essentially are a near forequarter amputation.[31] They are the upper extremity's counterpart of the traumatic near hemipelvectomy. In this injury, all connections from the body to the arm are severed, with only the skin remaining intact. The injury may be closed or open. The patient presents with a flail, pulseless arm associated with massive shoulder swelling. Soft tissue defects may be palpable. The chest x-ray shows lateral displacement of the scapula due to avulsion of the musculature about the shoulder. The subclavian artery is torn (although sometimes the level of the injury is at the axillary artery) with an associated avulsion of the subclavian vein. Traumatic aneurysm may also occur. A massive brachial plexus injury is present, usually consisting of a complete avulsion, although some cases with neuropraxias have been seen. There is bony disruption at the level of the acromioclavicular or sternoclavicular joints, or through a clavicle fracture (Figure 8–14).

As 67% of these patients present in hypovolemic shock,[7] they need immediate resuscitation. There is a 20% mortality rate based on the known cases. Following the resuscitation, the vascular injury must be immediately addressed, after which the brachial plexus should be explored to assess the degree of injury. If any plexus repairs are possible, these are done. The clavicle should be plated to reattach the arm to the thorax.

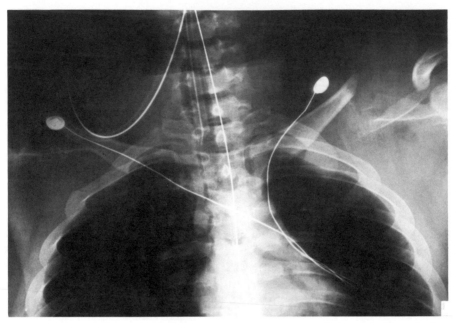

Figure 8–14. Left scapulothoracic dissociation. Note widely separated clavicle fracture and laterally displaced scapula in relation to the chest wall. Medial border of left scapula lines up with the lateral thorax instead of the normal relationship of the lateral border of the scapula and thorax as seen on the patient's right.

REFERENCES

1. Adams FL. *The Genuine Works of Hippocrates*. New York, NY: William Wood & Co; 1886.
2. Anderson K, et al. Treatment of clavicular fractures. *Acta Orthop Scand*. 1987;57:71–74.
3. Chapman MW, ed. *Operative Orthopaedics*. Philadelphia, Pa: JB Lippincott; 1988.
4. Chervu A, Quinones-Baldrich WJ. Vascular complications in orthopedic surgery. *Clin Orthop*. 1988; 235:275–288.
5. Crenshaw AH, ed. *Campbell's Operative Orthopaedics*. 7th ed. St. Louis, Mo: CV Mosby; 1987.
6. Ebraheim NA, et al. Scapulothoracic dissociation (closed avulsion of the scapula, subclavian artery, and brachial plexus): a newly recognized variant, a new classification and a review of the literature and treatment options. *J Orthop Trauma*. 1987;1:18–23.
7. Ebraheim NA, et al. Scapulothoracic dissociation. *J Bone Joint Surg*. 1988;70-A:428–432.
8. Galpin RD, et al. A comparative analysis of operative versus nonoperative treatment of grade III acromioclavicular separations. *Clin Orthop*. 1985;193:150–155.
9. Hardegger F. Die Behandlung von Schulterblattbrüchen. *Unfallheilkunde* 1984;87:58–66.
10. Hardegger F, et al. The operative treatment of scapular fractures. *J Bone Joint Surg*. 1984;66-B:725–731.
11. Hawkins RJ, et al. The three-part fracture of the proximal part of the humerus. *J Bone Joint Surg*. 1986;68-A: 1410–1414.
12. Hawkins RJ, et al. Anterior dislocation of the shoulder in the older patient. *Clin Orthop*. 1986;206:192–195.
13. Hawkins RJ, et al. Locked posterior dislocation of the shoulder. *J Bone Joint Surg*. 1987;69-A:9–18.
14. Hawkins RJ, Kiefer GN. Internal fixation techniques for proximal humeral fractures. *Clin Orthop*. 1987; 223:77.
15. Hierholzer G, Hax PM. Scapulafrakturen—Entstehung, Einteilung, Diagnose. *Hefte Unfallheilkunde* 1982; 160:87–99.
16. Henry JH, Genung JA. Natural history of glenohumeral dislocation—revisited. *Am J Sports Med*. 1982; 10:135–137.
17. Hill HA, Sachs MD. The grooved defect of the humeral head. A frequently unrecognized complication of dislocations of the shoulder joint. *Radiology*. 1940;35:690–700.

18. Hovelius L. Anterior dislocation of the shoulder in teen-agers and adults. *J Bone Joint Surg.* 1987;69-A: 393–399.
19. Kofoed H. Revascularization of the humeral head. *Clin Orthop.* 1984;179:175–178.
20. Lee CK, Hansen HR. Post-traumatic avascular necrosis of the humeral head in displaced proximal humeral fractures. *J Trauma.* 1981;21:788–791.
21. Lindholm TS, Elmstedt E. Bilateral posterior dislocation of the shoulder combined with fracture of the proximal humerus. *Acta Orthop Scand.* 1980;51:485–488.
22. McLaughlin HL, ed. *Trauma.* Philadelphia, Pa: WB Saunders; 1959.
23. McMurray TB. Recurrent dislocation of the shoulder. *J Bone Joint Surg.* 1961;43-B:402.
24. Mowery CA, et al. Recurrent posterior dislocation of the shoulder: treatment using a bone block. *J Bone Joint Surg.* 1985;67-A:777–781.
25. Neer CS II. Displaced proximal humeral fractures, part I. Classification and evaluation. *J Bone Joint Surg.* 1970;52-A:1077–1089.
26. Neer CS II. Displaced proximal humeral fractures, part II. Treatment of three-part and four-part displacement. *J Bone Joint Surg.* 1970;52–A:1090.
27. Neer CS II. Nonunion of the surgical neck of the humerus. *Orthop Trans.* 1982;6:389.
28. Neviaser RJ, et al. Concurrent ruptures of the rotator cuff and anterior dislocation of the shoulder in the older patient. *J Bone Joint Surg.* 1988;70–A:1308–1311.
29. Newell ED. Review of over 2000 fractures in past 7 years. *South Med J.* 1927;20:644.
30. Norwood LA, et al. Clinical presentation of complete tears of the rotator cuff. *J Bone Joint Surg.* 1989;71-A: 499–505.
31. Oreck SL, et al. Traumatic lateral displacement of the scapula: a radiographic sign of neurovascular disruption. *J Bone Joint Surg.* 1984;66–A:758.
32. Post M. Current concepts in the treatment of fractures of the clavicle. *Clin Orthop.* 1989;245:89–101.
33. Poulson S. Reduction of acute shoulder dislocations using the Eskimo technique: a study of 23 consecutive cases. *J Trauma.* 1988;28:1382–1383.
34. Rockwood CA Jr, Green DP. *Fractures in Adults.* 2nd ed. Philadelphia, Pa: JB Lippincott; 1984.
35. Rowe CR, Zarins B. Chronic unreduced dislocations of the shoulder. *J Bone Joint Surg.* 1982;64-A: 494–505.
36. Schatzker J, Tile M. *The Rationale of Operative Fracture Care.* Berlin, Germany: Springer–Verlag; 1987.
37. Stimson BB. *A Manual of Fractures and Dislocations.* 2nd ed. Philadelphia, Pa: Lea & Febiger; 1947.
38. Stimson LA. An easy method of reducing dislocations of the shoulder and hip. *Med Record.* 1900;57: 356–357.
39. Tanner MW, Cofield RH. Prosthetic arthroplasty for fractures and fracture-dislocations of the proximal humerus. *Clin Orthop.* 1982;179:116.
40. Thompson DA. The significance of scapular fractures. *J Trauma.* 1985;25:974.
41. Weaver JK. Skiing-related injuries to the shoulder. *Clin Orthop.* 1987;216:24.
42. Zimmerman LM, Veith I. *Great Ideas in the History of Surgery: Clavicle Shoulder, Shoulder Amputations.* Baltimore, Md: Williams & Wilkins; 1961.

9

Fractures of the Humerus and Forearm; Elbow Fractures and Dislocations

JAMES P. KENNEDY, M.D.

HISTORY: Fractures of the humeral shaft were once common sources of nonunion, and numerous operative procedures were devised to treat these nonunions.[43] Caldwell,[7] in 1933, developed the hanging arm cast technique which then became the standard of treatment and greatly reduced the incidence of nonunion. This technique, though successful, can be difficult for both the patient and physician. Recent fracture bracing techniques are becoming more popular, as they are equally successful and much more manageable for the patient.

INTRODUCTION

Generally, most fractures requiring operative treatment in the multiple trauma victim do best when operated on early. Those of the upper extremity are no different. Immediate or early operative fixation helps decrease stiffness and swelling locally, plus contributes to the overall well-being of the patient by allowing rapid mobilization out of bed.

Many upper extremity fractures that do quite well treated by closed means when they occur as isolated injuries will be treated operatively in the trauma patient. The need for unencumbered stable arms for crutch or walker ambulation, or the inability to control a reduction in the agitated uncooperative patient will lead to the operative stabilization of these otherwise "nonoperative" fractures.

HUMERUS SHAFT FRACTURE

Fractures of the humerus are among the most common of upper extremity fractures, and will be seen in approximately 1% of all multiple trauma patients.[6] Simple low-energy

136

transverse fractures often occur in the elderly as the result of a fall onto the arm. Higher energy comminuted fractures are the result of direct trauma to the region.[16] Spiral fractures are produced by indirect rotation forces directed up the arm.

In most instances of isolated shaft fractures, nonoperative treatment will give quite good functional results. The goal of treatment is a pain-free union resulting in a mobile, functioning extremity. The joints in the upper extremity have wide arcs of motion so that the hand can be positioned efficiently in space. The high degree of mobility at the shoulder and elbow will compensate for some angular deformity. The surrounding cuff of muscle will hide any minor deformity and contribute to a good cosmetic result.

Assessment

The fractured humerus will present with pain, swelling, and bony crepitus. Vascular injuries which are commonly seen with supracondylar fractures are infrequently seen with shaft fractures, as only 3% of shaft fractures are associated with a vessel injury.[30]

Neurologic injury is more common, being seen in 5% to 10% of humerus fractures.[43] The most common injury is a radial nerve palsy, usually seen in oblique fractures of the distal third of the shaft (the Holstein-Lewis fracture). The radial nerve is tethered at this site by the lateral intermuscular septum as it crosses from the posterior to anterior compartment of the arm. Wide displacement at the time of injury can cause a stretch injury to the nerve. The nerve may also be lacerated by the sharp fracture ends, contused or stretched by the fracture displacement, or entrapped within the fracture itself (Figure 9–1). Severe injuries with significant soft tissue damage may also present with nerve lesions from contusion (Figure 9–2).

The entire humerus is radiographed to rule out concomitant injury to the shoulder and elbow joints. Obtain forearm films as well if the injury mechanism or physical exam suggests the possibility of a forearm fracture, as the presence of an ipsilateral forearm fracture with the humerus fracture (resulting in a floating elbow) will affect how the injury is treated.

Treatment

The traditional form of treatment for humeral shaft fractures has been the hanging long arm cast.[43] This treatment, difficult to manage in the isolated fracture, is nearly impossible to successfully use in the bedridden trauma victim. Unlike other casts, a hanging arm cast is not designed to immobilize the fracture and maintain it in a reduced position, but rather the weight of the cast supplies traction to maintain the position of the fragments through gravity. Indeed (for proximal fractures especially), the fracture site may not even be contained within the cast. For this technique to properly function, the patient must remain in the upright position at all times, including sleeping in a chair. In the upright posture, gravity maintains the reduction which is controlled by a complicated adjustment of the hanging position of the cast. This technique will not work for the patient who cannot maintain an upright position due to other injuries.

Even for isolated injuries the technique is cumbersome and difficult for the patient. A common mistake is to use a standard cast which is too heavy for this application and will

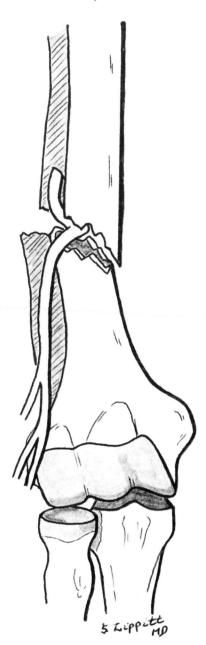

Figure 9–1. Distal humeral shaft fracture with entrapped radial nerve.

result in distraction of the fracture—the major cause of nonunion following closed treatment.[45] Spiral and oblique fractures (Figure 9–3) will maintain bone-to-bone contact if some distraction occurs; transverse fractures will not. Due to this short area of cortical bone contact, transverse fractures unite slowly with a high nonunion rate even in ideal circumstances.[30]

A preferable method of closed treatment for shaft fractures is a sugar-tong splint for

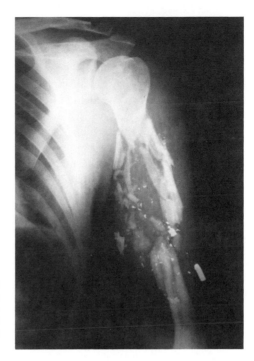

Figure 9–2. Humeral shaft fracture with radial nerve palsy. A battlefield injury from a high-powered Kalashnikov rifle, the explosive nature of the injury resulted in the nerve palsy from the concussion of the shock wave traveling through the soft tissues.

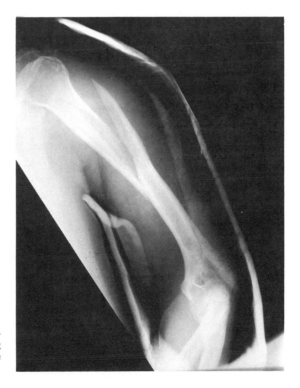

Figure 9–3. Spiral fracture of humerus immobilized in sugar-tong splint until swelling diminishes enough to allow fracture cuff to be applied.

7 to 10 days until the acute swelling and pain dissipate, followed by a Sarmiento[44] humeral cuff fracture brace and a sling as needed for comfort. Made of lightweight plastic materials, these cuffs are comfortable and well tolerated by the patient. The brace works on the principle of hydrostatic forces. The pressure applied by the cuff increases the hydrostatic pressure in the muscle envelope surrounding the fracture to the point where the fracture is immobilized. Good to excellent results can be expected in most patients treated in this manner for isolated fractures.[51]

Fracture care is made more complicated by the presence of chest injuries or chest tubes; and a splint, cuff, or any cast short of a shoulder spica simply cannot control a fracture in the obtunded or head-injured patient who is agitated. The multiple trauma victim usually needs operative stabilization of the fracture—sometimes more so to allow the treatment of other injuries than that of the fracture itself. Operative stabilization of the fracture will also allow early range of motion of the elbow and shoulder to prevent stiffness.

Any fracture that cannot be held in position with less than 20° of anterior angulation, 30° of medial angulation, or 3 cm of shortening warrants operative fixation.[9] Angulation of this magnitude will almost always occur with the hanging cast treatment in the very obese or women with large breasts. Angulation of the humerus is caused by the body displacing the forearm anteriorly when it is placed across the chest. This is not as great a problem with the humeral fracture cuff, as the cuff provides a greater amount of stability for the fracture, and often will better control the position in these difficult situations.

Bilateral upper extremity injuries are justification for rigid operative fixation of at least one side to give the patient one good extremity for eating and personal hygiene. Floating elbows (ipsilateral humeral shaft and forearm fractures) suffer a high rate of nonunion due to difficulty in controlling motion at both fracture sites. The elbow joint is prone to stiffness, and as there are two injuries in the vicinity of the joint, a floating elbow is susceptible to posttraumatic stiffness from immobilization.[9]

Most open fractures in the trauma victim are best treated by internal stabilization with plate and screw fixation[8] or unreamed nails upon presentation. Even though the fracture is open, with aggressive irrigation and debridement, low rates of infection occur due to the good vascularity of the humerus from its surrounding cuff of muscle. If a vascular repair has been required for either an open or closed fracture, rigid bony stabilization through plate and screw fixation is needed to protect the repair. Severe open fractures such as the comminuted Type IIIb fracture may be better treated with external fixation.

If the radial nerve is not initially functioning upon presentation, isolated fractures still may be treated closed with expectation for good return of nerve function[37] as the neuropraxia is usually due to a traction injury. This may take up to several weeks or even months.[27] In only 12% of patients with radial nerve palsies is it due to a nerve laceration, and these will do well following late repair at 3 to 4 months.[37]

Follow nerve function closely by exam throughout the course of treatment and with electrical studies at 4 to 6 weeks if there is no improvement. Splint the wrist-drop until the palsy resolves to prevent flexion contracture. Passive range of motion should also be used to guard against wrist and finger stiffness. If no neurologic return is noted clinically or by EMG studies by the time the fracture is fully healed, exploration may be indicated for nerve repair or grafting.[21] In cases where the nerve is initially intact, then stops functioning following reduction, it probably has become entrapped within the fracture site. In spite of this, the palsy will still often resolve. Exploration may be warranted as above for those cases which do not show early improvement. The nerve is always exposed and explored in any operative case such as open fractures and fractures in the face of multiple other injuries where internal fixation is being performed to ensure it is not surgically injured and to evaluate it if a preoperative palsy is present.[37]

OPERATIVE TECHNIQUE

Plate and screw fixation is the usual operative treatment for humeral shaft fractures (Figure 9–4). It is well suited for those fractures that demand rigid stability such as fractures with associated nerve or artery repair, intra-articular fractures, segmental fractures, or open fractures. Only the most severe Grade III open fractures are best treated by other means.

Semirigid nonreamed nails are a good choice for the head-injured or multiple trauma patient[18] when the humerus must be quickly fixed if the patient's condition does not allow enough time for plate and screw fixation (Figure 9–5). Multiple nails are inserted to fill the canal for increased rigidity and better rotational control. More rigid nails, such as those developed for the treatment of open tibia fractures, can be used with good results in the humerus as well.

The nails are inserted using a small entrance incision splitting the deltoid, being careful to protect the axillary nerve. Closed technique with the image intensifier eliminates the need for surgical approaches and subsequent soft tissue healing.[11] A proximal entrance site is used for fractures of the distal third of the humerus, and the distal portal for all other fracture patterns.[5,6] Neither the rotator cuff nor the olecranon fossa can be violated if optimal results are to be obtained.[11] A poorly placed proximal nail will lead to rotator cuff

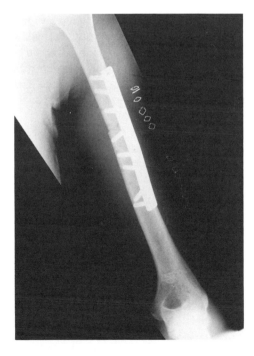

Figure 9–4. Plate and screw fixation of humeral shaft fracture.

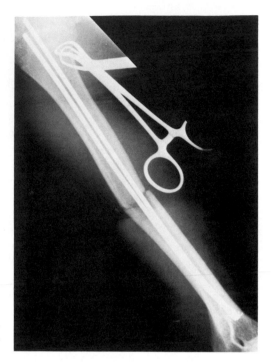

Figure 9–5. Flexible nail fixation of humeral shaft fracture in patient with head injury.

tendinitis and may impinge on the acromion; distally a triceps tendinitis may be induced, or impingement on the olecranon may occur blocking elbow extension.

The larger, more rigid unreamed tibial nails may be used in a similar fashion (Figure 9–6)—especially for open fractures. Reamed intramedullary nails, inserted under closed technique, may also be used in the humerus. These are best suited for those patients who must ambulate on crutches postoperatively[5] and need stronger internal splinting. Flexible nails and plates with screws cannot be loaded in this fashion until after bony healing begins. Both the reamed and unreamed nails offer the advantage of increased strength as well as the ability to cross lock the nail with screws to control rotation.

The cortical bone of the diaphyseal humerus may not heal well, leading to a delayed or nonunion. Therefore keep soft tissue stripping to a minimum no matter which fixation techniques are chosen. Bone graft fractures are opened if there is comminution or bone loss; open fractures may be grafted on a delayed basis at the time of delayed primary closure of the wound.

DISTAL HUMERUS FRACTURES

The supracondylar fracture of the humerus, commonly seen in children as the result of a fall on the outstretched hand, is less frequently seen in the adult, with only 20% of cases occurring after closure of the physes.[49] Intra-articular fractures are more commonly seen in the adult[46] and are the result of more significant trauma. The olecranon when the elbow is in flexion,[42] or the coronoid when the elbow is in extension,[46] acts as a wedge driving up through the articular surface of the humerus.

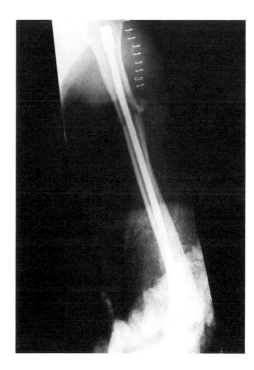

Figure 9–6. Rigid nonreamed humeral nail.

These intracondylar fractures can be technically very challenging to treat. The fractures frequently are distal with little or no nonarticular surfaces available on the fragments for the attachment of blood supplying soft tissues, or for the placement of screws (Figure 9–7). This, coupled with comminution or loss of bony contiguity from impaction, makes these fractures difficult to reassemble, and the poor distal bone stock makes rigid fixation more difficult to achieve.

Assessment

Distal humeral fractures typically present with massive soft tissue swelling about the elbow. Deformity is usually masked by the swelling. Neurovascular compromise is not uncommon[35,43] due to the close proximity of the radial, median, and ulnar nerves with an incidence as high as 17%.[24]

Laceration of the brachial artery can occur especially with those fractures with an extension deformity as only the brachialis separates the artery from the anterior humerus. Compartment syndrome in the forearm must also be anticipated and guarded against.[8,43]

Treatment

Treatment of distal humerus fractures in the multiple trauma patient is generally the same as that for isolated injuries. Although some recommend that closed treatment can be successful for the rare nondisplaced fractures,[43] others[8,45] feel that better results will be achieved

ELBOW DISLOCATION

Dislocation of the elbow can occur in any direction, although 80% to 90% are posterior or posterolateral.[43] In children, the elbow is the most commonly dislocated joint; in adults, only the shoulder is more frequently dislocated.[35] The radius and ulna usually displace together in the same direction; rarely they may dislocate divergently.

Falls onto the outstretched arm account for the majority of dislocations.[35] There are two theories for the mechanism of dislocation. The first hypothesizes hyperextension as the mechanism, stating that as the elbow hyperextends, the olecranon impinges on the humerus acting as a fulcrum. With further extension, the anterior capsular structures and collateral ligaments tear, resulting in disruption of the joint.[47] The second theory states that the dislocation occurs from axial loading with the elbow in slight flexion. The resultant force then drives the proximal radius and ulna posteriorly.[36]

Dislocation of either the radius or ulna alone may occur as an isolated event. Most commonly an isolated dislocation of one bone will occur in association with a fracture of the other bone which destabilizes the elbow enough to allow the dislocation. As will be seen, the presence of the dislocation in these instances often dictates how the fracture is treated.

Fractures about the elbow commonly occur in association with a dislocation. Chip fractures are usually present from ligamentous or capsular avulsions. The radial neck will suffer a compression fracture in up to 10% of cases, there will be avulsion fractures involving the medial or lateral epicondyles in approximately 10%, and avulsions of the coronoid occur in 10% as well.[35]

Evaluation

Gross deformity of the extremity will be evident, as will a mechanical block to motion. A careful neurovascular examination is mandatory. Just as in the supracondylar fracture, compromise of the brachial artery can occur in about 5% of cases,[28] usually from compression. Median and ulnar nerve lesions may also occur, with the ulnar nerve more commonly involved.[35] Radial nerve lesions have not been reported.[43]

Routine AP and lateral elbow films will demonstrate the direction of dislocation for planning of reduction and reveal any major associated fractures. Less evident fractures may not be identifiable due to the distorted anatomy. The post-reduction elbow films in addition to confirming an adequate reduction, are necessary to diagnose some of these associated fractures.

Treatment

The treatment of elbow dislocations is the same as that for any dislocation—early atraumatic reduction. In the multiple trauma or comatose patient, this can often be done without any additional analgesia. In the conscious alert patient, analgesics or muscle relaxants are helpful.

Almost all dislocations can be successfully reduced by closed techniques,[43] especially if there are no associated fracture fragments to potentially block reduction. Traction in line with the forearm, elbow flexion, and manipulation of the olecranon to ease it back into place is the most common reduction technique used for the posterior dislocation. Hyperextension to unlock the coronoid is sometimes needed as well. A method similar to the Stimson maneuver for shoulder or hip dislocation may also be employed. With this method, the patient is placed prone with the elbow flexed 90° over the edge of the bed with 5 to 10 pounds of weight supplying traction at the wrist. If the dislocation does not spontaneously reduce, the olecranon may be manipulated into place.

Another convenient technique is for the physician to interlock fingers with the patient and place his elbow in the patient's antecubital fossa. The elbow will then reduce by the physician extending his wrist and applying traction distally with his elbow (Figure 9–10).

Open reduction is required only rarely for cases that are irreducible due to soft tissue interposition, or for dislocations treated late. More commonly, open reduction will be necessary to remove an interposed fractured medial epicondyle. This is most apt to occur in the pediatric patient with open physes.[38]

After the reduction, examine the elbow through a full range of motion to be sure that there is no mechanical block to motion from intra-articular fragments, and to see where the elbow is unstable. Intra-articular fragments must be surgically removed from the joint. Establishing the "safe zone"—that is, the arc of motion within which the elbow is stable— is helpful for rapid mobilization. Generally the position of immobilization must be that of flexion greater than 90°. As the elbow is notorious for early stiffness, start motion within the

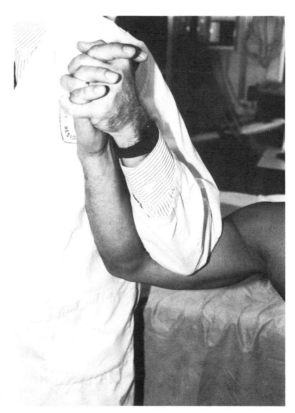

Figure 9–10.   Hand-to-hand method of elbow reduction.

first week. Active motion may be begun immediately within the confines of the "safe zone."

Late instability or recurrent dislocation is rare[35,43] due to the interlocking stability afforded by the configuration of the ulna and trochlea. Poor results are more often associated with stiffness either from lengthy immobilization[32] or heterotopic ossification than from chronic instability.

RADIAL HEAD AND NECK FRACTURES

Treatment of intracapsular proximal radius fractures is generally the same whether they occur in the multiple trauma patient or as isolated injuries. If surgical intervention is required, it is best done early to avoid heterotopic bone formation and permit early motion. Early range of motion is necessary regardless of treatment for best functional results.

Roughly one half of radial head and neck fractures are due to a direct blow to the area with the other half resulting from an indirect force applied across the joint.[39] Indirect forces are often the result of a fall onto the outstretched hand producing an axial compression across the joint and subsequent collapse of the head or neck.

Fractures of the radial head or neck account for one third of all elbow fractures,[29] and make up 2% to 5% of all fractures.[35]

Evaluation and Assessment

The treatment of these fractures is in some ways comparable to that of femoral neck fractures. The vascular anatomy is similar, and if the fractures are displaced, they should be addressed within the first 24 hours for best results. The radial head and neck are entirely contained within the joint capsule without soft tissue attachments. Fractures within these synovial confines may therefore devascularize the fragments. As the only source of blood to the radial head is the intraosseous supply, if this is disrupted due to the fracture, the possibility of avascular necrosis or nonunion will result.

On examination, pain, swelling, and a hemarthrosis are present. Ten percent of radial head fractures are associated with an elbow dislocation (Figure 9–11), and 10% of elbow dislocations have an associated radial head fracture.[35] With a radial head or neck fracture, it is important to make sure that an Essex-Lopresti injury is not present. This injury, consisting of the radial fracture and a distal radioulnar disruption, is discussed further below.

Radiographic examination will reveal the presence and nature of the fracture. Nondisplaced fractures are often difficult to see. A "clinical" radial head fracture may be presumptively diagnosed by the presence of pain on direct palpation of the radial head or with pronation and supination, and the presence of a posterior fat pad sign on x-ray.

Treatment

Nondisplaced fractures are generally stable and can be treated by a short period of immobilization followed by range of motion in 2 or 3 days. Acutely, the hemarthrosis

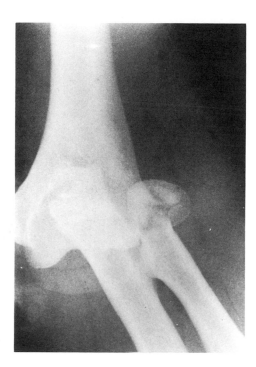

Figure 9–11. Elbow dislocation with comminuted radial head and neck fracture.

causing painful capsular distention may be aspirated. Injecting the joint with local anesthetic will also help with pain relief. Displaced fractures will sometimes need reduction. As the radial head is a non–weight-bearing joint, there is more leeway for accepting nonanatomic reductions. Although the radial head and ulna are in constant contact, the radial head contacts the capitellum only at 135° of flexion[35,43] or greater, so some mildly displaced fractures may not interfere with elbow function.

The "Rule of Threes" has been used to determine which fractures require reduction and fixation. Fractures with greater than 30° of angulation, more than 3 mm of articular displacement, or involving more than one third of the joint surface[13] require reduction. Recently, this has been updated to include 2 mm of articular displacement.[35] Perhaps a better method is to assess the nature of the fracture—that is, the "fracture personality"—to see if function has been impaired.[45] If so, reduction and fixation are undertaken. This philosophy does not require the memorization of "rules."

To assess the personality of the fracture, aspirate the hemarthrosis and inject local anesthetic into the joint if necessary to examine the joint without pain. The elbow is then placed through a full range of motion. If the arm cannot be extended to within 10° of full extension, or if there is more than a 30° loss of the pronation/supination arc, function will be impaired and reduction is warranted.[35]

The surgery for these injuries can be quite difficult. The fragments are small in size and the tight quarters of the surgical approach limit the amount of exposure possible. Soft tissue stripping can further increase the risk of avascular necrosis. Small screws are required, and if a fragment that is completely articular must be fixed, recess the screw heads below the articular surface (Figure 9–12A,B). If small plates are used, they must be placed

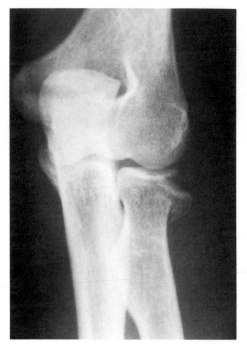
A

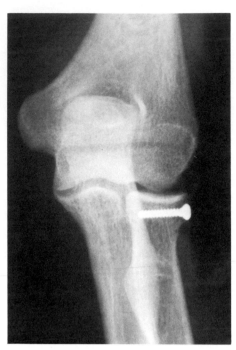
B

Figure 9–12. A, B: Displaced radial head fracture requiring open reduction and screw fixation.

so as not to interfere with pronation or supination. Larger fracture fragments can be thus stabilized; fragments too small for fixation often must be excised. In cases where the radial head is completely shattered, it may not be possible to reconstruct it. Traditionally, excision of the entire head within 24 hours of injury[35] has given the best results. This is especially true for the trauma patient so that early motion can be instituted to prevent stiffness from heterotopic ossification. Recently it has been shown that delayed excision as a salvage procedure for isolated injuries with persistent pain will also give good relief.[3]

Radial head excision can be performed with the expectation of good results and only minimal, pain-free shortening of the radius if the elbow's ulnar collateral ligaments and the distal radioulnar joint are intact.[35] If there is an Essex-Lopresti injury, excessive radial shortening will occur leading to chronic wrist pain. In case of injury to the ulnar side of the elbow, late instability can be a problem as well. If a simple radial head excision cannot be performed because of the above reasons, excision with the insertion of a silastic prosthesis will maintain stability and prevent undue shortening.[35] Due to the risk of subsequent silicone synovitis, this prosthesis should then be removed for most patients at 8 to 12 months when the risk of radial shortening has passed.

MONTEGGIA FRACTURE, GALLEAZI FRACTURE, ESSEX-LOPRESTI FRACTURE

Logic tells us that due to the presence of two bones in the forearm, both will often be injured together. This was first described by Paul of Aegina in the mid-600s.[1] Direct trauma such as a blow may be absorbed by only one bone causing an isolated injury. Any indirect force applied to the forearm will be transmitted into both radius and ulna, and if sufficiently strong, will cause injury at both locations. Therefore, whenever an injury is diagnosed by physical or radiographic evidence involving the elbow, radius, ulna, or wrist, the remaining structures in the forearm must be carefully scrutinized for injury as well.

The student of orthopaedics curses its propensity to identify fractures by eponyms. The following eponymic fractures occur about the elbow, and although it is not so important to know the name of the man they are associated with, it is important to recognize the injury complex and its ramifications for treatment. If these injuries are not recognized, but are treated as simple fractures or dislocations, late problems such as pain and instability will be common.

Monteggia Fracture

First described by Monteggia[34] in 1814, this injury is characterized by a fracture of the proximal ulnar shaft with an associated dislocation of the radial head. The mechanism is either one of a direct blow to the elbow region, or the indirect axial compressive forces and pronation that occur with a fall onto the outstretched hand. Radial nerve palsies occur quite often with an incidence of up to 20%.[35] The posterior interosseous is generally the branch involved.

Four types of Monteggia fractures occur, and are described based upon the position of the fragments.[43] Generally, the angulation of the fractured ulna follows the direction of the dislocated radial head (Figure 9–13). Anterior dislocation of the radial head and anterior

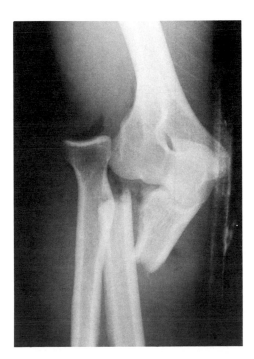

Figure 9–13. Monteggia fracture. This is an open injury—note air density about radial head and capitellum.

angulation of the ulnar shaft fracture (Type I) is the most common, making up one half to three quarters of cases.

The reduction of the radial head is rendered unstable by the presence of the ulnar fracture. This injury is especially dangerous in cases where the radial head may have reduced itself spontaneously by the time the patient is examined. In cases of isolated fracture of the ulnar shaft, always examine the radial head for pain and possible instability. This is most true for the patient whose injury mechanism is not consistent with a nightstick fracture (discussed below).

Whereas an isolated nightstick fracture of the ulnar shaft may be treated by closed means if it is in good position, Monteggia fractures in adults must be operatively stabilized in order to maintain the radial head reduction.[45] This is followed by four weeks of immobilization in a position of radial head stability—at least 110° of flexion and moderate supination for anterior dislocations, and 70° of flexion for posterior dislocations. Monteggia fractures can usually be treated closed in children with the above guidelines for positioning,[43,50] but only if an anatomic stable reduction of the ulna can be maintained.

Galleazi Fracture

First described in 1934,[20] the Galleazi fracture consists of a fracture of the distal radial shaft associated with disruption of the distal radioulnar joint (Figure 9–14A) and is sometimes called the reverse Monteggia fracture. This fracture has also been called the "Fracture of Necessity"[43] due to the fact that surgical fixation is necessary.

Just as the dislocated radial head is unstable in the Monteggia fracture, the distal radioulnar joint cannot be held stabilized with nonoperative treatment of the Galleazi fracture. Open reduction and internal fixation of the radial shaft is necessary to maintain stability of the distal radioulnar joint and achieve a good result (Figure 9–14B). Postoperatively, immobilize the forearm in a position of distal radioulnar joint stability— supination for dorsal dislocations of the ulna, and pronation for volar.

Essex-Lopresti Fracture

The Essex-Lopresti fracture is a "new" and a relatively rare lesion. First described in 1951,[14] it consists of a radial head fracture with associated disruption of the distal radial ulnar joint. A result of a longitudinal force, the entire radius is driven proximally with a tear in the interosseous membrane (Figure 9–15).[12] This totally destabilizes the radius, and if not properly treated, radial shortening will ensue.

This lesion is often missed at the time of initial examination. Palpation at the wrist for pain and radial shortening is the key to recognition of the injury. In the obtunded patient, reliance must of necessity be based on the radiographic exam. Unfortunately, films showing the entire forearm are usually obtained. Due to the divergent incident beam and the resulting distortion, the film will often not show proximal radial migration.[12] In cases of displaced radial head fractures, a wrist series is required. Comparison films of the opposite normal wrist can be helpful in diagnosing radial shortening due to the variance in the position of the distal radius and ulna from patient to patient.

The importance in recognizing this lesion lies in the form of treatment. Often, the

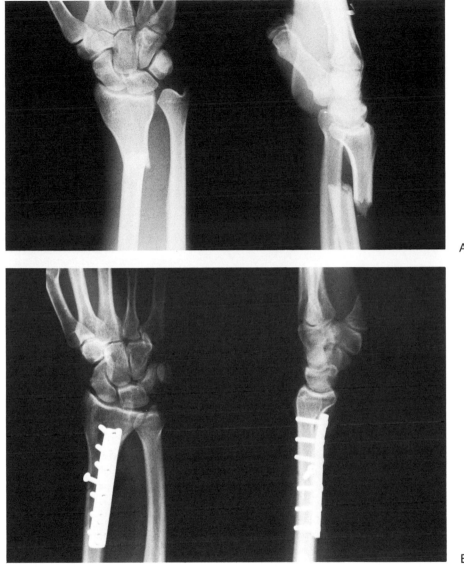

Figure 9–14. **A:** Galleazi fracture with volar dislocation of ulna on lateral view (right) and shortening of radius with disruption of distal radial-ulnar joint on AP view. **B:** Anatomic reduction following internal fixation.

radial head is damaged severely enough to require its excision. If this is done, severe shortening of the longitudinally unstable radius will rapidly occur with instability and wrist pain. In order to get a good result, the radial head must be stabilized by reduction and fixation (if possible) to allow soft tissue healing of the radiocapitellar and distal radioulnar joints as well as the interosseous membrane. If reconstruction of the head is not possible, a silastic implant should be temporarily used to maintain the position and length of the radius.[12,35]

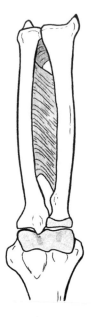
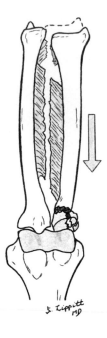

Figure 9–15.   Mechanism of Essex-Lopresti fracture. Axial force causes tearing of interosseous membrane and unstable radial head or neck fracture. Unless properly stabilized, the radius will shorten causing chronic·wrist pain.

OLECRANON FRACTURES

Introduction

Fractures of the olecranon may be either extra-articular or intra-articular. Extra-articular fractures occur at the tip of the olecranon and represent triceps avulsion lesions occurring from a sudden forceful synergistic contracture of both the elbow flexors and extensors.[35] Intra-articular fractures can occur by this same mechanism as well, but more commonly are precipitated by a direct blow to the region.

Early treatment of olecranon fractures utilized splinting in extension. Although this produced union, it resulted in a stiff elbow in the dysfunctional extended position.[25] Subsequently, the injury was treated in a position of midflexion with early motion. This prevented the extension deformity, but resulted in bony nonunion due to distraction of the fragments from the pull of the triceps leading to an elbow which was weak in extension.[10] This "Catch-22" situation led to the development of operative fixation for these displaced fractures. Lister performed the first open reduction and internal fixation of a fracture using his newly developed aseptic techniques on just such a displaced olecranon fracture in 1884.[25] Lister's original wire loop fixation has over the years been modified to the tension-band techniques that are in standard use today.

The two key factors in the treatment of these injuries are the restoration of the joint surfaces and maintaining an intact triceps mechanism that will allow early motion and result in an elbow that will be strong in extension.

Assessment

The patient will present with pain and swelling about the elbow. Displaced fractures will often have a palpable bony defect where the pull of the triceps has opened up the fracture site (Figure 9–16). These patients will be unable to actively extend the elbow.

The triceps mechanism must be tested for extra-articular fractures or nondisplaced intra-articular fractures to determine if it is intact. An intra-articular local anesthetic can be used if necessary. If the patient can extend the elbow against gravity, the triceps mechanism is functionally intact. Forced or resisted extension should not be attempted as this could complete a partial triceps rupture. The obtunded or multiple trauma patient often will not be able to cooperate with this type of examination, but observation will often demonstrate spontaneous triceps function, or withdrawal from pain can be tested.

Management

If the triceps mechanism is intact, the extra-articular fracture may be treated symptomatically with early passive range of motion to prevent stiffness. Whether small fractures heal with a bony or fibrous union is of little consequence. In unusual cases of late symptoms, the fragment can be excised.

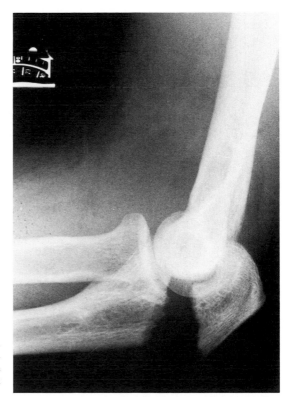

Figure 9–16. Intra-articular olecranon fracture. Displacement occurs from pull of triceps mechanism. This patient would have weakness of the extensor mechanism on physical exam.

For cases of extra-articular fracture in which the triceps function has been lost, early surgical repair is necessary. Large fragments can be internally fixed to obtain bone-to-bone healing. Occasionally the fragments are too small to be amenable to fixation. In these instances excise the fragments and suture the tendon into the raw cancellous bony surface.

Nondisplaced intra-articular fractures are generally stable if the triceps aponeurosis is intact to hold the fragments together. These fractures may be treated with immobilization in a position of midflexion with early passive motion guarding against flexion past 90° until bony union begins.[35] To be considered nondisplaced, there must be less than 2 mm of distraction at the fracture site,[13] and the position must not change with flexion up to 90°.[48]

Displaced fractures have had the triceps aponeurosis torn at the fracture site and are therefore unstable. As for all intra-articular fractures, best results are obtained with early fixation (within 24 hours). The multiple trauma patient is best treated immediately.

Various methods are available to internally fixate olecranon fractures. The tension band wire and pin technique, tension band wire with intramedullary screw, or plate and screw fixation are all possible depending on the nature of the fracture (Figure 9–17). The key is anatomic reduction and stable fixation to permit immediate motion for articular cartilage healing.

Some fractures, especially in the badly injured trauma patient, are so comminuted that reconstruction is not possible. These injuries are known as "sideswipe" injuries from the days before automobile air conditioning. They occurred from the driver's elbow hanging out the window at the time of an accident, and are often associated with other fractures in the arm.

For severely comminuted fractures, a portion of the olecranon may be excised, as first

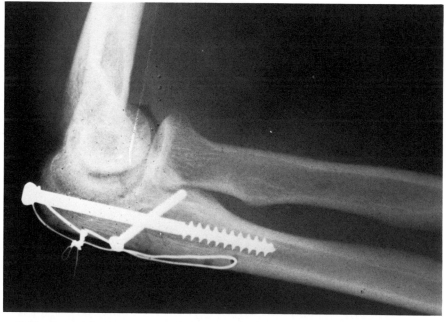

Figure 9–17.   Internal fixation of olecranon fracture. Tension band wire with intramedullary screw. Additional lag screw has been placed across the fracture as well.

reported by Fiolle in 1918[17] based on his experiences in World War I. This is especially true for the elderly or low-demand individual. The triceps tendon is reattached to the remaining ulna to obtain tendon to bone healing and preserve elbow function. The coronoid must remain intact, as the ulnar collateral ligaments insert here and are necessary to maintain elbow stability. McKeever and Buck following World War II[31] stated that 80% of the entire olecranon may be excised with good results so long as the coronoid remains intact.[35,43] Recently, this has been challenged. The proximal ulna has been found to be more important for stability than previously thought.[2] Although no new recommendations exist, it would be wise to leave as much of the olecranon intact as possible if excision is to be undertaken, and make every attempt to reconstruct the olecranon for high demand, active individuals.

Coronoid Fractures

Isolated coronoid fractures are avulsion fractures and usually occur in association with elbow hyperextension and dislocation.[43] These can mostly be treated by closed methods. If the fracture is through the base involving a significant portion of the coronoid, open reduction and internal fixation is necessary. Closed treatment of these fractures has been unsatisfactory 80% of the time due to stiffness and heterotopic ossification.[41]

More comminuted coronoid process fractures also occur in the severe "sideswipe fractures" that involve the entire proximal ulna. Internal fixation of the coronoid should be part of the operative fixation of the olecranon in these instances.

FOREARM FRACTURES

The forearm is a complicated structure consisting of five joints (distal radial ulnar, proximal radial ulnar, radial carpal, radial capitellar, and ulnar trochlear). In addition, there is a complex double sigmoid bow to the radius. This arrangement is necessary to position the hand in space for fine motor function. For this reason, anatomic reduction of the adult forearm is mandatory. The forearm fracture which is so commonly seen in the young child secondary to a fall can be given more leeway in its reduction due to the remarkable remodeling that occurs with growth.[40,50]

The vast majority of forearm shaft fractures in adults occur as a result of motor vehicle accidents.[43] These are not uncommonly open fractures due to the high energy involved and the subcutaneous location of the ulna throughout its length, and that of the radius distally. The forearm is also frequently fractured when the victim is attempting to fend off blows during an altercation or in a reflexive attempt to protect the head from falling objects. Most of the remaining fractures are the result of falls.

Evaluation

Upon evaluating the patient with a fractured forearm, the possibility of injury to the surrounding joints must also be considered as discussed above to properly diagnose and treat the Galleazi, Monteggia, and Essex-Lopresti fractures. The fractured forearm will exhibit swelling. Deformity from angulation at the fracture is common. Instability and crepitus may be noted on exam. Neurovascular lesions are uncommon with straightforward shaft fractures.[9,43]

Compartment syndrome may complicate this injury, so the patient with a significant soft tissue injury must be carefully evaluated. Abrasions and lacerations about the forearm are carefully inspected. Due to the subcutaneous position of the ulna and the lack of thick muscle mass in the distal forearm, these insignificant-appearing skin injuries may indicate the presence of an open fracture and can therefore alter the treatment plan.

Treatment

Some feel isolated nondisplaced stable adult forearm fractures may be treated by closed methods[9] in selected individuals. Patients treated in this manner must be watched very carefully. Others[45] believe that every adult forearm fracture which involves both bones requires internal fixation. In the multiple trauma victim, it is generally agreed that these injuries cannot be treated closed due to the almost assured displacement that will occur in the agitated patient or those with mental status changes. In rare instances, consideration should be given to operating on the child's forearm fracture when multiple other injuries are present, or in the presence of high grade unstable open fractures.[50] Otherwise, children's forearm fractures are routinely treated by closed reductions if necessary and a period of casting.

The forearm fracture should be quickly operated on if at all possible, before swelling occurs.[9] By doing so, a potential compartment syndrome may be prevented simply by the operative approach. This permits evacuation of the hematoma and hemostasis, and the surgical approach performs a fasciotomy. Even in cases where compartment syndrome is not a high risk, do not close the forearm fascia upon completion of the procedure for fear of potential compartment syndrome postoperatively. In cases where the fracture cannot be operated upon quickly, swelling may be too great to allow skin closure[45] even in the absence of a compartment syndrome.

The standard for operative fixation of forearm shaft fractures is plate and screw fixation (Figure 9–18).[9,43,45] Comminuted fractures, segmental fractures, those with bony loss, or fractures with extensive soft-tissue stripping will benefit from bone grafting. The diaphyseal cortical bone will not heal well without grafting if conditions are not ideal.

Open fractures of the forearm, if properly addressed through open fracture techniques (see Chapter 7), may be internally fixed on presentation in most cases.[33] Severe Grade III fractures of the forearm are unusual, and are usually the result of industrial or farm accidents. These contaminated injuries should be treated with external fixation. Less severe open fractures have a less than 3% infection rate[8] following open reduction and internal fixation due to the good blood supply of the forearm.

Nightstick Fracture

Isolated shaft fractures of the radius are unusual, and, if seen, there is a high probability that one of the fracture-dislocation injuries already discussed is present. Isolated fractures of the ulnar shaft, however, are common.

Due to its subcutaneous position, the shaft of the ulna is vulnerable to direct violence.

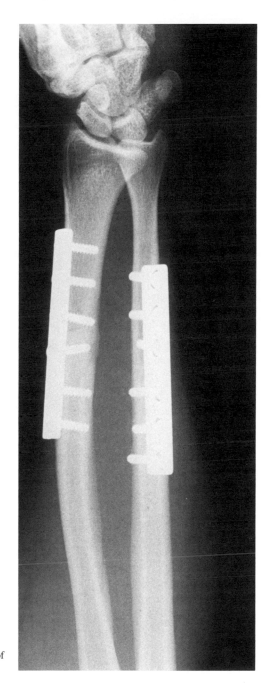

Figure 9–18. Plate and screw fixation of radius and ulna.

Isolated ulnar shaft fractures are commonly known as the nightstick fracture from the injury which is received while trying to fend off a blow with the upraised arm.

Nondisplaced nightstick fractures can be treated by closed means with the knowledge that these diaphyseal cortical fractures heal slowly[43] and may require late bone grafting to stimulate union. Displaced fractures require reduction and fixation. It is probably best to treat even nondisplaced fractures in the multiple trauma victim with internal fixation due to the encumbrance of a long-arm cast and the difficulty with nursing care of the other injuries. Also, immobilization is sure to lead to stiffness of the elbow in the multiple trauma victim, especially if heterotopic ossification occurs.

REFERENCES

1. Aegina P, Adams F, trans. *Fractures and Dislocations*. London: New Sydenham Society; 1846.
2. An K, et al. The effect of partial removal of proximal ulna on elbow constraint. *Clin Orthop*. 1986;209: 270–279.
3. Broberg MA, Morrey BF. Results of delayed excision of the radial head after fracture. *J Bone Joint Surg*. 1986;68-A:669–674.
4. Broberg MA, Morrey BF. Results of treatment of fracture-dislocations of the elbow. *Clin Orthop*. 1987;216:109–119.
5. Browner BD, Edwards CC. *The Science and Practice of Intramedullary Nailing*. Philadelphia, Pa: Lea & Febiger; 1987.
6. Brumback RJ, et al. Intramedullary stabilization of humeral shaft fractures in patients with multiple trauma. *J Bone Joint Surg*. 1986;68-A:960–970.
7. Caldwell JA. Treatment of fractures in the Cincinnati General Hospital. *Ann Surg*. 1933;97:161.
8. Chapman MW. The role of intramedullary fixation in open fractures. *Clin Orthop*. 1986;212:26–34.
9. Chapman MW, ed. *Operative Orthopaedics*. Philadelphia, Pa: JB Lippincott; 1988.
10. Deliyannis SN. Comminuted fractures of the olecranon treated by Weber-Vasey technique. *Injury*. 1973–1974;5:19–24.
11. Distefano MC, Sallis JG. Closed intramedullary nailing of the humerus: a modified technique. *J Ortho Trauma*. 1987;1:245–256.
12. Edwards GS Jr, Jupiter JB. Radial head fractures with acute distal radioulnar dislocation. *Clin Orthop*. 1988; 234:61–69.
13. Eriksson E, et al. Late results of conservative and surgical treatment of fracture of the olecranon. *Acta Chir Scand*. 1957;113:153–166.
14. Essex-Lopresti P. Fractures of the radial head with distal radio-ulnar dislocation. *J Bone Joint Surg*. 1951; 33-B:244.
15. Evans EM. Supracondylar Y fractures of the humerus. *J Bone Joint Surg*. 1953;35–B:381.
16. Fenyo G. On fractures of the shaft of the humerus. *Acta Chir Scand*. 1971;137:221.
17. Fiolle DJ. Note sur les fractures de folecrane par projectiles de guerre. *Mars Med*. 1918;55:241–245.
18. Foster RJ, et al. Internal fixation of fractures and non-unions of the humeral shaft. *J Bone Joint Surg*. 1985; 67-A:857–864.
19. Gabel GT, et al. Intraarticular fractures of the distal humerus in the adult. *Clin Orthop*. 1987;216:99–108.
20. Galleazi R. Uber ein besonderes Syndrom bei Verletzungen im Bereich der Unterarmknochen. *Arch Orthop Unfallchir*. 1934;35:557–562.
21. Garcia A Jr, Maeck BH. Radial nerve injuries in fractures of the shaft of the humerus. *Am J Surg*. 1960; 99:625.
22. Henley MB, et al. Operative management of intra-articular fractures of the distal humerus. *J Orthop Trauma*. 1987;1:24–35.
23. Holstein A, Lewis G. Fractures of the humerus with radial-nerve paralysis. *J Bone Joint Surg*. 1963;45-A: 1382–1388.
24. Hördegen KM. Neurologische Komplikationen bei kindlichen supracondylären Humerusfrakturen. *Arch Orthop Unfallchir*. 1970;68:294.
25. Howard JL, Urist MR. Fracture-dislocation of the radius and the ulna at the elbow joint. *Clin Orthop*. 1958; 12:276–284.
26. Hughston JC. Fractures of the distal radial shaft. Mistakes in management. *J Bone Joint Surg*. 1957;39-A: 249–264.
27. Kettlekemp DB, Alexander H. Clinical review of radial nerve injury. *J Trauma*. 1967;7:424.

28. Linscheid RL, Wheeler DK. Elbow dislocations. *JAMA*. 1965;194:1171–1176.
29. Mason MB. Some observations on fractures of the head of the radius with a review of one hundred cases. *Br J Surg*. 1954;42:123.
30. Mast JW, et al. Fractures of the humeral shaft. *Clin Orthop*. 1975;112:254–262.
31. McKeever FM, Buck RM. Fracture of the olecranon process of the ulna. *JAMA*. 1947;135:1–5.
32. Mehlhoff TL, et al. Simple dislocation of the elbow in the adult. *J Bone Joint Surg*. 1988;70-A:244–249.
33. Moed BR, et al. Immediate internal fixation of open fractures of the diaphysis of the forearm. *J Bone Joint Surg*. 1986;68-A:1008–1017.
34. Monteggia GB. *Instituzioni Chirurgiche, V*. Milan, Italy: Maspero; 1814.
35. Morrey BF. *The Elbow and Its Disorders*. Philadelphia, Pa: WB Saunders; 1985.
36. Osborne G, Cotterill P. Recurrent dislocation of the elbow. *J Bone Joint Surg*. 1966;48–B:340.
37. Pollock FH, et al. Treatment of radial neuropathy associated with fractures of the humerus and forearm. *J Bone Joint Surg*. 1981;64-A:239–243.
38. Purser DW. Dislocation of the elbow and inclusion of the medial epicondyle in the adult. *J Bone Joint Surg*. 1954;36–B:247.
39. Radin EL, Riseborough EJ. Fractures of the radial head. *J Bone Joint Surg*. 1966;48–A:1055–1061.
40. Rang M. *Children's Fractures*. 2nd ed. Philadelphia, Pa: JB Lippincott; 1983.
41. Regan W, Morrey B. Fractures of the coronoid process of the ulna. *J Bone Joint Surg*. 1989;71-A:1348–1354.
42. Reich RS. Treatment of intracondylar fractures of the elbow by means of traction. *J Bone Joint Surg*. 1936;18:997.
43. Rockwood, CA Jr, Green DP. *Fractures in Adults*. 2nd ed. Philadelphia, Pa: JB Lippincott; 1984.
44. Sarmiento A, Latta LL. *Closed Functional Treatment of Fractures*. New York, NY: Springer; 1981.
45. Schatzker J, Tile M. *The Rationale of Operative Fracture Care*. Berlin, Germany: Springer-Verlag; 1987.
46. Smith FM. *Surgery of the Elbow*. Philadelphia, Pa: WB Saunders; 1972.
47. Thomas TT. A contribution to the mechanism of fractures and dislocations in the elbow region. *Ann Surg*. 1929;89:108.
48. Thompson TKF, Scham SM. A posteromedial approach to the proximal end of the ulna for the internal fixation of olecranon fractures. *J Trauma*. 1969;9:594–602.
49. Wade FV, Batdorf J. Supracondylar fractures of the humerus: a twelve year review with follow-up. *J Trauma*. 1961;269:1.
50. Weber BG, Brunner Ch, Freuler F, eds. *Treatment of Fractures in Children and Adolescents*. Berlin, Germany: Springer-Verlag; 1980.
51. Zagorski JB, et al. Diaphyseal fractures of the humerus—Treatment with prefabricated braces. *J Bone Joint Surg*. 1988;70-A:607–610.

10

Wrist Fractures and Dislocations

JAMES P. KENNEDY, M.D.

HISTORY: The understanding of the kinematics and pathophysiology of the wrist historically lagged behind other areas of the body. It was not until the middle of the 1500s that Vesalius[6] identified and numbered the various carpal bones. Referring to the carpals by number and not name[13] remained popular well into the 1800s—a fact probably well appreciated by medical and anatomy students of the day. Although the anatomy was known at an early date, as late as 1833 Sir Charles Bell described the wrist with the statement, "In the human hand, bones of the wrist are eight in number and they are so closely connected that they form a sort of ball, which moves on the end of the radius."[2]

The classic descriptions of many of the distal radial and ulnar injuries were made in the 1800s, but it was not until after the advent of radiography that precise diagnoses and understanding of fracture patterns began. Some early descriptions of the kinematics of the wrist were made at the turn of this century,[3] however it was not until the last twenty to thirty years that a good understanding of the complex movements and interrelationships of the carpals and radiocarpal joints has occurred.

INTRODUCTION

The wrist is frequently injured in the polytrauma patient due to its vulnerability. The hands tightly gripped on a steering wheel or handlebars, falls onto the outstretched arm, and reflexive movements in an attempt to protect the head and face all place the wrist at risk. It is also a frequent site for isolated injuries due to sporting activities and falls.

Although a wrist fracture or dislocation may not be as dramatic as one occurring in the pelvis or femur, it should be given just as much attention. It is not uncommon for a carpal subluxation to be missed, forgotten about, or ignored as an "insignificant injury" while more exciting problems are being treated. A 10% impairment in the dominant hand and wrist can be a much greater disability than a similar impairment in the lower extremity.

If not treated properly, even a minor injury can lead to a useless hand if stiffness, contracture, neurologic loss, or posttraumatic arthritis occurs. For these reasons, the wrist injuries must be given close attention with prompt treatment and aggressive rehabilitation.

Assessment

A high index of suspicion must be maintained to diagnose wrist injuries in the trauma patient who may have mental status changes due to other injuries, or unable to communicate because of the placement of an endotracheal tube or the administration of sedatives. The knowledge of a mechanism of injury (such as a high energy fall onto the hand) as well as the presence of signs such as deformity, swelling, ecchymosis, lacerations and abrasions, or bony crepitation prompts radiologic investigation of the wrist.

The physical exam must also include a detailed neurovascular examination. A median nerve or ulnar nerve compression are commonly produced with displaced wrist injuries. These are most often seen with carpal dislocations and displaced distal radius fractures. Lacerations of the median nerve can be produced with high energy fractures of the distal radius which are dorsally displaced. The nerve is tented over the jagged end of the proximal fragment which acts like a guillotine and often produces an open fracture as well.

True compartment syndrome commonly seen in the forearm is not seen distally at the wrist. Little muscle tissue is present at this level to bleed from injuries. Although the metaphyseal bone of the distal radius can bleed significantly in comminuted fractures, the poorly developed fascial compartments here are not filled with muscle as in the forearm so the perpetuating mechanism of muscle ischemia and swelling does not occur. Bleeding can occur into the carpal canal, however. Bounded by the carpal bones dorsally, and the transverse carpal ligament volarly, it is rigid and absolutely unforgiving. An acute carpal tunnel syndrome requiring emergency release therefore can be produced due to resulting pressure on the median nerve. Close observation for the development of such a problem must be maintained.

A thorough exam of the musculotendinous units (described in Chapter 11) as well as all the nerves and vessels traversing the wrist must be performed whenever any injury penetrating from within or without is present anywhere in the distal forearm, wrist, or hand. Many trauma patients will not be able to cooperate with such a directed exam, so the burden of proof will rely on surgical exploration at the time of irrigation and debridement.

Routine biplanar x-rays will be sufficient for the initial investigation of wrist injuries. Bony fractures, dislocations, and ligamentous instabilities causing disruption of normal anatomy and requiring immediate intervention will be diagnosed. Treatment can also be planned based on these initial films.

The radial styloid projects distally an average of 12 mm giving the distal face of the radius approximately 23° of angulation on the AP film (Figure 10–1). This varies somewhat from individual to individual. Intercarpal distances, that is, the joint spaces between the carpals, are symmetric in the normal wrist. On the lateral film, the articular face of the radius is inclined volarwards at an angle of 11° to 15°[3,8,25] (Figure 10–2). A line drawn down the axis of the radius should roughly bisect the lunate and capitate without deviation. The scapholunate angle is formed by the axis of the scaphoid intersecting with this normal radial-lunate-capitate axis (Figure 10–3). The scapholunate angle averages 47°, but can vary from 30° to 60°.[17,30] When the radial-lunate-capitate axis is altered due to either an acute or chronic ligamentous instability, the scapholunate angle can be determined by a line

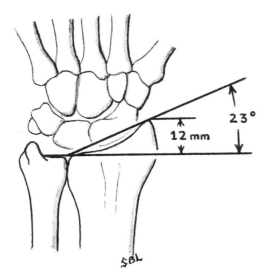

Figure 10–1. The radial styloid normally projects distally a distance of 12 mm so that the articular face forms an angle of 23°.

drawn perpendicular to the line connecting the two poles of the lunate (Figure 10–4). Comparison films of the opposite normal wrist are often helpful due to anatomic variability.

If there is suspicion for injury, but initial films appear normal, no harm will come to the patient if the wrist is temporarily splinted. Later, when the patient is stabilized and able to cooperate with an exam, if this suspicion remains, more sophisticated investigations such as deviation views, obliques, clenched fist films, tomography, arthrography, cine-röntgenograms, or magnetic resonance imaging can be undertaken. These studies will reveal the "more minor" chip fractures, soft-tissue injuries, or dynamic instabilities which although not requiring emergent treatment on presentation must be properly addressed to prevent long-term disability.

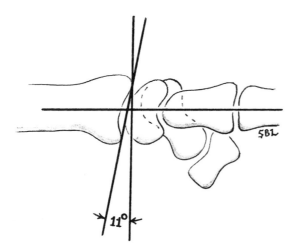

Figure 10–2. The articular surface of the distal radius faces volarwards at an angle of 11°.

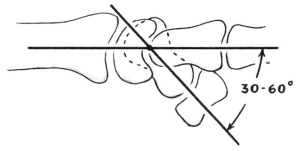

Figure 10–3. The scapholunate angle ranges between 30° and 60°. It is formed by the axis of the scaphoid and the radial-lunate-capitate axis. This angle is increased in early stages of perilunate instabilities.

Treatment

Although specifics of treatment will be discussed for each particular injury, there are some principles which are common throughout. Once the injury has been diagnosed and characterized, an initial reduction is performed on badly displaced fractures and dislocations to restore alignment and relieve any pressure on neurovascular structures. This can be

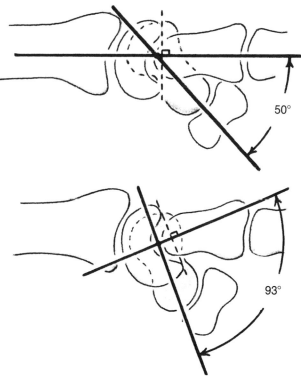

Figure 10–4. With alteration of the radial-lunate-scaphoid axis, the lunate axis is determined by a line (solid) drawn parallel to the line connecting the two poles of the lunate (dashed). Here, due to the "tipping" of the lunate, the scapholunate angle is markedly increased.

performed quickly in the operating room under anesthesia while the patient is being prepared for other emergency surgery, or in the emergency department with either intravenous sedation and analgesia or with a hematoma block. Temporary splints are applied to stabilize the extremity preventing further injury from shifting bone and to give pain relief. Some dislocations cannot be reduced by closed means and will require open reduction at the initial surgical setting. Although not necessary as a life-saving emergency procedure, joint restoration is necessary as soon as possible once the patient is stabilized—preferably within the first 24 hours.

Acute carpal tunnel syndrome or any neurovascular compromise requires immediate attention. An acute carpal tunnel syndrome is diagnosed by elevated carpal canal pressures which are measured by the techniques discussed in Chapter 20. If paresthesias do not improve following a reduction, immediate surgical decompression is warranted.[11] Open injuries are a high priority in the surgical sequence and are treated with the protocol described in Chapter 7. The principles of intravenous antibiotics, irrigation, aggressive debridement, and stabilization of bones and soft tissues must be adhered to.

Dislocations are reduced and stabilized with bony fixation to protect the ligamentous repairs. Fractures must be reduced and stabilized to restore normal joint alignment. Fixation techniques include the use of screws, plates, pins, and external fixators alone and in combination. Articular fractures demand anatomic reduction and rigid stabilization to prevent loss of reduction, early range of motion, and improved cartilaginous healing of the articular surface.

High energy fractures requiring surgical reduction and fixation are commonly seen about the wrist in the trauma patient. Although more minor injuries can be treated with the same closed methods used when these fractures occur as isolated entities, often even these can benefit from open treatment.

Allowing the patient the freedom of movement after internal fixation can be very helpful when bilateral upper extremity fractures are present. An otherwise totally dependent patient can then be independent or assist in his personal hygiene, eating, and activities of daily living. Multiple ipsilateral upper extremity injuries when treated with closed techniques will result in a greater degree of stiffness. Surgical treatment of a wrist fracture will speed and improve the rehabilitation of the forearm or elbow fracture.

DISTAL RADIUS FRACTURES

Eponyms abound in the wrist as nowhere else in the body. The differences between the Colles, Smith, volar Barton, dorsal Barton, and chauffeur fractures are difficult enough to remember. When one considers that a Colles' fracture is also known as the Pouteau, the Smith as the Goyrand or the reverse Colles', and the chauffeur's as the "backfire" or Hutchinson's; includes all of the subclassifications of the different fractures; and then realizes the overlap (ie, a Smith Type II is the same as a volar Barton's), it is easy to understand why the uninitiated often resort to calling every distal radius fracture by the generic term, "Colles'."

To avoid confusion, it is always best to describe the fracture with the terms every first-year orthopaedic resident is taught—fracture orientation, displacement, angulation, distraction/impaction, degree of comminution, intra- vs extra-articular—if there is any question on the proper eponym.

Colles'/Pouteau's Fracture

Claude Pouteau[24] first proposed in the late 1700s that many of the injuries to the wrist were fractures of the distal radius and not dislocations and subluxations of the wrist joints as it was commonly believed up until that time.[23] This theory was unpopular and not widely known outside France. The great Irish surgeon, Abraham Colles, independently described this same fracture in 1814.[5]

Resulting from a dorsiflexion injury (the mechanism for 90% of wrist injuries),[25] such as a fall on the outstretched hand, the fracture may or may not involve the articular surface. The distal fragment is displaced dorsally and the fracture is angulated with its apex in a volar direction (Figure 10–5). Shortening due to comminution (the result of high energy or osteoporosis) is common. Failure to reduce the fracture produces the classic "talon de fourchette" or silver fork deformity first described by Alfred Velpeau.[19] The Colles' fracture can be graded by Frykman's[10] classification based on the involvement of the articular surfaces of the radiocarpal and distal radioulnar joints (Table 10–1).

Smith's/Goyrand's/Reverse Colles' Fracture

Goyrand in 1832[14] and Robert Smith in 1847[27] described a variant of the Colles' fracture in which the distal fragment displaces volarly and angulates with the apex dorsal (Figure 10–6). The opposite of a Colles' fracture is produced, explaining the sometimes-used term, "reverse Colles' fracture."

Thomas[29] has classified the Smith fracture into three types (Table 10–2). Smith's

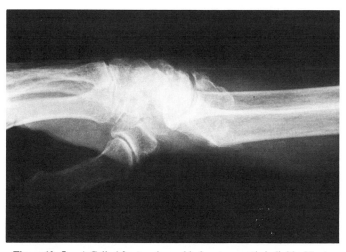

Figure 10–5. A Colles' fracture in an elderly osteoporotic individual (note the calcification of the ulnar artery). The fracture is shortened and angulated with the apex in the volar direction.

Table 10–1   Frykman Classification of Colles' Fractures[10]

	DISTAL ULNAR FRACTURE	
RADIUS FRACTURE	Absent	Present
Extra-articular	I	II
Intra-articular radiocarpal joint	III	IV
Intra-articular distal radioulnar joint	V	VI
Intra-articular radiocarpal + distal radioulnar joint	VII	VIII

Type I is a transverse fracture with volar and proximal displacement, Smith's Type II an articular fracture also known as a volar Barton's fracture (see below), and Smith's Type III is an oblique fracture of the distal radius which is tilted volarly but not displaced.

Barton's Fracture

John Rhea Barton described fracture-dislocations of the wrist in 1838.[1] He felt these were often confused with extra-articular fractures. Forces transmitted through the carpus shear off the lip of the radius supporting the carpus leading to the dislocation. Depending on the position of the hand at the time of injury, the dorsal lip is fractured leading to a dorsal

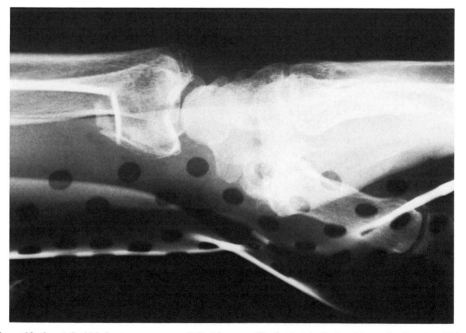

Figure 10–6.   A Smith's fracture, or reverse Colles' fracture. The fracture is displaced in a volar direction. There is comminution of the volar cortex which often causes these fractures to angulate with the apex dorsal. (Note the radiolucent splint to immobilize the extremity while x-rays are being obtained.)

Table 10–2   Thomas Classification of Smith's Fractures[29]

Type I	Transverse radial fracture
	Volar and proximal displacement
Type II*	Volar lip intra-articular fracture
	Volar displacement
	Volar dislocation of carpus
Type III	Oblique radial fracture
	Volar tilting

*volar Barton's fracture.

dislocation, or the volar lip leading to a volar dislocation (Figure 10–7). The volar Barton's is also known as a Type II Smith's fracture or Lentenneur's fracture.[25]

Chauffeur's/Backfire/Hutchinson's Fracture

First described as a common injury from hand-cranking automobile engines,[18] we have Charles Kettering's invention of the electric starter to thank for the relatively few cases of chauffeur's fracture seen today. An intra-articular fracture of the radial styloid, a triangular fragment is produced by an avulsive force through the radiocarpal ligaments. This

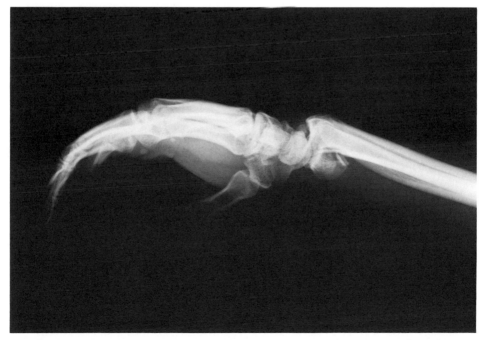

Figure 10–7.   A volar Barton's (or Smith's Type II) fracture. The volar lip of the radius is fractured. The carpus then subluxes volarwards due to the loss of its volar buttress.

commonly resulted from the forceful jerk produced when the engine "backfired" while being cranked, hence its other name. Although no single person's name is commonly associated with this fracture, it has been described as Hutchinson's fracture,[25] but is not widely known as such.

Treatment

Nondisplaced articular or nonarticular stable fractures of the distal radius need only be protected through immobilization with a short arm cast for 4 to 6 weeks followed by a period of rehabilitation to restore motion.

Displacement or angulation of fractures of the distal radius is the rule. Although restoration of the tilt of the articular face of the distal radius to its volar direction is desirable, restoration to neutral is acceptable.[25] The length of the radial styloid is also best restored to prevent distal ulna impingement on the carpus or radial drift of the hand due to loss of the buttressing effect of the styloid on the carpus. Comparison views of the uninjured wrist can be helpful as the length of the distal radius in comparison to the distal ulna varies from patient to patient.

Nonarticular fractures can be treated through closed reduction using traction and manipulation to restore the normal length and attitude of the distal radius. Splints or casting are used to maintain the reduction. Ten degrees to 15° of ulnar deviation will help maintain radial styloid length and approximately 10° of wrist flexion to control the angulation. Volar flexion is used for Colles' fractures, dorsal flexion for Smith's. Three-point molding of the plaster completes the immobilization. All but the most stable fractures require 3 to 4 weeks of immobilization in a long-arm cast to control pronation and supination, followed by a period of short-arm casting. Immobilization is maintained for a total of 6 weeks. A removable splint for protection can be used following cast removal until motion and strength are restored.

Comminuted fractures may settle or reangulate following an initially acceptable reduction due to the lack of good bone-to-bone contact. Such fractures can be remanipulated in their "sticky" stage at which point the early fracture callus will afford some stability. If comminution is present to an extent that a reduction and casting will predictably fail, other stabilization techniques discussed below should be used.

If an elbow or forearm injury is present necessitating early mobilization of the elbow, the patient will benefit from percutaneous surgical stabilization of the distal radius fracture to permit elbow movement. This also gives the added benefit of protected early movement at the wrist at 7 to 10 days.

Articular fractures demand anatomic reduction, and in many instances need some form of fixation to maintain the reduction. Simple displaced articular fractures without comminution and consisting of a single fragment can often be manipulated in a closed fashion then percutaneously stabilized with crossed percutaneous K-wires inserted across the fracture for 6 to 8 weeks.[4] Alternatively, a Rush pin can be contoured and inserted through the radial styloid as an intramedullary splint (Figure 10–8). This gives good results and has the advantage of not needing to be removed, but cannot control two or more separate articular fragments. An additional K-wire or two is necessary in these cases. With either technique, the superficial branches of the radial nerve must be avoided to prevent paresthesias or a painful neuroma.

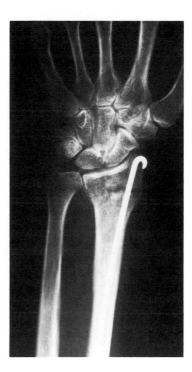

Figure 10–8. This Colles' fracture has been stabilized through the insertion of a percutaneous Rush rod through the radial styloid. The Rush rod provides enough stability to begin early range of motion within the first few post-operative days.

Fractures consisting of more than two fragments often cannot be manipulated with closed techniques into an acceptable reduction. This is almost always true if there is more than one articular piece. In these instances, an open reduction is often required. If a limited open reduction can be performed, several percutaneous K-wires may be sufficient to hold the reduction if good bone stock is present. The "joy-stick" technique can be used to avoid an open reduction in some cases. This method employs the insertion of K-wires percutaneously into the fragments. The wires are then used to manipulate the fragments into position then are driven across the fracture to stabilize it (Figure 10–9). Image intensification is mandatory.

Internal fixation with plate and screws is another option. These have the advantage of more rigid fixation if good bone stock is present allowing an early and wider range of motion program. Fracture patterns associated with carpal instability such as Barton's fractures require rigid fracture fixation to restore carpal stability. Place the plate on the volar surface of the radius under the pronator quadratus for a volar Barton's fracture and on the dorsal surface for the dorsal variant. Attempt to place some soft tissue such as extensor retinaculum between the dorsal plate and the extensor tendons to prevent late tendon erosion.

Some fractures are too comminuted to permit either K-wire or plate and screw fixation. Others may have severe soft tissue injuries or swelling precluding open treatments. In these instances, an external fixator can restore alignment to the distal radius and prevent collapse through ligamentotaxis. Soft tissues—capsule and ligaments—remain attached to the fracture fragments. By distracting through these tissues with a fixator anchored into the shaft of the radius proximally and into the second and third metacarpals distally, an

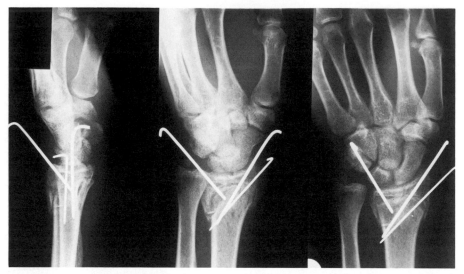

Figure 10–9.   A comminuted displaced intra-articular fracture of the distal radius in a 20 year old. The fracture was reduced in a closed fashion with manipulation and percutaneous K-wire "joy-sticks." Due to good bone stock, the K-wire fixation was adequate to allow early range of motion exercises at one week post-fixation.

acceptable reduction can be achieved (Figure 10–10). If not, manipulation of the fragments through a limited opening or with a K-wire joy-stick can be performed when necessary.

To apply the fixator, two 4 mm half pins are inserted into the diaphysis of the distal radius. These are placed through an incision[3] with direct exposure of the bone to prevent injuring the superficial branches of the radial sensory nerve which are at risk during percutaneous insertion. The distal pins are placed percutaneously into the index meta-carpal from its radial aspect. The proximal of these two is placed into the base of the index metacarpal and enters into the third metacarpal as well without violating the interosseous space and tethering the intrinsics. This pin then has purchase into four cortices. The last pin is placed more distally into only the index metacarpal.[26] The fixator remains in place for 6 to 8 weeks following which rehabilitative exercises are begun to restore motion.

DISTAL ULNA INJURIES

Injuries to the distal ulna fall into three main categories: 1) ulna styloid fractures, 2) distal radioulnar joint (DRUJ) disruptions, and 3) disruptions of the triangular fibrocartilaginous complex (TFCC).

Styloid Fracture

Ulnar styloid fractures commonly occur along with the distal radial fractures, but can also occur as an isolated injury. Nondisplaced fractures usually heal well with immobilization for

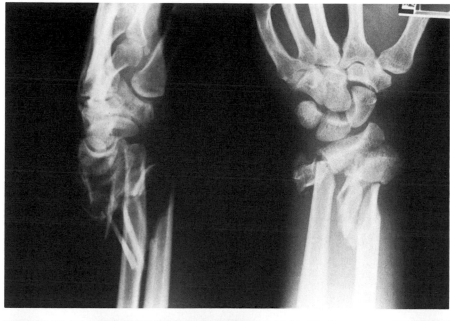

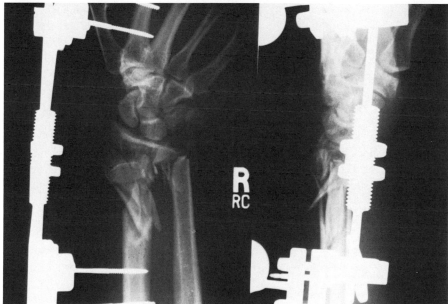

Figure 10–10. **A:** A severely comminuted distal radial fracture. This young motorcycle rider was injured in an accident. The impact caused axial loading of the radius from the hand gripping the handle bars. **B:** Distraction with an external fixator has restored adequate position to the distal articular face of the radius. Severe soft tissue swelling precluded an open reduction on this patient. By avoiding soft tissue stripping of the fragments, they remained vascularized and readily healed.

4 to 6 weeks. Displaced fractures can be associated with a more significant soft tissue injury to the TFCC or ligaments of the carpus. These soft tissue injuries often will heal with casting of the fracture. The displaced styloid fracture can heal with a fibrous union on x-ray. Most of these remain asymptomatic. If symptoms persist following casting, reconstruction of the area can be undertaken.

DRUJ

The DRUJ can be disrupted from a Galleazi fracture of the radial shaft (discussed with forearm injuries in Chapter 9) or following a distal ulnar fracture. Fractures of the distal radius or the proximal Essex-Lopresti fracture of the radial head can injure the joint as well. Dislocations of the joint are easily missed if true lateral radiographs are not obtained. Also, some individuals have a dorsally prominent distal ulna that can appear subluxed. Again, comparison films of the opposite wrist will help in this determination.

A dislocated DRUJ is treated by reduction and stabilization of any associated fracture. Once the joint is restored, immobilize it in a position of stability to prevent late subluxation. Although it is technically incorrect to speak of a "dorsal" or "volar" dislocation of the distal ulna since the ulna remains stationary while the radius rotates about it, convention describes DRUJ disruptions in this manner. Dorsal dislocation of the ulna occurs in pronation and volar in supination. The position of stability is the opposite of these mechanisms. Thus, immobilize the dorsal dislocation in supination and the volar in pronation. Immobilization for six weeks will allow soft tissue healing and the return of stability. A long arm cast to control the elbow is necessary to maintain pronation or supination.

TFCC

The distal ulna does not articulate directly with the carpus, but through the intervening triangular fibrocartilaginous tissue, the TFCC. Often described as a "meniscal homologue" due to its similarity to a knee meniscus, tears of the TFCC can lead to ulnar sided pain, clicking, or weakness of the wrist. These injuries can be difficult to accurately diagnose without wrist arthrography, or more recently, wrist arthroscopy. Although significant injuries, treatment of TFCC tears in the trauma patient is best done on a delayed basis unless the surgeon is performing an approach to this region for other reasons such as open injuries, unstable fractures and dislocations, or neurovascular compromise.

Carpal Fractures

Although isolated fractures can occur in any of the carpals, they are infrequently seen in the trauma patient with the exception of scaphoid fractures. Isolated fracture patterns occur from lower energy forces such as a fall onto the outstretched hand or when the hook of the hamate fractures in the golfer who misses a swing. When carpal fractures occur in the polytrauma victim who receives high energy forces, it is important not to miss a perilunate instability. This is especially true with seemingly minor dorsal chip fractures of the triquetrum,[3] or when fractures of carpals other than the scaphoid are present.

Scaphoid Fractures

Of the bones about the wrist, only the distal radius is fractured more frequently than the scaphoid.[15] The two pitfalls associated with scaphoid fractures are missed diagnosis and inadequate immobilization. Nondisplaced fracture lines frequently are not visible on the initial radiographs.[3,25] In cases of "clinical fractures" characterized by tenderness in the snuffbox dorsally or at the distal pole of the scaphoid volarly, treat the patient presumptively with a cast. If a fracture is present, it will be readily visible on x-ray following resorption of the fractured ends which occurs as part of the healing process within three weeks.[3] Tomograms or bone scans will diagnose the fracture earlier if prompt diagnosis is necessary.

The second pitfall is inadequate immobilization of a diagnosed fracture. The majority of the blood supply enters the scaphoid through its distal pole in a retrograde fashion.[28] Fractures through the relatively avascular proximal pole can take 20 weeks or longer to heal[25] and frequently go on to a nonunion. Distal fractures through the well-vascularized region almost always heal quickly within 4 to 6 weeks.

Treatment

Unstable fractures require fixation; stable fractures can be treated by casting. Six radiographic views commonly are obtained to determine instability. These are the routine AP and lateral films, AP films in full radial and ulnar deviation, and lateral films in full flexion and extension. Signs of instability are displacement of a fracture fragment, motion at the fracture on the six-view x-ray series, presence of a ligamentous carpal instability pattern (discussed below), and shortening or angulation at the fracture.[25]

Stable nondisplaced fractures are placed in a thumb-spica cast with the wrist in slight palmar flexion, the thumb abducted away from the palm, and the forearm in neutral pronation/supination. Fractures of the middle or proximal thirds should be placed in a long-arm cast for the first six weeks due to the relative avascularity at the fracture site. A short-arm spica cast is then used until the fracture is united. Distal third fractures can be treated with a short spica from the outset.[12]

Unstable fractures or those with more than 1 mm of displacement will benefit from reduction and fixation. Fixation with K-wires had been the rule until recently. Screw fixation of the scaphoid is difficult due to the problem of screw heads protruding from the articular surface. Traditional screws must be countersunk so that the head is buried beneath the surface of the articular cartilage. Newer headless screws designed for the scaphoid have been popularized and are rapidly becoming the standard.

CARPAL INSTABILITY PATTERNS

The bones of the carpus are joined together by ligaments, the most important of which are intracapsular. The volar ligaments are more significant than those of the dorsal wrist. An area of weakness exists volarly overlying the capitolunate joint known as the space of Poirer[8,16,20,25] (Figure 10–11). This ligamentous anatomy leads to the pattern of ligamentous failure seen with intercarpal dislocations.

Carpal ligamentous injuries are usually a result of hyperextension, ulnar deviation, and intercarpal supination.[21] A progression of ligamentous failure then occurs, leading to a

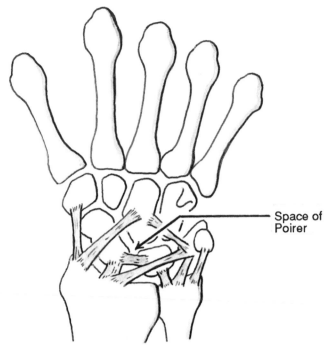

Space of
Poirer

Figure 10–11.   The volar ligaments of the wrist. A weak area, the space of Poirer exists over the scaphocapitate joint.

spectrum of dorsally unstable injuries[22] centered about the lunate. It is convenient to think of these occurring in a circular fashion about the lunate with a progressive "peeling away" of bones starting at the scaphoid (9:00), leading to the capitate (12:00), then the triquetrum (3:00), and finally, completion of the cycle at the lunate (6:00) (Figure 10–12).

The first stage of instability is scapholunate dissociation. The interosseous scapholunate ligament is torn, resulting in rotatory instability of the scaphoid and widening of the scapholunate joint (Figure 10–13). Further loading will lead to Stage II injury of either failure of the radiocapitate ligament (Figure 10–14) or an avulsion fracture of this ligament off the radial styloid. A midcarpal dislocation between the capitate and lunate results. Stage III occurs when there is ligamentous disruption of the triquetrolunate joint on the ulnar side of the wrist (Figure 10–15), and Stage IV is total perilunar instability with complete disruption of all ligaments from the forearm to the scaphoid, capitate, and triquetrum (Figure 10–16).

Traumatic perilunate dislocations usually occur dorsally. The lunate remains located in respect to the radius, all remaining carpals are out of their normal positions (Figure 10–17A,B). Alternatively, all the ligaments connecting to the lunate may be torn producing a lunate dislocation—usually volar. The remaining carpals stay in their normal relationship to the distal radius.

Perilunate fracture-dislocations can occur as well—depending on whether failure occurs through bone or ligament (Figure 10–18A,B). Transscaphoid perilunate dislocations are often seen as the scaphoid spans both the proximal and distal carpal rows. Fracture occurs at the wrist due to the concentration of motion forces here.

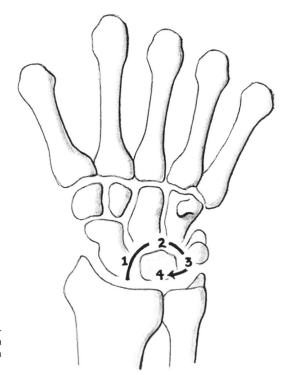

Figure 10–12. The sequential failure of ligaments about the lunate in a circular direction from the scaphoid to the triquetrum with progressive stages of perilunate instability.

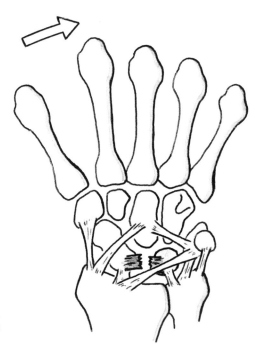

Figure 10–13. Stage I perilunate instability. The interosseous scapholunate ligament has torn, causing a scapholunate gap.

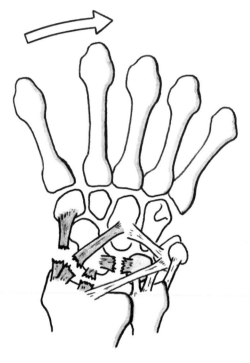

Figure 10–14. Stage II perilunate instability. Further ligamentous injury has caused subluxation between the lunate and capitate resulting in a midcarpal dislocation.

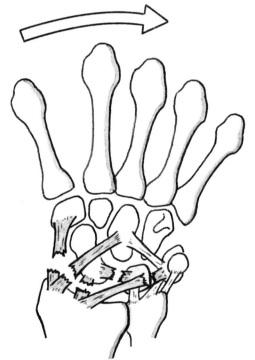

Figure 10–15. Stage III perilunate instability with the addition of dislocation at the triquetrolunate joint.

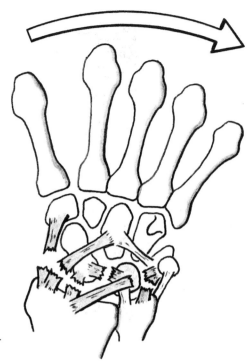

Figure 10–16. Stage IV perilunate instability—complete perilunate dislocation.

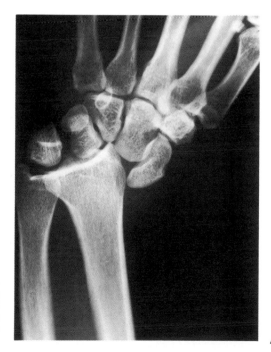

Figure 10–17. A: A perilunate dislocation. The remaining carpals have peeled away from the lunate and distal ulna and radius. The carpus and hand have displaced radialwards and locked on the radial styloid. (Figure continued on next page.)

A

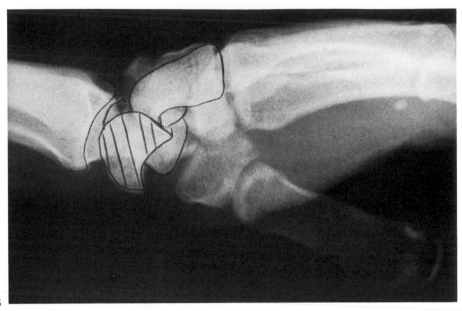

B

Figure 10–17, cont.   B: On the lateral view, the lunate (shaded) is seen in its normal position. The scaphoid is dislocated dorsally. The capitate is absent from the concavity of the lunate.

Assessment

The high-grade variants are easily recognized by the gross deformity of the wrist and the "jumble" of bones on the x-ray. Obvious deformity accompanied by significant swelling due to the associated soft tissue injury occurs and neurovascular compromise is common. Median nerve symptoms, especially, can be seen due to stretching or pressure on the nerve from the displaced bones. The lesser grades of injury can present as a wrist "sprain" and may not be appreciated for the ligamentous disruptions they represent unless a high index of suspicion and vigilance for subtle radiographic abnormalities are maintained.

Widening of the normally symmetric intercarpal joint spaces is a sign of instability. Early stages of instability occurring first at the scapholunate joint are diagnosed by the "Terry Thomas sign"[9] (named after the gap-toothed British actor) of widening greater than 2 mm at the scapholunate joint on the AP view (Figure 10–19). The scaphoid then tilts volarly giving it a foreshortened appearance on the AP. On the lateral view, the scapholunate angle is increased with the scaphoid lying nearly perpendicular to the long axis of the radius.

Treatment

Gross dislocations are reduced as promptly as possible to relieve pressure on neurovascular structures. A period of 10 to 15 minutes of Chinese fingertrap traction with a counterweight of 10 to 15 pounds is often necessary. Regional block or general anesthesia are often

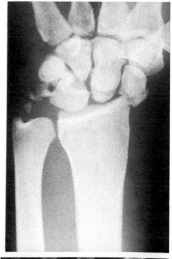

A

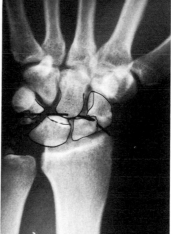

B

Figure 10–18. **A:** A trans-scaphoid trans-triquetral perilunate fracture dislocation. This pre-reduction film is hard to interpret due to the "jumble of bones." **B:** Following a closed reduction to relieve neurovascular compromise, the injury pattern is evident. The heavy dashed line shows the disruption in a circular fashion about the lunate. The line of failure began through the waist of the scaphoid, traversed the scaphocapitate joint, then exited through the triquetrum. There is also a fracture of the ulnar styloid. **C:** Open reduction has been performed to allow anatomic reduction and pinning of the scaphoid fracture. An additional pin across the lunato-capitate joint completes the stabilization. The triquetrum is anatomically reduced and does not need to be pinned.

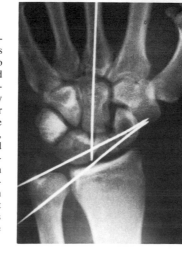

C

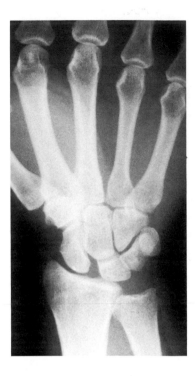

Figure 10–19. Stage I perilunate instability—scapholunate dissociation. Note the
"Terry Thomas Sign" or gapping between
the scaphoid and lunate.

required for these reductions. "Minor" adjustments can then be done later after more vital
injuries have been addressed.

   Early stages of injury consisting of minor subluxations and rotations can sometimes be
treated in a closed fashion if anatomic reduction can be achieved through positioning of the
hand. The wrist is then immobilized in slight palmar flexion.[8] The problem with this
treatment has been the "paradox of reduction" of scapholunate rotatory subluxation.[21]
Palmar flexion is necessary to approximate the torn ends of the critical volar ligaments to
prevent chronic instability from their healing in a lengthened position. Palmar flexion,
however, causes increased displacement of the scaphoid. If extension is used to reduce the
scaphoid, the ends of the torn ligament are not approximated.

   When the carpals can be reduced but not held reduced, percutaneous pinning for six
weeks in the reduced position is necessary. Early stages of subluxation that cannot be
satisfactorily manipulated in a closed fashion, the higher grades of instability (the dislocations), and instabilities associated with fracture patterns are best treated by open means.

   Two approaches through both volar and dorsal incisions offer the best opportunity to
debride flakes of articular cartilage, remove interposed soft tissues from the joint spaces,
achieve an anatomic reduction of all fractures and dislocations, and repair torn ligamentous
structures. The disrupted areas of fracture and dislocation are pinned and splinted 4 to 6
weeks until ligamentous healing has occurred (Figure 10–18c).

CARPOMETACARPAL JOINT DISLOCATIONS

Carpometacarpal (CMC) joint dislocations occur secondary to an axial force directed along the metacarpals such as that which occurs when striking an object with the fist. The bases of the metacarpals generally displace in a dorsal direction. They are usually stable once reduced and casted due to the tight fitting arrangement of these joints; however, late dislocations have been known to occur.

Small chip fractures off the bases of the metacarpals or the distal carpal row are often seen as a result of CMC ligamentous avulsions. Avulsions off the triquetrum are a tip-off to look for perilunate instability.

CMC dislocations are generally easily reduced by longitudinal traction applied to the metacarpal through its corresponding finger and with pressure applied by the thumb to the base of the metacarpal. Cases of multiple CMC dislocations are more unstable due to significant soft tissue disruptions and are stabilized with percutaneous pins into an adjacent stable metacarpal or the distal carpal row. A short arm cast for six weeks is sufficient to allow ligamentous healing.

REFERENCES

1. Barton JR. Views and treatment of an important injury of the wrist. *Med Examiner*. 1838;1:365.
2. Bell C. *The Hand: Its Mechanism and Vital Endowments as Evincing Design*. London, Engl: W Pickering; 1833.
3. Chapman MW (ed.). *Operative Orthopaedics*. Philadelphia, Pa: JB Lippincott; 1988.
4. Clancy GJ. Percutaneous Kirschner wire fixation of Colles' fractures. *J Bone Joint Surg*. 1984;66–A:1008.
5. Colles A. On the fracture of the carpal extremity of the radius. *Edinburgh Med Surg J*. 1814;10:182.
6. Dameron T. Traumatic dislocation of the distal radioulna joint. *Clin Orthop*. 1972;83:55.
7. Ellis J. Smith's and Barton's fractures: a method of treatment. *J Bone Joint Surg*. 1965;47–B:724–727.
8. Evarts CM (ed.). *Surgery of the musculoskeletal system*. New York, NY: Churchill Livingstone; 1983.
9. Frankel VH. The Terry Thomas sign. *Clin Orthop*. 1977;149.321–322.
10. Frykman G. Fracture of the distal radius including sequelae—shoulder-hand-finger syndrome, disturbance in the distal radio-ulnar joint, and impairment of nerve function: a clinical and experimental study. *Acta Orthop Scand*. 1967;108(suppl):1–155.
11. Gelberman RH, et al. Carpal tunnel pressures and wrist position in patients with Colles' fractures. *J Trauma*. 1984;24:747.
12. Gellman H, et al. Comparison of short and long thumb-spica casts for non-displaced fractures of the carpal scaphoid. *J Bone Joint Surg*. 1989;71–A:354–357.
13. Goddard PB. *The Dissector or Practical and Surgical Anatomy*. Philadelphia, Pa: Lea & Blanchard; 1844.
14. Goyrand G. Memoirs sur les fractures de l'extrémité inferieure de radius, qui simulent les luxations du poignet. *Gazette de Medicine*. 1832;3:664.
15. Green D (ed.). *Operative Hand Surgery*. New York, NY: Churchill Livingstone; 1982.
16. Lewis OJ, et al. The anatomy of the wrist joint. *J Anat*. 1970;106:539–552.
17. Linscheid RL, et al. Traumatic instability of the wrist; diagnosis, classification and pathomechanics. *J Bone Joint Surg*. 1972;54–A:1612–1632.
18. Lund FB. Fractures of the radius in starting automobiles. *Boston Med Surg J*. 1904;151:481.
19. Malgaigne JF. *A Treatise on Fractures*. Packard JH (trans.). Philadelphia, Pa: JB Lippincott; 1859.
20. Mayfield JK, et al. The ligaments of the human wrist and their functional significance. *Anat Rec*. 1976;186:417–428.
21. Mayfield JK. Mechanism of carpal injuries. *Clin Orthop*. 1980;149:45–54.
22. Mayfield JK. Patterns of injury to carpal ligaments. *Clin Orthop*. 1984;187:36–42.
23. Peltier LF. Fractures of the distal end of the radius—an historical account. *Clin Orthop*. 1987;187:18–22.
24. Pouteau C. *Oeuvres posthumes de M. Pouteau: memoire, contenant quelques relfexions sur quelques fractures de l'avant-bras, sur les luxations incomplettes du poignet et sur le diastasis*. Paris, France: Ph-D Pierres; 1783.
25. Rockwood CA Jr, Green DP, ed. *Fractures in Adults*. 2nd ed. Philadelphia, Pa: JP Lippincott; 1984.

26. Seitz WH, et al. Biomechanical analysis of pin placement and pin size for external fixation of distal radius fractures. *Clin Orthop*. 1990;251:207–212.
27. Smith RW. *A Treatise on Fractures in the Vicinity of Joints and on Certain Forms of Accidental and Congenital Dislocations*. Dublin, Ireland: Hodges & Smith; 1847.
28. Taleisnik J, Kelly PJ. The extraosseus and intraosseus blood supply of the scaphoid bone. *J Bone Joint Surg*. 1966;48–A:1125–1137.
29. Thomas FB. Reduction of Smith's fracture. *J Bone Joint Surg*. 1957;39–B:463–470.
30. Vance RM, et al. Scaphocapitate fractures. Patterns of dislocation, mechanisms of injury, and preliminary results of treatment. *J Bone Joint Surg*. 1980;62–A:271–276.

11

Hand Injury

EUGENE KILGORE, M.D.

HISTORY[1,2]: As early as the 10th century, Avicenna (980–1037) of Boukhara, in Persia, advocated surgical suturing of tendons, but this practice did not reach the west until much later. This delay in the development of hand surgery was due primarily to Galen (130–201), who had mistaken tendons for nerves. He stated that interfering with these structures could only result in pain and convulsions. Galen's influence plus medical conformism resulted in this erroneous teaching being passed on until the 18th century when Galen's dogma was officially refuted in the Sorbonne.

Duchenne de Boulogne in France (1867) was the first to describe the action of each muscle in the hand but his work was initially ignored.

At the turn of this century, extensive experimental and clinical studies were done by the Germans—Lange, Kirschner, Rehn and Biesalski—with the result that principles of hand surgery, particularly repair of tendon injuries, were established.

The first major advance in modern surgery of the hand was the publication of Allen B. Kanavel's book, Infections of the Hand, *in 1912.[3] It was the culmination of almost ten years of systematic studies of the applied anatomy of the fascial spaces of the hand. These studies, as they were applied to clinical practice, revolutionized the treatment of hand infections.*

INTRODUCTION

One third of all injuries involve the upper extremity—numbering 16 million a year in the United States. This results in 50,000 inpatient hospitalizations, 6 million emergency department visits, and 12 million visits to physicians' offices each year. Sixteen million days are lost from work yearly. The total cost of these upper extremity disorders in the United States in 1980 was estimated by Kelsey to be over 10 million dollars.[4] The majority occur during wage-earning years.

ANATOMY[5]

All references to the forearm and hand should be made to the radial and ulnar sides (not lateral and medial) and to the volar (or palmar) and dorsal surfaces. The digits should be identified as the thumb, index finger, long finger, ring finger, and small finger, or referred to as rays I, II, III, IV, and V.

Skin is the elastic outer sleeve and glove of the arm and hand. Sacrifice of its surface area or elasticity by debridement and fibrosis can severely curtail range of motion and constrict circulation. In the adult hand, the dorsal skin stretches about 4 cm in the longitudinal and in the transverse planes when the fist closes, and the palmar skin stretches a similar amount when the palm is flattened and spread. The long finger can easily have 48 cm^2 of skin cover, and the whole hand (exclusive of digits) 210 cm^2.

Fascia anchors palmar skin to bone to make pinch and grip stable; the midlateral fibers of "Cleland's and Grayson's ligaments" (Figure 11–1) keep the skin sleeve from twisting about the digit. In the form of sheaths and pulleys, fascia holds tendons in the concavity of arched joints to convey mechanical efficiency and power. The fascial sleeve of the forearm, hand, and digits must sometimes be slit along with skin to prevent or relieve congestion (eg, compartment syndrome). Any fascial compartment of the hand provides a space for infection or an avenue for its dissemination.

Each finger ray has four joints (MC, MP, PIP, and DIP) of which the MP and PIP are the most important for function. The thumb has only three joints (MC, MP, and IP), and every effort must be made to preserve at least two. The position of the wrist stretches and governs the efficiency of extrinsic muscle contraction. The wrist is the "key joint" of the hand, governing motion of the digits, and must be included in the immobilization process required for any major digital problem. The stability of the digital joints and their planes of motion are governed by the length of the ligaments and the anatomy of their articulating surfaces. The longitudinal and transverse arches of the hand are architectural prerequisites to gripping, pinching, and cupping and are maintained by the active contraction and passive tone of intact intrinsic muscles. The arches create the position of function. When the arches are collapsed, the hand assumes the position of injury or the clawed hand. Loss of these arches is most often initiated by edema. They may be preserved by splinting in the position of function, elevation without constriction, and early restoration of active and vigorous joint motion.

Each MP and IP joint has a distally anchored volar trap-door called the volar plate (Figure 11–2). With joint flexion it serves to increase the moment arm and therefore the power of extrinsic flexor tendons. In addition, each joint has collateral ligaments stabilizing the joint in either side (Figure 11–2, top).

The extrinsic flexor tendons are contained in fibrous sheaths to prevent bow-stringing and preserve mechanical efficiency as the digits furl into the palm. Pulleys (hypertrophied sections of the sheath) resist the points of greatest tendency to bowstring. Sheaths are inelastic and relatively avascular. Therefore, they crowd and congest any swollen, inflamed, or injured tendons and curtail glide by friction, constriction, and the generation of inelastic adhesions. "No-man's-land" is the zone from the middle of the palm to just beyond the PIP joint, wherein the superficialis and profundus lie ensheathed together and recovery of glide is so difficult after wounding (Figure 11–3). Across the wrist, the dense volar carpal ligament closes the bony carpal canal (carpal tunnel) through which pass all eight finger flexors as well as the flexor pollicis longus and median nerve. The ulnar bursa is the continuation of the synovium around the long flexors of the small finger through the carpal tunnel, encompassing the other finger flexors which interrupted their separate bursae at the midpalmar level. The radial bursa is the synovium around the flexor pollicis longus continued through the carpal tunnel. These two bursae may intercommunicate. Parona's space is that tissue plane over the pronator quadratus in the distal forearm deep to the radial and ulnar bursae.

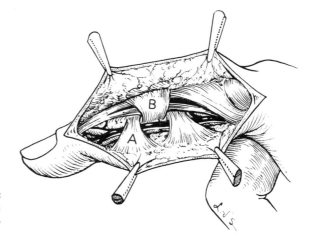

Figure 11–1. **A:** Cleland's ligaments. **B:** Transverse retinacular ligament. (From Way. *Current Surgical Diagnoses and Treatment*, 8th ed. Reprinted with permission.)

The extensor tendons are ensheathed in six compartments at the wrist beneath the extensor retinaculum (Figure 11–4), which predisposes to adhesions. Its role as a pulley is not vital and can be dispensed with.

The nerves of greatest importance to hand function are the musculocutaneous, radial, ulnar, and median. The importance of the musculocutaneous and radial nerves combined is forearm supination and of the radial nerve alone is innervation of the extensor muscles. The

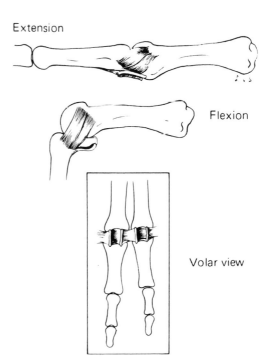

Figure 11–2. Volar plate, M-P joint and collateral ligaments. (From Way. *Current Surgical Diagnoses and Treatment*. 8th ed. Reprinted with permission.)

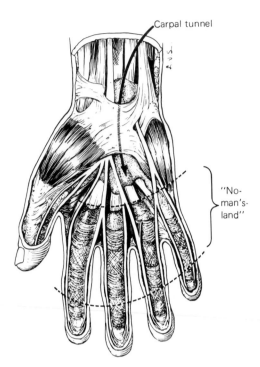

Carpal tunnel

"No-man's-land"

Figure 11–3. Carpal tunnel of the wrist. (From Way. *Current Surgical Diagnoses and Treatment*, 8th ed. Reprinted with permission.)

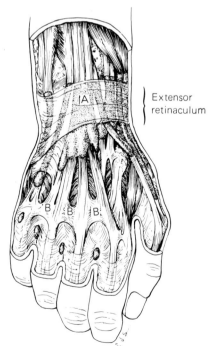

Extensor retinaculum

Figure 11–4. Extensor retinaculum of the hand. (From Way. *Current Surgical Diagnoses and Treatment*, 8th ed. Reprinted with permission.)

ulnar nerve innervates 15 of the 20 intrinsic muscles. The median nerve, by its sensory innervation, is "the eye of the hand"; through its motor innervation, it maintains most of the long flexors, the pronators of the forearm, and the thenar muscles. Figure 11–5 shows the sensory distribution of the ulnar, radial, and median nerves.

PHYSIOLOGY[6]

The prime functions of the hand are feeling (sensibility) and grasping. Sensibility is most important on the radial sides of the index, long, and ring fingers, and on the opposing ulnar side of the thumb, where one must feel to effectively pinch, pick up, and hold things. The ulnar side of the small finger and its metacarpal, upon which the hand usually rests, must register the sensations of contact and pain to avoid burns and other trauma.

Mobility is critical for grasping. The upper extremity is a cantilevered system extending from the shoulder to the fingertips. It must be adaptable to varying rates and kinds of movements. Stability of joints proximally is essential for good skeletal control distally.

The specialization of the thumb ray has endowed humans with superior aptitudes for defense, work, and dexterity. The thumb has exquisite sensibility and is a highly mobile structure of appropriate length, with a well-developed adductor (prime flexor) and thenar (pronating) musculature. It is the most important digit of the hand, and every effort must be made to preserve its function.

The position of function of the upper extremity favors reaching the mouth and perineum as well as comfortable, forceful, and unfatiguing grip and pinch. The elbow is held at or near a right angle, the forearm neutral between pronation and supination, and the wrist extended 30° with the fingers furled to almost meet the opposed (pronated) tip of the thumb. This is the desired stance of the extremity if stiffness is likely to occur, and it should be adopted when joints are immobilized by splinting, arthrodesis, or tenodesis.

Opposite to the position of function is the position of rest, in which the flexed wrist extends the digits, making grip and pinch awkward, uncomfortable, weak, and fatiguing. The forearm is usually pronated and the elbow may be extended. This habitus is assumed, without intention, after injury, paralysis, and the onset of painful states; it is also called the *position of the injury*. Stiffening in this attitude jeopardizes function.

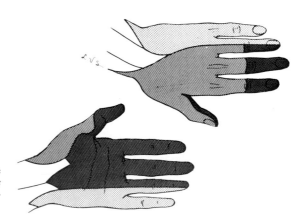

Figure 11–5. Sensory innervation of the hand. *Light shading*: Ulnar nerve. *Cross hatching*: Radial nerve. *Dark shading*: Median nerve.

EVALUATION[7]

The *history* for diagnostic reasons, and for proper treatment planning, is essential. It is important to learn the time of onset of the patient's problem and the details of his chief complaints (subjective and objective factors).

With wounds, the interval from wounding to treatment dictates the need for antibiotics for the risk of infection. It also indicates the extent of the healing process that has already taken place. After three to four weeks it may be impossible to reduce a fracture and after two to four months to retrieve a divided flexor tendon. At this stage it is necessary to go into the details of the history of the development of the disorder and the mechanism of the injury. In evaluating the risk of infection it is important to know where, how, and when a wound occurred. If it occurred in soapy dishwater the risk is small compared to its having occurred in a barnyard.

In considering a fracture there must be some history of violence. Hence we should know the forces involved and their direction.[8] The history must reflect the physical findings. An abrasion with a crust and dry gangrene of a fingertip are not acute injuries. The location and amount of injury created by broken glass puncture wounds are far less predictable than are those created by local incision with a knife. The innocuous wound of entrance of a high-pressure injection injury of the hand may belie the severity of the problem initiated. The importance of historical detail is obvious when comparing the location of the stumps of the flexor tendon injured in a fall on the outstretched palm to their location when the injury is sustained in grabbing a knife.

In an acute injury showing progressive neurological impairment, some form of decompression may be urgent. In contrast to this, the stiffness of the digit that has had every modality of treatment without any change in a period of 2 to 3 months is permanent.

A diagram is indispensable to good recording of certain hand problems, and is often far more succinct and definitive than the written word. It shows the topography of subjective and objective problems.

The *examination* of the patient should begin by focusing attention on the total patient, the neck, both upper extremities, and finally the involved part of the hand. This pertains to acute and chronic cases and should be modified only in the presence of hemorrhage, marked pain, circumstances of severe mangling, and the like. The surgeon should allow ample time within the bounds of good treatment to become aware of coexisting psychological and physical problems and their magnitude. Good light and a well-ventilated room with proper help and equipment are needed for an adequate efficient examination.

With acute problems, the need of facilities for comfort is often more pressing than in the case of chronic disorders. Having the patient supine will generally accomplish this, and will obviate syncope and its hazards. Clothing and jewelry should be completely removed from the upper extremity.

The *priorities* for evaluating the acutely injured hand are: (1) the control of hemorrhage, (2) the extent of viability (vascular integrity), (3) the appreciation of motor and sensory nerve function, (4) the maintenance of skeletal alignment and joint function, (5) the control of pain by suitable systemic, regional, or local analgesia, and (6) the evaluation of the wound and the injuries within it.

The initial control of bleeding should be attempted by direct pressure by sterile pads pressing against the bleeding point. More definitive control can then follow with a sphygmomanometer as an arterial tourniquet. This should be padded with cast padding and secured with more cast padding or adhesive tape. The tubing should be directed toward the shoulder, the extremity elevated, and the tourniquet inflated rapidly to 250 to 300 mm Hg. The tubing should then be clamped at the cuff by a large hemostat and the inflation valve released. Tolerance of the tourniquet under these circumstances is excellent in the average patient for at least 20 to 30 minutes. The use of the tourniquet serves as an effective psychological distraction. If not done previously, the wound should now be rendered anesthetic by suitable field or nerve block with 1% lidocaine without epinephrine. The skin can now be suitably cleansed and the extremity draped. The final control of the bleeding point can then be discretely done by precise identification and ligation. This usually requires the use of a magnifying loupe, extension of the wound, and removal of clots. Ligatures should be nonreactive, eg, nylon. This technique avoids iatrogenic injury to uninjured nerves and other structures.

At this point it is possible to survey the extent of injury and to determine the best facilities for treatment. Complex injuries, flexor tendon, nerve and difficult bone and joint problems, as well as some extensor tendon injuries, should generally be referred to the operating room.

Specific attention is then directed to the skin, its color, temperature, and perspiration. Scars, contractures, wounds, and other lesions are noted, as is the character of the fingernails. The radial and ulnar pulses are palpated, and where appropriate an Allen's test is done. Abnormal pulsations or bruits are recorded.

The neuromuscular evaluation must specifically identify the integrity of the three major nerves and of the individual musculotendinous units. The integrity of the *radial nerve* is tested by forceful wrist extension and extension of the metacarpophalangeal joints and by pinprick within the dorsum of the thumb web. The *ulnar nerve* is tested by forceful spreading of the fingers and flexion of distal joint of the ring and little fingers and by pinprick over the eponychium of the little finger. The *median nerve* is tested by forceful flexion of the wrist and of the interphalangeal joints of the thumb and index finger and by pinprick over the eponychium of the index and long fingers. A test should be made of the distal phalangeal flexors and of the independence of action of the superficialis tendons, the independent extensors of the thumb, index, and little fingers, and of the wrist flexors and extensors. Consistency of findings by repeated evaluations is essential for accurate diagnosis. The time frame for this may be minutes, hours, or days, depending on the circumstances. A critical test of sensory function of the median nerve is the blindfold coin-discrimination test in which the patient is asked to identify coins while blindfolded.

Where appropriate, points of tenderness must be elicited and the mechanism of pain reproduced by active and passive stress-testing of muscles, tendons, ligaments, and joint surfaces. The instability of ligaments and the existence of crepitation and trigger phenomena must be established by appropriate testing.

An adjunct to the history and physical examination consists of *roentgenographic* studies. Musculoskeletal injury generally requires initial and follow-up roentgenograms to aid in diagnosis and treatment. Where results are inconclusive it is often helpful to have comparable views of the opposite extremity and to obtain views in multiple planes. Many scaphoid fractures have been missed because of failure to get a plane of exposure that passes exactly parallel to the plane of the fracture.

Special examinations—tomography, magnification views, cineroentgenography, arthrography, bone scan, CT scan, and MRI—can aid in the diagnosis of certain difficult problems. The Doppler ultrasound probe can be used to assess arterial patency when clinically it is doubtful.

PREOPERATIVE PREPARATION[9]

Surgical Facilities

An operating table, arm board, good light, a magnifying loupe, specialized fine instruments, a pneumatic gauged cuff, and surgical assistance are essential for hand surgery. Inexperience, haste, and fatigue are serious handicaps.

Preparation for Surgery

The patient should be supine and comfortable, with a well-padded pneumatic tourniquet on the arm. Many surgeons sit, but it is better to elevate the table and stand so that the surgeon can readily shift his position as circumstances require. However, microsurgery of nerves and vessels is done sitting.

If pain is not severe, anesthetic paralysis of the whole upper extremity should be withheld until the skin preparation and draping are completed since the patient's cooperation greatly facilitates these procedures. Skin preparation consists of one paint brush coating of 1% to 2% iodine, which is then neutralized with alcohol. These solutions should be kept out of the wound and off of the tourniquet and its padding. Sterile waterproof draping is applied, and general or regional anesthesia can be administered.

The freshly injured or infected extremity may then be passively elevated and the tourniquet inflated (to 300 mm Hg for adults or to 150 to 250 mm Hg for infants and persons with very thin arms). Uncontrolled bleeding may necessitate tourniquet control before the anesthesia and skin preparation. In elective surgical cases which are not infected, the extremity is usually exsanguinated by manual compression or an elastic roll (eg, Esmarch bandage) before inflation of the tourniquet. The patient will generally tolerate tourniquet ischemia on the unanesthetized upper arm for 20 to 30 minutes. When the arm is anesthetized, the tissue tolerance for ischemia is 2 to 2½ hours. The tourniquet manometer should be tested for accuracy before use since paralyses have occurred as a result of excessive tourniquet pressure. The tourniquet may be released and reinflated after the reactive hyperemia subsides in procedures demanding prolonged tourniquet time.

Anesthesia

General anesthesia (or axillary block or IV 0.5% lidocaine block) is preferred for procedures which last for over 20 to 30 minutes. Premedication with morphine sulfate and scopolamine (when not contraindicated by allergy or glaucoma) is ideal for its tranquilizing and analgesic effect.

Lidocaine (1% to 2%) without epinephrine injected slowly through a fine needle (eg, #26-30 gauge for the digit) is used for local blocks (into the wound) or nerve blocks (axillary, radial, ulnar, median, or digital nerve). Excessive amounts which will congest the nerve, the hand, or the digit should be avoided. The skin and fat should still be soft and pliable after the injection. The most that should be injected at the base of an adult digit is 2.5 mL. Large caliber needles may cut nerve tissue and should not be used.

SURGICAL TECHNIQUES[10]

Anything that touches the wound must be aseptic and both chemically and mechanically atraumatic. Starch powder should be wiped off of sterile gloves. Sponging should be by dabbing, not wiping. Instruments must be in the best condition and should consist of a selection of fine plastic surgery hooks, retractors, forceps, clamps, scissors, needle holders, atraumatic sutures, and Kirschner wires and drill. Nonreactive material should be stipulated for sutures and ligatures. Catgut should be avoided except for the closure of skin wounds of infants (eg, 6-0 or 7-0 catgut). Monofilament nylon is preferred. The tissues must be kept moist, preferably with lactated Ringer's solution. Hemostasis must be complete.

The fundamental principles of treatment involve the following: (1) Dissect with at least 2× magnification utilizing tourniquet ischemia, and a needle point electrocautery for hemostasis. (2) Dissect from normal tissue into abnormal. (3) Keep the tissues dissected under tension. (4) Keep the margins of the wound suspended by hooks or stay sutures. (5) Once through the dermis with a scalpel, use short-bladed, sharp, fine scissors for dissection and identify and coagulate or ligate all vessels that need to be divided. (6) Spread the tissue gently before cutting, and then cut with precision only the tensed white fascial or fibrous tissue. This will prevent the inadvertent severing of nerves or vessels, which are identifiable by their soft and lax consistency, and will reduce trauma to fat which is the vital cushion of the hand.

Good irrigation is essential. Gross dirt on the skin should be washed off with soap and water. Skin stains do not necessarily have to be washed off. If the skin is coated with oil, grime, or tar, ether or benzine may be necessary to remove it, but such solutions must be kept out of the wound. Dried blood is most easily removed with hydrogen peroxide. An open wound may be irrigated with lactated Ringer's solution with or without antibiotics.

Debridement is required to remove blood clots, nonviable tissue, and foreign bodies which will constitute dead space. Thus, living tissue can be coapted and grafted tissue can be nourished by capillary invasion. It is occasionally necessary to debride without tourniquet ischemia so that the level of viability can be determined by the scalpel. The surgeon should know when and how to save debrided tissue for primary or secondary use in reconstructive surgery. The objective of debridement in the primary care of injuries is to preserve function by preserving circulation and curtailing edema and infection. Closing a wound with irregular but viable margins or with primary or delayed split thickness grafting is far preferable to trimming the edges and forcing the closure with tight sutures. Stained but viable tissue and minute fragments of foreign material should not be removed unless the foreign material is known to be caustic.

Evaluation and repair demand identification of the anatomic relationships. Incisions often must be extended beyond scar or blood-discolored tissue. This should be done without injury to the blood supply, nerves, and tendons, and should not predispose to secondary disabling contractures (eg, scars crossing at right angles to flexion skin creases) (Figure 11–6).

After debridement and exposure, the surgeon's experience and facilities will determine how much to repair deep to the skin. Skilled primary reparative or reconstructive hand surgery will go far to spare function, time, and expense. Unskilled efforts may do just the opposite. Generally speaking, skeletal distortion should be gently corrected, and if the tissues are not congested and the circulation is good, structures that are easily identifiable and clearly matched should be approximated. Unstable bone alignment often requires some

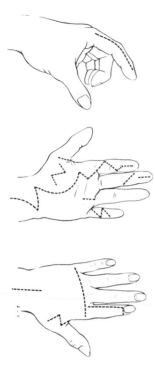

Figure 11–6.   Incisions for the hand and fingers.

form of internal fixation. Sutures of nylon vary in caliber from 8-0 to 11-0 for digital nerves and from 4-0 to 6-0 nylon for tendons, ligaments and skin.

Given satisfactory skeletal stability, the circulation has first priority, skin and fat second, tendons (eg, long flexor tendons) third, and nerves the last priority in primary repair. One must avoid overloading the already injured tissues with the trauma of surgery itself.

Primary repair is that which is done within the first 24 to 72 hours. If circumstances of wounding suggest heavy contamination (eg, a tooth-, a farmyard-, or a sewer-inflicted wound), it is probably best to instill antibiotics and drain the wound and repair nothing primarily. When contamination is minimal but the circulation is impaired (eg, much swelling)—or if over 8 hours have passed without any surgical toilet or splinting—then it is best to prepare, dress, splint, and elevate the part and administer prophylactic broad-spectrum antibiotics. If within the first 2 weeks there is no evidence of inflammation and the tissues are soft and pliable, delayed primary repair may be considered.

Secondary repair is that which follows the first 2 weeks after injury and is usually undertaken after resolution of the swelling and induration that followed the injury.

Wound drainage and closure requires attention. A loosely fitting drain prevents the accumulation of serum and blood and forestalls the development of "dead space" and infection or cicatrix. Therefore, drainage should be selectively used in contaminated wounds and severe compound crushing wounds. Drains should be inserted in such a way as to favor gravity drainage from the elevated extremity.

Wounds should never be closed with tension. If tension is unavoidable, it is best to leave the wound open or to graft it. When tension has already built up and if uncontrollable throbbing pain has developed, it should be treated by adequate slitting of the skin and slitting the fascia of all tight compartments.

Most wounds of the hand can be closed with one layer of interrupted or running everting skin sutures. Interrupted sutures are preferred if motion is to start early.

Prophylaxis against infection involves prophylaxis against tetanus and against streptococcal and staphylococcal infections. If the wound is contaminated (not necessarily clinically infected), it should be irrigated with penicillin or bacitracin solution at surgery and systemic antibiotics should be given for 48 to 72 hours afterward. The systemic drugs of choice for gram-positive organisms are penicillin, methicillin, erythromycin, or cephalosporin; for gram-negative organisms, kanamycin or gentamicin. Antibiotics must not be regarded as a substitute for the more important fundamental principles of surgical technique and protection of circulation (especially venous return).

DRESSING AND SPLINTS[9]

The *dressing* should serve to keep the soft tissues at rest and prevent the development of "dead space" by gentle compression that does not obstruct venous return. Sopping wet dressings facilitate drainage of blood and serum. A single layer of fine mesh gauze smoothed out flush with the wound prevents granulation tissue from invading the dressing and facilitates the search for sutures when the dressing is removed. On top of this should be placed wet, loose-meshed gauze which should be tailored to lie flat without folds and ridges. Up to this point nothing is wrapped circumferentially around the digit, hand, or forearm. Over this should then be placed a carefully tailored sheet of sponge rubber or plastic (eg, Reston) to prevent congestion by the dressing. This in turn is held in place with circumferentially wrapped, loose-meshed gauze (eg, Kling, Kerlix, Tubegauz) or cast padding. Care should be taken not to wrap the part too snugly.

Immobilization is mandatory initially in most cases of hand trauma, bearing in mind that prolonged immobilization involves a risk of stiffness. The position in immobilization must never be at the extreme of joint extension or flexion but must generally serve its need, ie, to relieve tension on a tendon or nerve suture line. Whenever possible, immobilization should be in the position of function. This favors circulation and promotes comfort as well as early reestablishment of unimpaired function. It is the posture assumed when the hand holds a small drinking glass and is most readily achieved by putting a soaking-wet roll of gauze (eg, Kerlix) in the palm between the thumb and fingers and molding it to them. Loosely wrapped dry cast padding covered with a volar plaster splint (12 to 16 thicknesses, 1 to 2 inches wide and 6 to 8 inches long) from the midpalm across the wrist to the midforearm and held in place with one 3 to 4 inch wide roll of circumferentially wrapped plaster makes a light and effective splint which is generally much more trustworthy than a forearm splint secured with a wrapping of bias stockinette or elastic roll. Congestion is avoided by keeping the elbow flexed during the wrapping and the rigid component of splintage well distal to the antecubital flexion crease.

After extensive hand trauma, infection, or surgery, a softly padded boxing-glove forearm cast is preferred. One may put only part of the hand in such a cast—eg, the thumb alone, or a combination of any 2 or 3 adjacent fingers. Generally speaking, such splinting is preferred for even severe fingertip injuries (eg, amputation or crush). The wrist must be immobilized to adequately splint any part of the hand. Flat splints (eg, tongue blade) and single digit splinting for an extensive injury impose a risk of distortion and stiffness and often fail to relieve pain. Infants and irresponsible adults usually need a long arm cast rather than a forearm cast. The elbow is immobilized at 90 degrees.

The duration of splinting will vary with the problem and the age of the patient. Repair of nerves and tendons and fractures of phalanges and metacarpals usually require immobilization for 3 to 4 weeks, whereas ganglionectomy and fingertip grafting require only 6 to 8 days of casting.

POSTINJURY AND POSTOPERATIVE CARE

Control of Circulation and Pain

The hallmark of postinjury or postoperative management includes the following orders: (1) comfortably elevate the hand to heart level; (2) no snug sleeve or jewelry; (3) keep the dressing and/or cast dry; (4) call if there is unrelenting throbbing pain or other serious problem; (5) take appropriate pain medication (eg, Tylenol with codeine); (6) be seen by the surgeon or his representative in adequate follow-up period (eg, which may be hours or 1 to 4 days depending on the circumstances); and (7) take prophylactic antibiotics in most cases of open injury or lengthy surgery for at least 3 days.

It is essential that the hand be constantly elevated in comfort above the heart. In serious cases where microcirculation is threatened by tissue trauma and congestion, sludging and microthrombosis may be curtailed by administering 1 unit of low molecular weight dextran (Dextran 40) daily. There must be no compression or constriction by clothing, jewelry, dressings, casts, or even skin or fascia. Throbbing and brawny induration must be mechanically (not medicinally) relieved—if necessary, by slitting skin and fascia. Chronic (eg, "fixed") edema may be overcome by wearing an elastic glove (eg, surgeon's glove), exercises, and elevation.

Dressings and Splints[11]

There must never be any snugness of a dressing or splint or it will favor swelling, pain, hemorrhea, and even infection. A comfortable dressing and splint may be left undisturbed for 4 to 7 days, but changed early on if uncomfortable. Drains are generally removed at 2 to 4 days unless there is infection.

Movement

The patient must understand that motion inside a splint is undesirable even though possible and that vigorous movement of any part of the upper extremity may disrupt the tissues being splinted. On the other hand, gentle movement of all unsplinted joints helps the circulation of the whole upper extremity. When immobilization is discontinued, active exercise should be started on an organized routine (eg, 4 times daily for 15 minutes). The frequency and duration of rehabilitative exercises of the injured part should steadily increase. The more the patient can do on his own and the less he needs the crutch of physical therapy, the better.

Chronic Stiffness

Pain is often the chief deterrent to overcoming stiffness caused by tight scar tissue and contracted ligaments. This can sometimes be relieved around joints by the intra-articular and periarticular injection of a small amount of lidocaine mixed with triamcinolone. Passive stretching is also possible by the use of dynamic splints carefully adjusted and tailored to the needs of the specific problem, but these must be worn intermittently rather than continuously and should not be permitted to cause pressure sores, nerve injury, or edema. In selected intractable cases, arthrolysis, tenolysis, or modification of skin scars may be required.

Care of the Paralyzed Hand

During the recovery stage following anesthesia or nerve injury, the patient must take care not to injure anesthetic skin by burns or cuts, or pain-free joints by sprains and subluxations. Splints should be used to keep paralyzed muscles from being overstretched and uninvolved muscles from overcontracting without antagonism. An example is the cock-up splint for the wrist and metacarpophalangeal joints in radial nerve palsy.

REFERENCES

1. Tubiana R. Historical survey. In: *The Hand*. Philadelphia, Pa: WB Saunders; 1988: chap 1.
2. Mason ML. Fifty years' progress in surgery of the hand. *Int Abstr Surg*. 1955;101:541.
3. Kanavel AB. *Infections of the Hand*. Philadelphia, Pa: Lea & Febiger; 1912.
4. Kelsey JL, Pastides H, Bisbee GE Jr. *Musculoskeletal Disorders: Their Frequency of Occurrence and Their Impact on the Population of the United States*. New York, NY: Neale-Watson Academic Publishers; 1978.
5. Kaplan EB. *Functional and Surgical Anatomy of the Hand*. 2nd ed. Philadelphia, Pa: JB Lippincott; 1965.
6. Brand P. *Clinical Mechanics of the Hand*. St. Louis, Mo: CV Mosby; 1985.
7. Kilgore ES Jr, Graham WP III. *The Hand: Surgical and Nonsurgical Management*. Philadelphia, Pa: Lea & Febiger; 1977.
8. Hankin FM, Peel SM. Sports related fractures and dislocations of the hand. *Hand Clin*. 1990;6:429.
9. Newmeyer WL. *Primary Care of Hand Injuries*. Philadelphia, Pa: Lea & Febiger; 1979.
10. Buck-Grameko D, Hoffman R, Neumann R. *Hand Trauma: A Practical Guide*. Stuttgart, Germany: Thieme Inc; 1986.
11. Fess EE, Gettle KS, Strickland JW. *Hand Splinting: Principles and Methods*. St. Louis, Mo: CV Mosby; 1981.

12

Management of Specific Hand Injuries

EUGENE KILGORE, M.D.

HISTORY: No important progress was made in hand surgery as a result of World War I. In the interval between World War I and World War II, hand surgery developed steadily but slowly. During that time the significant advances could be attributed only to the repeated efforts of a relatively few surgeons in North America and overseas. After infections were better understood, the basic principles of treatment of open hand injuries remained to be established. Halsted's precepts regarding tissue handling in relation to wound healing were quickly adopted by certain surgeons who eventually became noted in the field of hand surgery. In 1921 Bunnell introduced the term atraumatic technique, *which was to become the byword of hand surgery throughout the world.[1]*

In 1944, Major General Norman T. Kirk, the Surgeon General, sought to alleviate the haphazard situation which existed regarding military hand casualties. He requested that Sterling Bunnell of San Francisco be appointed as a special civilian consultant to the Secretary of War in order to develop hand surgery in the Army. By early 1945, military casualties with severe hand injuries were referred to certain general hospitals that had hand surgery services that were designated as autonomous units.[2]

The first edition of Bunnell's comprehensive textbook, Surgery of the Hand, *was published in 1944.[3] It was adopted immediately as an official text by the Army and was widely distributed throughout military medical installations.*

The problem of attaining uniformly satisfactory results following primary or secondary tendon procedures continues as a major challenge. Peacock and Cameron have experimented with the use of homologous composite grafts of the entire digital flexor tendon mechanism. Hunter, Carroll, and others have approached the problem by clinical use of artificial tendon implants. Investigations by Potenza, Peacock, Madden, and others on the biological control of scar tissue represent a major breakthrough toward solving the complex problems of wound healing in relation to gliding function.[4]

INTRODUCTION

The specific injuries which involve the hand are multiple and frequently occur in combination with one another. Although most of these injuries can be managed successfully by the average general, orthopaedic, or plastic surgeon, many can tax the skills of the most expert hand specialist.[5] Tendon, nerve, and amputations which would benefit from replantation are such examples. However, soft-tissue injuries and fractures also may present demanding problems. The key to successful hand surgery is not simply restoring anatomy, it is maintaining or restoring function. If function is lost in the process of restoring anatomy, then therapy can be considered unsuccessful.

CONTUSION AND COMPRESSION INJURIES

A crushing or compressive force to the forearm, hand, or digit causing skeletal or soft-tissue injury can result in severe stiffness and even impairment of nerve function. Impaired circulation in such cases results from bleeding and serous effusion, then swelling, and finally venous obstruction and microvascular thrombosis caused by tissue tension. This can lead to irreversible ischemic fibrosis, as in Volkmann's ischemic paralysis and contracture. This process can occur in any fascial compartment of the upper extremity—even that of any of the intrinsic muscles or digital fat pads. It can usually be prevented by attending promptly to throbbing pain and relieving it mechanically. Brawny (rocky hard) congestion must be prevented even if it means slitting the skin and fascia extensively. It is both useless and harmful to try to squeeze infiltrated blood out of tissues, though clearly defined clots can occasionally be extracted.

SKIN AVULSIONS

Most wounds should be inspected and closed under tourniquet control. A magnifying loupe should be available. If a full thickness of skin has been lost, the wound may be primarily closed with a skin graft. If oozing is too great, grafting should be delayed for 1 or 2 days. Split-thickness grafts are the most certain to take, but a full-thickness graft may be prepared by defatting an avulsed piece of skin or by taking some from the hairless portion of the groin. Very long reverse flaps and flaps that have been significantly traumatized are preferably defatted and applied as free full-thickness grafts or replaced by a split-thickness graft. Immobilization is crucial to the healing of lacerations and grafts.

TENDON INJURIES

Any laceration must be assumed to have divided a tendon until proved otherwise by inspection of the wound under tourniquet ischemia with prior or simultaneous systematic testing of all tendons as they are actively tensed. An abnormal digital stance created by a tendon injury can often be demonstrated by extreme passive flexion or extension of the wrist. Penetrating glass and metal wounds can damage tendons far in excess of what is apparent and at sites far removed from the skin wound. Tendon rupture occurs from a sudden stretching force, and tendon adherence due to adhesions (tenodesis) is common after all forms of trauma or infection.

Treatment

Because of the complexity of restoring tendon and joint function after injury or other impairment, most problems of the flexor or extensor musculotendinous systems should be referred to the hand specialist for definitive treatment.

The restoration of function after division of tendons requires surgical judgment and skill and the subsequent perseverance of the patient in the rehabilitation effort. Tendon repair must not be at the expense of mobility of uninjured tendons and joints. The surgeon may appropriately elect no treatment, tenorrhaphy, tendon transfer, tenodesis, or arthrodesis. The state of the wound and the complexity of the injury are the principal issues one must weigh in choosing primary tenorrhaphy (within 24 to 72 hours) or secondary tenorrhaphy. When wounds are untidy, contaminated, lacking skin and fat cover, or complicated by fracture or ischemia, formal tenorrhaphy may have to be delayed for weeks or months until the tendon bed is favorable to healing and glide. However, interim tacking of the tendons—together, to tendon sheath, or to bone—to maintain muscle fiber length may be done as a preliminary procedure. Tenorrhaphy may be done primarily or secondarily by direct suture, by tendon graft, or by tendon transfer, followed by immobilization for 3 to 4 weeks. Cases referred to the specialist should receive primary wound toilet, closure, splinting, and prophylactic antibiotics. Joints must be freely mobile and skin- and fat-cover healthy and pliable before tenorrhaphy or tendon transfer is undertaken.

The handling of tendons and their fibro-osseous sheaths should be atraumatic. Sponges, forceps, clamps, and needles all invite adhesions where they contact these structures. The long flexor tendons require pulleys for mechanical efficiency and to prevent bow-stringing; however, in order to make certain that this pulley system does not choke and prevent excursion of a tenorrhaphy callus, enough fibro-osseous sheath must be removed to correspond with the expected amplitude of the callus, or the tendon(s) should be transposed superficial to the retinaculum.

The technique of suturing a tendon must be meticulous. The amount of suturing required depends on the amount of separation of the proximal stump from its distal attachment and the force necessary to hold the suture line. Retraction of the proximal stump may be prevented while placing the tendon suture by skewering the stump with a straight needle. Atraumatic nonreactive 4-0 to 5-0 sutures (eg, monofilament nylon) should be used and can be threaded (see Figure 12–1) in a mattress, figure-of-eight, or once or twice crisscrossing fashion through the tendon stumps. The rim of a tendon juncture may be reinforced and evened up by a 6-0 or 7-0 running over-and-over suture. Nylon sutures are usually buried except when anchoring a tendon into bone, in which case the suture ends may pass through the bone and overlying epithelial layer (eg, fingernail) to be tied over a cotton dental roll and then withdrawn in 3 to 4 weeks. When the size of 2 tendons to be joined is disproportionate, the smaller one may be woven once or twice through the larger one.

Immobilization should be in a position that takes tension off the tendon wound without putting any joints in extreme flexion or extension. The wrist is most often the principal joint to be positioned.

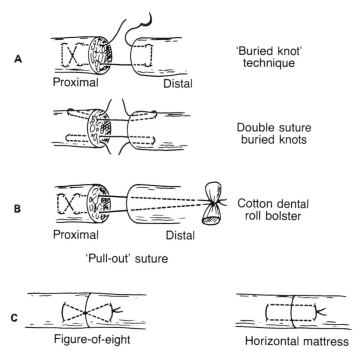

Figure 12–1. Methods of tenorrhaphy. **A:** for larger caliber tendons; **B:** for distal tendons near site of insertion; **C:** for thin tendons, or those with limited separation. (From Schrock. *Handbook of Surgery*. 9th ed. Reprinted with permission.)

Extensor Tendon Injuries[6]

If injury to an extensor is recognized immediately and proper treatment is given, the prognosis for recovered function is usually more favorable than is the case with flexor tendon.[7] This is because there is less sheath to contend with and, over the digit, less glide (eg, 1 to 15 mm). The danger with extensor hood over the digit lies in the fact that it is very complex and at first may fully compensate for a major interruption only to decompensate insidiously later, due to inadequate treatment.

Exposure (often by proximal and distal extension of the wound) is important for the proper assay and repair of the injury. Because retraction of the proximal stump may be physically negligible but functionally significant, reapproximation of ends and immobilization are usually essential.

Positioning alone may satisfactorily restore the continuity. If not, buried 4-0 to 6-0 monofilament nylon sutures are placed as figure-of-eight, horizontal mattress, or (on the dorsum of the hand and forearm) crisscross weaving sutures. Immobilization should be maintained for 3 to 6 weeks.

Mallet (Baseball) Finger. (Figure 12–2) is a flexion stance of the distal joint resulting from separation of the attachment of the extensor to the distal phalanx. Bone or tendon may be separated, and active extension may be partially or completely lost. It occurs most often from jamming the end of the digit. A dorsal or volar padded splint across the distal joint for 6 to 8 weeks may be all that is needed in fresh cases. Hyperextension and excessive skin pressure must be avoided. If the mallet results from a laceration, the tendon should be

in this area is untidy or when several weeks or months have elapsed since the injury, a tendon graft is generally preferred in zone 2. Secondary tendon repair (more than 2 weeks after injury) is frequently possible in zones 3, 4, and 5.

When multiple tendons are divided in one zone, it may be preferable to repair only the more important ones. This is especially true in injuries in zone 2, where the profundus is usually the preferred one to be repaired.

Lateral digital incisions may be made to connect the ends of the flexion creases, or volar incisions may cross the fat pads obliquely in a zigzag fashion. Zigzagging is also preferred for opening the palm or wrist. Damage to neurovascular bundles must be avoided (see Figure 11–6).

Priority should be given to repairing flexor tendons before repairing nerves. When dealing with a very bloody palm or digit with both nerve and flexor tendon injury, neurorrhaphy often demands such excessive surgical dissection to even identify a nerve that it is contraindicated as a primary procedure.

Movement of digits within 3 weeks after flexor tenorrhaphy, if permitted at all, must be done very guardedly. If controlled early motion is initiated, it is primarily applicable to repairs of the profundus in zones 1 and 2. At intervals each day the finger is held *passively* in flexion at all of its joints while the PIP and DIP joints are *actively* extended. The MP joint is always kept in flexion. This action invokes contraction of the lumbrical, not the long flexors, and promotes passive glide of the profundus without straining its suture. This must be carefully supervised. After 3 weeks, active motion of the repaired tendon may progress in a graded fashion.

The results following tenorrhaphy depend on the mobility of joints, the remodeling of scar tissue so that it yields to the glide of tendons, adequate strength of muscles, and perseverance by the patient. It often takes many months—even up to a year—to regain maximal tendon excursion and joint motion and for the collagen of scar tissue to attenuate and adapt. The patient must be encouraged to persevere and must be made aware of the difficulty and sometimes impossibility of recovering completely normal excursion. Progress may be gauged by serial records of the distance by which digital tips fail to reach points in space (eg, a straight line in extension or the midpalm in flexion). If there is no sign of improvement during a period of 4 weeks of close supervision beginning 2 to 3 months after surgery, further spontaneous improvement is most unlikely.

NERVE INJURIES

The interruption of nerve conduction following injury may be merely physiologic (ie, neurapraxia) or it may be anatomic. The distinction can be made by repeated examination in the first few hours after an open injury and before any anesthetic is administered if the neurapraxia is transient.[9] Treatment of nerve injuries are discussed further in chapter 6.

FRACTURES

Fractures can usually be reduced with gentle traction and compression. The wrist and digits should be generally maintained in the position of function after reduction. Unstable alignment may require internal fixation to hold reduction. At all costs, avoid extremes of joint position. Forceful pressure of external splints and plaster should be avoided also.

Constant digital traction is hazardous because it leads to joint stiffness. To minimize stiffness, immobilization should be maintained for the shortest time consistent with adequate control of pain and tissue repair.

Elevation of the forearm and removal of all jewelry and snug clothing are essential to control edema. The patient's own responsibilities in this regard must be repeatedly explained. When swelling is excessive, it must be reduced and the soft tissues rendered pliable as soon as possible. Reduction of the displaced fracture or dislocated joint sometimes makes the soft tissues pliable again. A releasing incision of skin and fascia may be needed to overcome brawny induration. It can be closed later with a split-thickness skin graft.

Open injuries involving bones and joints require prophylactic antibiotics systemically and often in the wound or joint as well.

Fractures of metacarpals and proximal and middle phalanges tend to bow and to rotate. Rotation of a finger causes it to cross over an adjacent finger during flexion, thus blocking digital excursion, fist making, and grasp. Rotation is avoided by having the injured finger flexed alongside an adjacent finger.

Dorsal and volar bowing is caused by the pull of intrinsic and extrinsic flexor and extensor forces. These forces can be most effectively neutralized by immobilizing the wrist and the digits in the position of function. Reduction of bowing has the risk of added predisposition to joint stiffness and tenodesis incident to excessive manipulation or surgery. Therefore, if the bowing is less than 20 to 30 degrees, this risk must be weighed carefully, for such deformity may not be functionally significant. Significant angles of bowing of phalanges must, however, be corrected by either closed or open methods. Angulation of up to 40 degrees can be tolerated in some metacarpal neck fractures.

The immobilized MP joints must be maintained in functional flexion. In the case of the ring and small fingers, this function means between 60 and 80 degrees of flexion. Malleable and rigid ready-made volar splints cannot be applied without a threat to this important angle of MP joint flexion or (equally harmful) a threat of too much compression of the soft tissue or a rotary deformity at the fracture site.

After closed or open reduction, a preferred method of immobilization is to furl the digits over a volar roll of soft gauze, which allows the position of function to be maintained. The forearm and pertinent digits are then wrapped in loosely applied cast padding followed by a light circumferential plaster cast, keeled for strength across the extended wrist.[10] This immobilization is usually maintained for 3 weeks, although with rigid internal fixation it may be for only a few days. The patient should be seen every 2 to 3 days so that the cast can be removed for guarded active and passive joint motion under supervision of the surgeon.

Two basal metacarpal fractures deserve special mention. Benett's intra-articular fracture is an impaction of the thumb metacarpal, causing an oblique fracture into the MC joint between the volar base and the dorsal base. The latter frequently subluxates dorsally. The ideal treatment when there is displacement is reduction by centrifugal pulling on the thumb and pressure volarward on the base of the metacarpal followed by fixation with a Kirschner wire. If satisfactory realignment is not achieved, open reduction is advocated. A spiral or displaced fracture of the base of the fifth metacarpal always deserves an immediate and repeated check on the function of the first dorsal interosseous muscle to establish the integrity of the deep motor branch of the ulnar nerve, which is easily injured by this fracture.

Distal phalangeal fractures are located at the tuft, shaft, or base. Pain is the prime reason for treatment, and it may be compounded if subungual hematoma is also present.

Decompression relieves pain. This can be done by drilling the nail with a 19-caliber hypodermic needle mounted on a syringe, or by burning a hole through the nail with the hot end of a safety pin or paper clip. This is quite painless if done gently, but in the anxious patient a digital nerve block may be required. Pain and swelling are best controlled by applying a well-padded forearm cast covering the injured finger with at least one adjacent finger or the injured thumb alone in boxing glove fashion. After 1 to 2 weeks, a digital guard can take the place of the cast.

Minute marginal digital joint fractures usually need no more than 1 to 2 days of immobilization. Stiffness and pain can be overcome by early mobilization. Fractures with involvement of one fourth to one third of the joint surface require careful reduction and immobilization for 3 weeks unless rigid internal fixation is resorted to, in which case guarded early motion may be initiated under supervision. In some cases, the fragment should be resected. Mangled joints should be set at a functional angle for fusion or, in select circumstances, the MP or PIP joints may be replaced by a silastic implant if tendons are functioning.

In closed or open crushing fractures with a lot of swelling, the prime consideration should be preservation of the circulation, particularly venous return. Anatomic reduction of the bone is of secondary importance. Leaving a wound open or even slitting skin and fascia to loosen the tissues may be the best way to aid the circulation and may also make it possible to secure alignment and the position of function. Reduction is often well maintained by molding a roll of very wet, loose gauze to the injured digits or whole hand and then applying a well-cushioned boxing-glove type of forearm cast to the appropriate digits or the whole hand. Internal fixation is advisable in selected cases.

Open reduction is the technique of choice in injuries that present a gaping wound with exposed fractures. It is also the preferred technique in the following circumstances: (1) when perfect reduction is important for subsequent function, as in intra-articular fractures, or when indicated for the removal of a potentially troublesome displaced small fragment; (2) if it allows reduction with less soft tissue trauma than by closed reduction; (3) to facilitate internal fixation in difficult reductions; or (4) to allow early movement and prevent stiffness.

DISLOCATIONS

Dislocations of the wrist and fingers are less frequent than fractures. Swelling may completely mask the bone displacement, but motion is usually limited and painful. X-rays may be indispensable to the diagnosis. In the case of the wrist, multiple views and comparison of right and left may be necessary.

Dislocations are most easily reduced by accentuating the position that produced the deformity with simultaneous centrifugal traction on the distal segment followed by firm pressing of the displaced bone into its anatomic position. A reduction snap may be heard and is often promptly followed by excellent range of motion. A postreduction x-ray should usually be taken.

Limited progressive mobilization is usually advisable to avoid stiffness. It may start within 3 to 4 weeks for the wrist and a week for the digits. A concomitant fracture or an open dislocation would interdict mobilization so early. Compound dislocations require prophylactic treatment with antibiotics.

Open reduction is indicated whenever closed reduction requires much force. A chronic dislocation may defy even an open reduction without lysis and division of soft tissue or resection arthroplasty.

The most common dislocation about the digits is dorsal displacement of the distal segment on the proximal one. When ligaments are intact, reduction may be difficult. The most difficult is the dislocated MP joint of one of the fingers, which normally requires open reduction. It traps the head of the metacarpal in a noose formed by the lumbrical radially, the flexor tendons and pretendinous palmar fascia band ulnarly, the volar plate and collateral ligaments on the dorsum distally, and the transverse palmar fascia on the volar aspect proximally. Volar exposure with section of the fascia proximally or dorsal exposure with splitting of the volar plate makes reduction quite easy, although section of the ulnar collateral ligament must sometimes be added.

Dislocation of an IP joint is most often reduced immediately by the patient or a bystander and requires little or no immobilization. Resistance to flexion means inadequate reduction. Failure of reduction can mean that the displaced phalangeal head has escaped sideways from under the hood of the extensor mechanism, which then closes in between the head and the base of the more distal phalanx and locks the deformity. Recurrence of the dislocation usually means that the volar plate has been torn off at its origin distally. All three of these difficulties require open procedures to restore normal anatomic relationships. Repair of the volar plate requires 3 to 4 weeks of immobility. One obliquely placed Kirschner wire provides sufficient fixation of the joint.

Chronic dislocations with erosion of the joint should be handled by replacing the joint with a silastic prosthesis if the surrounding tendons are functionally intact; otherwise, the joints should be fused in the position of function.

LIGAMENTOUS INJURIES

The ligaments of the MP and PIP joints are the most commonly injured. These vary from total ruptures to tears without any loss of stability. Either the ligament tears, or its bony attachment is avulsed, or both ligament and bone are torn. Those of the MP joint are usually due to violent abduction, whereas PIP ligaments rupture with equal proclivity on the radial or ulnar sides. Diagnosis may depend on stress x-ray view, often requiring a local lidocaine infiltration to block pain to show abnormal widening of a joint.

Except for the thumb, treatment of purely ligamentous injuries is seldom surgical. Splinting should often be brief to avoid excessive stiffness and pain, which may result. As long as there is intact intrinsic and extrinsic tendon function and the patient is careful to avoid further injury, early motion within 2 to 3 days of injury is often desirable. One finger can be splinted by loosely strapping it to an adjacent digit ("buddy-taping") for 2 to 4 weeks. The pain of these injuries is notoriously slow to resolve, irrespective of treatment.

Twisting injuries and falls may rupture the radial collateral ligament of the thumb by an adduction force, most commonly, however, the injury is an abduction force that tears the ulnar collateral ligament ("game-keeper's thumb"). Partial tears with limited instability may be treated by buddy-taping the thumb to the index finger for four weeks. Total tears should be sutured or reconstructed surgically.

If there is a sizable avulsed bone fragment in any of these injuries, it must be accurately reduced or, if it involves less than one fourth of the surface area of the PIP or MP joint, removed.

AMPUTATION

Sudden physical or functional loss of part or all of the hand or arm is a shocking experience that deserves special recognition and attention on the part of the surgeon. Psychologic and physical comfort should be given, and the patient must be spared alarming comments as well as any false hopes of replantation or salvage.

Amputation may be physical or functional. Injury and disease may functionally (though not physically) amputate by crushing, mangling, paralyzing, stiffening, causing pain, or otherwise destroying all or part of the hand beyond hope of useful recovery. In such cases, salvage may be impossible and surgical amputation is justified to improve the overall physical and psychologic effectiveness of the patient.

When surgery must be deferred, the injured part should be comfortably aligned and splinted without constriction. Bleeding should be controlled by compression or by ligation of the bleeder provided it is adequately exposed under tourniquet ischemia and loupe magnification to avoid injuring adjacent nerves. Wet dressings should be applied to open wounds to facilitate sequestration of blood and serum, and the extremity should be comfortably elevated. In the case of open injuries, prophylactic antibiotics should be given.

Complex injuries notoriously cause multilevel and multitissue involvement ("common wound"). All structures are congealed in the reactive process, culminating in a common scar (callus) with loss of structural independence.

The surgeon must individualize the treatment of complex hand injuries by considering such factors as age, occupation, hand dominance, economic status, cosmesis, emotional make-up, and general health. In other words, adequate salvage and maximal salvage are relative to the patient's needs, desires, and capacities. An extensive reconstructive effort is justified if, without it, there will be little or no function; but one must be careful not to destroy existing function and to spare the patient unwarranted disability, time, expense, and disappointment by heroic efforts that might fail. It is sometimes best to remove part or all of the hand in the interest of the patient's overall psychologic and functional competence and productivity.

A "nearly amputated," badly crushed, or mangled digit, hand, or arm may present a great challenge to good judgment and to the surgeon's technical skill in acting on a decision to attempt salvage. Viable structures and tissues can often be replanted or transferred to give maximal restoration of function, ie, the patient can serve as his or her own "*in vivo* tissue bank" if the surgeon keeps a functionally irretrievable digit or other forearm or hand structure alive, or as a free graft transfer, for use elsewhere in reconstruction.

Indications for Amputation

Irreversible ischemia is the only absolute indication for amputation. The other major indication is where salvage of the digit or part of it will threaten the overall function of the hand, the extremity, or the patient. Such may be the case with an overwhelmingly injured or infected finger that is hopelessly stiff or painful and may jeopardize the function of the other good fingers, or with malignant tumor (eg, malignant melanoma).

Degloving Injuries

These injuries are usually caused by having a ring torn violently from a digit, eg, in falling from a fence and simultaneously hooking the ring on a prong.[13] The skin, fat, and neurovascular bundles are ripped off, and flexor tendons may be avulsed along with the middle and distal phalanges. The other digits are usually not injured. The best treatment is usually to amputate. One has a choice of primary ray amputation through the metacarpal or amputation through the proximal phalanx. Salvage and reconstruction are possible only rarely and often involve a great deal of time, with several major surgical procedures and some jeopardy to the function of adjacent normal digits, as well as marked stiffness of the injured digit.

Amputation of Rays III and IV

Amputation of the long or ring finger causes a gap through which material and liquids in the cupped hand will escape. This gap can be closed by removing the metacarpal at its proximal third (ray resection) and allowing the adjacent metacarpal heads to be approximated; or by the central transplantation of an adjacent osteotomized metacarpal onto the stump of the resected metacarpal (ray transfer). When the index, long, and ring fingers are gone, rotation osteotomy of the fifth metacarpal may be needed so that the small fingertip can comfortably oppose the thumb.

Thumb Amputation

Because most human skills are hampered by loss of part or all of the thumb, preservation, replantation, reconstruction, or replacement of a thumb has great functional merit. The prime objectives are the preservation of length, the proper placement for opposition, and provision of a stable strut against which the fingers can flex with force. Ideally, there should be sensibility where the thumb and fingers meet in pinch, and this can be provided with a neurovascular island pedicle transfer from the least important side of one of the fingers (eg, ulnar side of rays IV, III, or II or radial side of ray V). Not so urgent (but desirable) attainments are motion and power, particularly to control all the planes of movement of the MC joint. If this exists, bone-strutted tube pedicle thumb reconstruction—or a digital transfer (pollicization) on a neurovascular pedicle—can compensate remarkably for any loss. An alternative procedure is the free transfer of the first or second toe.

Management of the Stump

The objective in treating an amputated part is to create a painless stump with soft tissue cover that will meet the functional needs of a patient and will have good sensibility and adequate stability and pliability. Digital amputation will either be transverse or will face obliquely to the dorsal, palmar, radial, or ulnar aspects of the digit. It may involve more than one phalanx.[8]

When sufficient stump cover is not available locally, it must be obtained from grafts and flaps.[11] The most predictable take is achieved by a thin (0.2 to 0.25 mm) split-thickness graft; this should always be the first choice if there is any doubt about blood supply, infection, or joint stiffness. Sutures are not needed except in large grafts; however, initial immobilization and elevation of the wrist as well as the digit are vital in achieving a take of the graft.

Primary and secondary advancement or pedicle grafts should be considered when it is necessary to give better skin cover over palmar-oblique surfaces of all digits, the radial-oblique surface of the fingers, and the ulnar-oblique surface of the thumb[11] when one does not want to shorten digital bone to obtain a transverse amputation surface or when it is necessary to cover the body of the hand.[12] Transverse digital stumps of infants will close by secondary intention with a result equal to or better than what can be achieved by surgery. In case of the body of the hand, vascularized free flaps of muscle or skin are sometimes indicated.

Indications for Replantation[14]

It is feasible to replant (revascularize) all or part of any amputated finger even to the level of the mid-distal phalanx, providing there is not excessive tissue destruction (eg, mangling). This requires intimate familiarity with microvascular techniques.[15] However, replantation may restore tissue perfusion but not always function, and the surgeon must consider each case carefully to decide whether replantation will benefit the patient and whether return of function can be achieved. Some patients may benefit from replantation for cosmetic reasons even if function cannot be restored. Factors to consider are age (especially physiologic age), hand dominance, occupation, social and economic responsibilities, motivation, and ability to undergo the rehabilitative process.

Replantation should never be considered if the patient has severe coexisting injuries (eg, head trauma), significant chronic illness, or life-threatening acute illness, or if the amputated part is excessively crushed or mangled. Replantation should seldom be considered if the patient is over 50 years of age; if the extremity is severely contaminated, was avulsed rather than cut off, or had significant preexisting malfunction; if cooling of the amputated part has been delayed for 6 hours or more; or if only one finger is lost (especially the index which is the most functionally and cosmetically disposable digit).

When the patient is referred to the replantation center, the amputated part should be immediately placed in a dressing inside a waterproof plastic bag that is surrounded with ice (not dry ice). The replantation surgeon should be notified immediately, and the patient should be told that the surgeon will determine the feasibility and advisability of replantation.

Ninety percent of replantations maintain viability. Failures occur in the first 2 weeks (50% in the first 4 to 5 days).[16]

FOREIGN BODIES

Foreign bodies should be removed only if they interfere with function, threaten further tissue injury, cause symptoms or anxiety, or result in dead space or infection. If removal is necessary, it is often facilitated by a period of observation and waiting (eg, 2 to 3 weeks) until congestion and bloody extravasation have cleared. In the meantime, the hand should be initially splinted, elevated, and, in some cases, drained. Prophylactic antibiotics should be given. Roentgenograms are sometimes diagnostic, for certain foreign bodies such as glass and splinters.

WRINGER, CRUSH, AND COMPRESSION INJURIES

In wringer injury, part or all of the extremity is dragged into and compressed by one or more machine-driven rollers. It is common in industries where rolls or sheets of material are drawn between rollers for threading, printing, or compressing purposes or where conveyor belts are used.

The arm is advanced until anatomic obstruction is met. Avulsion of skin and fat or a friction burn of the tissues (or both) may result. The thumb web is the first common obstruction, and the hand skin (more commonly, the loosely fixed dorsal skin) then becomes avulsed or burned. The next obstruction is the elbow, and the last the axilla.

Vessels, nerves, and muscles may be avulsed and bones may be dislocated or broken. The most common unrecognized complication is secondary congestion, which can lead to paralysis and severe muscle fibrosis (eg, Volkmann's contracture) and joint stiffness.

Most patients should be hospitalized, kept flat in bed with the extremity comfortably elevated, and observed hourly. Progressive throbbing pain leading to anesthesia and tightness of the skin and fascia sleeves of the finger, hand, or arm requires longitudinal slitting of skin and fascia. More than one muscle compartment may need decompression, and the pronator teres muscle and transverse carpal ligament must sometimes be sectioned to liberate the median nerve.

Skin avulsed by the wringer is usually in the form of a retrograde flap with imperiled circulation to it. One must judge the color by capillary filling of the flap; if this is poor or absent, debride all the fat from the flap and apply it as a full-thickness graft, or discard it completely in favor of a primary or delayed split-thickness skin graft. In most cases, fractures and dislocations should be reduced and aligned, but the overall circulation of the extremity is of more initial concern than definitive management of specific tissue and structural injuries. Abrasion burns are often third degree and, if so, require debridement and grafting when the integrity of the circulation is restored.

INJECTION INJURIES

These injuries are caused by the sudden introduction of substances under high pressure (ie, hundreds or thousands of pounds per square inch). The substances include air or other gases; liquids such as water, paint, oil, and a host of chemicals in various solutions; and solids and semisolids such as grease and molten plastic. Accordingly, these accidents occur principally in industry. Air pressure hoses in gasoline service stations, aerosol bombs, and sandblast hoses are typical sources of gas-driven injuries. Paint guns, oil and grease guns, and nozzles that inject molten plastic at high temperatures (eg, 260°C [500°F]) are among the most common other sources of these injuries.

The history is the most important clue to the severity of the injury and the need for immediate treatment. While operating a high-pressure device, an individual suddenly feels a strange sensation which ranges from very painful to not painful at all. The patient may present a totally normal appearing hand with perhaps an almost undetectable pinpoint injection site; or the hand may be discolored or pale and cold, and tensely swollen due to the injected material.

Sometimes the injection is limited to a single digit, but often the great pressure forces the material to spread widely throughout the hand and even into the forearm. The greatest problems stem from the following: (1) the chemical irritant effect on all tissues, causing vascular thrombosis and toxic inflammation and necrosis; (2) the primary congestion effect of the material, leading within minutes or hours to secondary congestion due to the inflammatory response, all of which first interrupts microvascular and venous flow and then leads to arterial arrest and gangrene; (3) thermal burns (eg, from hot plastic); and (4) inability to remove enough of the offending material to forestall a short-term or long-term cicatricial foreign body response, which ultimately leads to fibrosis so extensive that it destroys the functions of sensation and mobility.

The examination should include an immediate x-ray to demonstrate, if possible, the distribution of material or gas in the hand; and a careful evaluation of sensibility, tenderness, induration, crepitation, color, temperature, and mobility. All such cases require immediate and continued unrelenting scrutiny, even if the part seems completely normal. With evidence of retained foreign material causing swelling, ischemia, or progressive throbbing pain, the hand must be immediately explored if for no other reason than to release the tourniquet effect of the skin and fascia induced by the congestion. It is impossible to remove all of the foreign material when it is widespread and invasive. As much should be removed as can be done by gentle scraping and teasing—and resecting that which lies in bloodless tissue—as long as one does not further damage the viable tissues to the point of greater congestion or ischemia and interfere with the normal process of demarcation and sequestration.

In addition to appropriate decompression and debridement, the hand must be drained and covered with compresses of zinc oxide, silver sulfadiazine, Ringer's solution, 0.5% silver nitrate solution, or povidone-iodine. The hand must be held in the position of function and elevated, with the patient kept supine. Prophylactic antisludging agents (Dextran 40), corticosteroids, antibiotics, and antitetanus medication must be administered. In most instances, hospitalization is urgent.

The objective is to minimize loss of function, and the most important initial effort must be to preserve circulation and avoid infection. If only one digit is involved and its functional fate is hopeless, amputation may be the most expeditious means of treatment.

RESULTS OF TREATMENT OF TRAUMA TO THE HAND[17]

The factors influencing results after significant trauma to the hand are: (1) age; (2) severity of injury; (3) presence of pre-existing hand disabilities (eg, injury, arthritis, Dupuytren's fascitis, etc; (4) presence of major coexisting health problems, illness or injury affecting total body function; (5) motivation and compliance of the patient; and (6) expertise in clinical management of the hand from beginning to the end of treatment.

Under the age of four compliance is a major handicap after tenorrhaphy, and after the age of forty the propensity for scar formation and joint stiffness makes the prognosis for ideal recovery from musculoskeletal trauma and surgery more guarded.

REHABILITATION

The rehabilitation process should begin the same day the impairment starts. The right-handed patient with an injury causing major irreversible functional impairment to the right hand should begin training to left-handedness on day one, not weeks, months, or years later. From the onset to the finish, when there is full recovery or the degree of impairment is permanent and stationary, no single phase of the treatment process is more important than another.

The personnel who are most qualified to help in the rehabilitative process of the patient with the hand problems are those who have had specialized, in-depth training and whose prime, if not only, professional effort is limited to the discipline of hand care. Even though they may subspecialize (eg, the surgeon caring mostly for rheumatoid afflictions vs trauma, or the therapist having a particular expertise for tailoring splints vs massage and passive exercise), they should all be well-versed in the total spectrum of hand problems, their treatments, and the reactions of patients to their problems and their treatments. Furthermore, in this day and age, when the cost of hand disability and medical care has become so staggering, they must keep a watchful eye on the clock, the calendar and the cost. The surgeon should be good at what he does. He should teach the patient well, remember that simplicity is generally predictable and less costly, and complexity unpredictable and expensive. Finally, he should communicate, get all the facts, and when good treatment has reached an impasse in altering function, be able to stop it so that the patient can get on with life the way it is.

REFERENCES

1. Boyes JH. *On the Shoulders of Giants*. Philadelphia, Pa: JB Lippincott; 1976.
2. Bunnell S, ed. *Hand Surgery in World War II*. Washington, DC: Office of the Surgeon General; 1955. Department of the Army.
3. Bunnell S. *Surgery of the Hand*. Philadelphia, Pa: JB Lippincott; 1944.
4. Kilgore ES Jr, Graham WP III. *The Hand: Surgical and Nonsurgical Management*. Philadelphia, Pa: Lea & Febiger; 1977.
5. Buck-Grameko D, Hoffman R, Neumann R. *Hand Trauma: A Practical Guide*. New York, NY: Thieme Medical Publishers; 1986.
6. Marin-Braun F. Primary repair of extensor tendons with associated postoperative mobilization. *Plast Reconstr Surg*. 1990;86:615.
7. Newport ML, Blair WR, Steyers CM Jr. Long-term results of extensor tendon repair. *J Hand Surg*. 1990; 15A:961.
8. Potenza AD. Philosophy of flexor tendon surgery. *Orthop Clin North Am*. 1986;17:349.
9. Hunter JM, et al. *Rehabilitation of the Hand*. 2nd ed. St. Louis, Mo: CV Mosby; 1984.
10. Fess EE, Gettle KS, Strickland JW. *Hand Splinting: Principles and Methods*. St. Louis, Mo: CV Mosby; 1981.
11. Cook FW. Local neurovascular island flap. *J Hand Surg*. 1990;15A:798.
12. Quaba AA, Davison PM. A distally based dorsal hand flap. *Br J Plast Surg*. 1990;43:28.
13. Baek SM. A clinical study of degloving injuries of the hand. *Plast Reconstr Surg*. 1990;86:1247.
14. Kleinert HE, Jablon M, Tsai TM. An overview of replantation and results in 347 replants in 245 patients. *J Trauma*. 1980;20:390.
15. O'Brien BMcC. Reconstructive microsurgery of the upper extremity. *J Hand Surg*. 1990;15A:317.
16. Hetland VR. Functional results following hand replantation. *Acta Orthop Scand*. 1988;59(suppl 227):81.
17. Conolly WD, Kilgore ES. *Hand Injuries and Infections*. Chicago, Ill: Year Book Medical Publishers; 1979.

13

Pelvis Fractures

JAMES P. KENNEDY, M.D.

HISTORY: Pelvic fractures are a result of high energy directed against the pelvis. Joseph François Malgaigne, in his classic fracture text of 1847, "Traité des Fractures et des Luxations,"[24] stated that these injuries occurred from direct forces such as crushing of the pelvis between two carriages or from a wheel passing over the hip region. Just as the automobile has replaced the horse as a means of transportation, it has also replaced the carriage as the source of pelvis fractures.[25]

Early authors noted a high incidence of chronic pain following the standard nonoperative treatment of many pelvic fractures.[36] Mortality was high. Holdsworth first noted in 1948 that retroperitoneal hemorrhage was a major source of mortality and morbidity in these injuries.[15] He felt that hemorrhage was due to tearing of the iliolumbar artery, and noted hemorrhage "severe enough to cause alarm" in 16% of patients and an 8% mortality rate. Holdsworth recommended transfusing only enough blood to prevent hemorrhagic shock, but keeping the blood pressure not more than 100 mm Hg as his opinion was that there was no possibility of controlling the hemorrhage by surgery or pressure.

Sir Astley Cooper first suggested pelvic slings in his text of 1842 as a means of treatment of these major pelvic fractures,[9] a method later perfected by Böhler.[2] With this technique, the patient's pelvis was placed in a stout canvas sling. Ropes were attached to the sling with the ropes from the right side crossing over to be suspended on the left side of the patient, and vice versa so that the compression from the sling closed the pelvis. Sufficient weight was applied to the ropes to just lift the patient off the bed with the sling. Immobilization was maintained for 12 weeks. Pelvic sling treatment was still being advocated as late as 1973.[16]

Sir Reginald Watson-Jones[34] suggested another method of lateral recumbency and plaster. The lateral decubitus position was used to reduce the fracture by gravity. The fracture was then held in plaster. In practice, however, this method was somewhat cumbersome for nursing care.

Due to the extended length of bed rest required by both these latter two methods, a high rate of morbidity can be expected especially in the multiple trauma patient. In an attempt to more rapidly mobilize the patient with multiple injuries, alternative methods of treatment were sought.

The external fixator was first postulated for use in unstable pelvic fractures by Carabalona in 1973.[7] As will be discussed, this is a useful technique for rapid stabilization of the pelvis if the patient cannot undergo immediate internal stabilization, but a period of up to three weeks of bed rest can still be required if the external fixator is to be used as definitive treatment.[32] Not all fractures are amenable to treatment with an external fixator alone, and may need skeletal traction for a period of up to six weeks as well.

Only in the recent decades has the concept of operative reduction and fixation been extended to pelvic fractures to provide immediate stabilization and mobilization for these injuries. Levine[19] reported the first case of open reduction and internal plate and screw fixation of a fracture of the pelvis and acetabulum in 1943 for a fracture which was irreducible either by traction or transrectal manipulation. Although a good result was obtained, this method of treatment was used sporadically and only in isolated instances. In the 1960s, when the Judet brothers and Letournel published their results of open reduction and internal fixation which they had been doing routinely since the mid-1950s,[17] this technique became widely accepted.

INTRODUCTION

Pelvis fractures can vary tremendously in severity, treatment, and prognosis. They range from minor fractures which are treated symptomatically without even the need for hospitalization to severe major pelvic ring disruptions that may need emergent stabilization as a life-saving measure.

Pelvic fractures are common in the high-energy multiple trauma victim. They constitute 3% of all skeletal fractures.[35] Two thirds of all pelvic fractures are the result of auto accidents.[28] The incidence of pelvic fractures in fatal motor vehicle accidents is as high as 24%,[30] and approaches 50% for fatal pedestrian accidents.[4] Patients suffering from blunt trauma who have a Glasgow Coma Score of 10 or less show a 10% incidence of major pelvic fracture.[21] Due to this significant incidence, an AP pelvic x-ray is required in the initial evaluation of all trauma victims, regardless of mechanism of injury.[31]

ANATOMY

In order to withstand the forces of bearing the weight of the body in an upright posture, the pelvis has developed into a stable construct of the two innominate bones and sacrum joined together by strong ligaments forming a ring structure. The most significant ligaments are the posterior complex (Fig. 13–1) consisting of the iliolumbar, sacrotuberous, sacrospinous, and posterior sacroiliac ligaments.[33] The anterior sacroiliac ligament (Fig. 13–2) is functionally less important. Avulsion fractures of the bone at the site of attachment of any of these ligaments imply incompetence of the ligament, and often major pelvic instability.[23]

The sacroiliac ligament, the strongest ligament in the body,[29] serves to tie the sacrum into the pelvic ring. The posterior portion of the ligament resists internal rotation (Fig. 13–3), while the anterior complex helps resist pelvic external rotation or "springing" open of the pelvis. The iliolumbar ligament enhances the stability of the pelvis and sacrum to the lumbar spine by preventing cephalad-caudad shift of the hemipelvis. The sacrotuberous ligament also prevents this instability from vertical shear along with the iliolumbar ligament (Fig. 13–4).

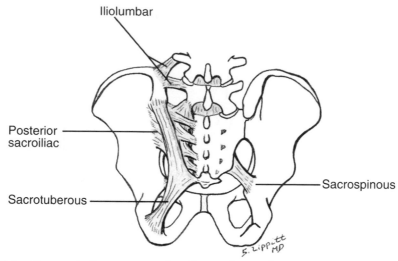

Figure 13–1. The posterior ligamentous complex. The posterior sacroiliac ligament is the prime stabilizer of the pelvis. The iliolumbar, sacrospinous, and sacrotuberous ligaments also contribute to pelvic stability.

Arranged at a 90° orientation to the sacrotuberous ligament, the sacrospinous ligaments prevent external rotation and springing open of the pelvis along with the weaker anterior sacroiliac complex (Fig. 13–5).

It can be trying to accurately assess the stability of pelvic fractures due to the difficulty of appreciating the three-dimensional complex structure of the pelvis on plain films which are often further obscured by overlying bowel shadows. An understanding of the bony and

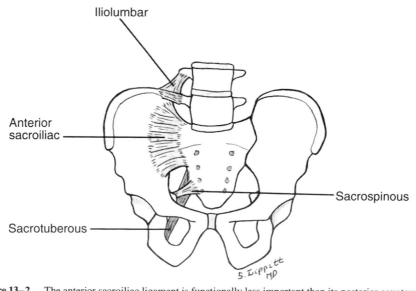

Figure 13–2. The anterior sacroiliac ligament is functionally less important than its posterior counterpart. Also illustrated are the sacrotuberous and sacrospinous ligaments as visualized from the front.

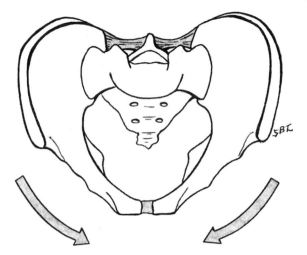

Figure 13–3. The posterior sacroiliac ligament resists internal rotation of the pelvis in lateral compression injuries.

ligamentous interaction in pelvic stability as well as how these structures fail when stressed will help to avoid missing pelvic injuries and in recognizing stable versus unstable patterns.

A final concept to remember is that the pelvis is a ring structure, and in order to have a disruption in one area, it is necessary to have a second failure elsewhere.[23] This can be likened to a pretzel, which also fails in more than one place when broken. This second

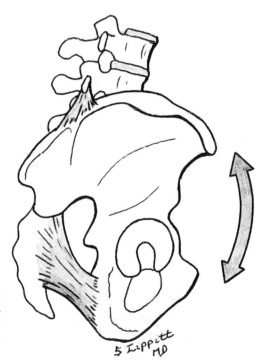

Figure 13–4. The sacrotuberous and iliolumbar ligaments, due to their cephaladcaudad orientation, resist vertical forces. If these ligaments fail secondary to vertical shearing forces, an unstable Malgaigne injury may result.

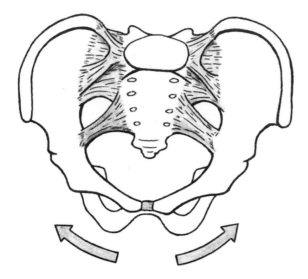

Figure 13–5. The anterior sacroiliac ligaments and sacrospinous ligaments, due to their horizontal orientation, resist external rotation or springing open of the pelvis. An anterior compression injury may lead to failure of these structures.

lesion may not be evident on x-ray, as the second "break" is often a ligamentous tear. Two studies have proven undetected posterior injuries occurred in every case of an anterior fracture when evaluated by bone scan[12] or at autopsy.[5]

PHYSICAL EXAM

The physical exam of pelvis injuries is directed primarily toward 1) localization and characterization of pain, and therefore that of the injury, 2) the neurologic exam, 3) the assessment of nonorthopaedic injuries to the region associated with or that affect the treatment of a pelvis disruption, and 4) inspection of the skin and soft tissues about the region.

The rigid ring structure of the pelvis has a propensity for hidden injury posteriorly. In the cooperative patient, it is very easy to slide an examining hand between the patient and the bed posteriorly to check for tenderness in the sacral and perisacral areas. Posterior pain provides presumptive evidence of a posterior injury. When performed early before swelling occurs, gentle palpation at the pubic symphysis, the sacroiliac joint, or at fracture sites may reveal gaps diagnostic of an unstable situation.

The pelvis should be gently stressed to assess instability. In the conscious patient, it is not necessary to attempt to demonstrate gross movement which is very painful. Stressing in this circumstance is purely to locate the site of injury by localizing pain. When suspicions of a posterior injury are aroused, appropriate x-rays are obtained to confirm the injury and to investigate the pelvis for instability. Once the patient is under anesthetic, more vigorous stressing can be done to demonstrate the degree of instability if needed.

A crucial part of the physical exam is the neurovascular assessment. The incidence of neurologic injury is high, as 5% of patients with pelvic fractures are left with permanent neurologic sequelae.[10] Nerve injury is seen especially with fractures of the sacral ala entering into the sacral foraminae or with fractures entering into the sciatic notch. The presence of a sciatic palsy should encourage early reduction and fixation to decompress the sciatic nerve when fractures into the sciatic notch are displaced. The sciatic nerve will often be found tented over a displaced fracture fragment or even caught between fracture fragments at the disrupted sciatic notch. A rectal exam is necessary to assess the lower sacral roots for damage.

Examination of the pelvic contents is directed not only to the diagnosis and treatment of genitourinary and rectal injury; but also toward how these injuries will affect the treatment of the pelvic fracture. Injury to these structures in communication with the fracture results in an open pelvic fracture.

Occult open fractures are characterized by hidden urethral tears, vaginal or perineal laceration, or rectal tears. Blood at the meatus is presumptive for a urethral injury. In the presence of blood at the meatus or an injury pattern involving the pubic area placing the urogenital structures at risk, a retrograde urethrogram is performed before attempting to pass a Foley catheter. An undiagnosed partial urethral tear may be converted to a complete tear by the catheter. The rectal exam demonstrating a high-riding prostate is also diagnostic. If no urethral damage is present, the Foley may be passed. When a tear is found, a suprapubic cystostomy may be necessary. In the patient requiring an anterior approach for internal fixation, it must be done at the time of the cystostomy. If not, the region will be contaminated by the cystostomy precluding approach from this direction at a later date.

In the female, blood at the urethra or vagina is presumptive for an occult open fracture as well. In these instances, speculum exam of the vagina is required to rule out vaginal laceration. A cystogram will evaluate the urethra, although due to a shorter urethra, urethral injuries in females are rare.[28]

If blood is found on the examining finger during the rectal exam to assess rectal tone and evaluate the prostate, sigmoidoscopy will confirm any injury and demonstrate the degree of rectal laceration present.

Last, but of great importance during the physical exam, is inspection of the skin. This is the step most frequently forgotten or ignored. The patient must be log-rolled to adequately inspect both the spine and sacral regions looking for areas of abrasion, laceration, or contusion. Surgical approaches may need to be planned about such areas to avoid subsequent wound healing problems. This is especially true posteriorly. The sacral area is often contused and hemorrhagic. Commonly, the soft tissues have been sheared off the bone from the force of the injury. Operative exposures posteriorly in these instances are in great danger of leading to flap necrosis and sloughing.

Radiography

In assessing the personality of a pelvic fracture, adequate x-rays must be obtained to diagnose the fracture pattern. This, coupled with the physical exam, will determine whether a stable or unstable pattern exists. Standard pelvic films alone can give an 88% accurate diagnosis of pelvic instability,[11] and when combined with the physical exam and stress films, accuracy should be greater than 95%. The stability of the pelvis along with the patient's overall condition dictates the type of treatment necessary for the fracture.

X-rays not only identify the fracture pattern but will help in assessing the stability of the injury. A single AP pelvis film is obtained in all patients who are victims of significant trauma as a matter of protocol[21]—the same as obtaining a cervical spine series. The AP pelvis will identify fractures and can also demonstrate ligamentous avulsions that contribute to instability (Fig. 13–6).

If a fracture is identified, Judet views taken at 45° of obliquity bilaterally may be helpful. Although most useful with acetabular fractures, they can further delineate the pattern of the pelvic fracture as well. The iliac oblique view shows the posterior column and the obturator oblique shows the anterior column of the pelvis (see Chapter 14).

When a sacroiliac complex injury is suspected, SI films can be helpful to compare widening of the injured joint with the normal joint. Widening also will be seen incidentally on the Judet obturator oblique view. The CT scan (Fig. 13–7) will confirm the amount of SI joint widening and is the definitive test for quantification and cases of questionable widening on plain films.

Perhaps of most importance in evaluating stability of the SI joints are the pelvic inlet and outlet views. Since the sacrum is positioned obliquely in the body, fractures of the sacroiliac area can be significantly displaced but the displacement may not be demonstrated on the AP view. As the superior end plate of the sacrum is inclined at an angle of 30° to 40°,[28] the inlet view, directed from the patient's head to the pelvis and taken at an angle of 60° from vertical[29] will approximate a perpendicular to this surface. This view then will show anterior and posterior shift of the hemipelvis in relation to the sacrum (Fig. 13–8). Likewise, the pelvic outlet view taken at an angle of 45° from the foot of the patient gives a true AP view of the sacrum and will demonstrate any cephalad-caudad migration (Fig. 13–9).

Significant pelvic instability is present with sacroiliac joint widening of greater than 1 cm, a pubic diastasis of greater than 2.5 cm (Fig. 13–10), sacral or iliac fractures showing

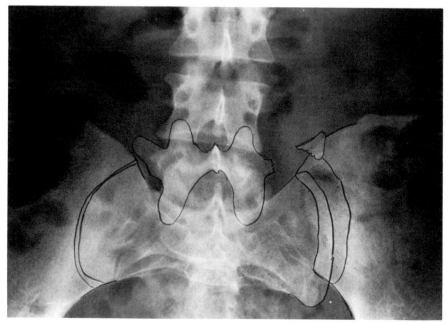

Figure 13–6.   AP x-ray of SI complex. Note left sacroiliac joint widening and vertical shift with associated L-5 transverse process avulsion fracture indicating an unstable injury pattern.

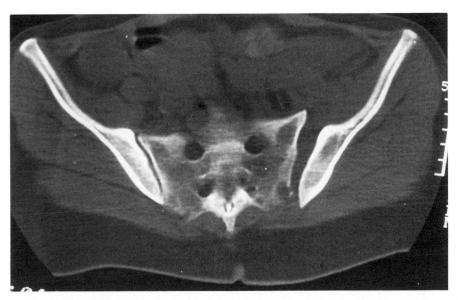

Figure 13–7. CT scan demonstrating widening of right SI joint. The anterior sacroiliac ligament has failed in tension first, the injury then continued posteriorly. Note the large hematoma present in the iliacus and psoas.

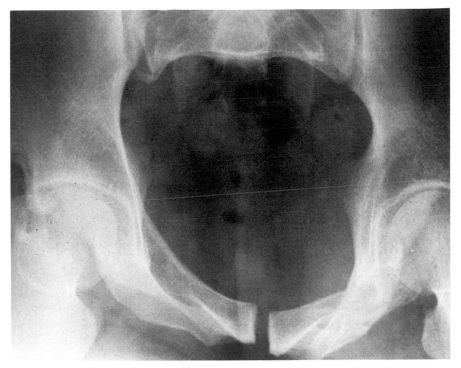

Figure 13–8. Inlet view. Note posterior displacement of right hemipelvis and opening of SI joint. The right pubic ramus is also correspondingly posteriorly displaced.

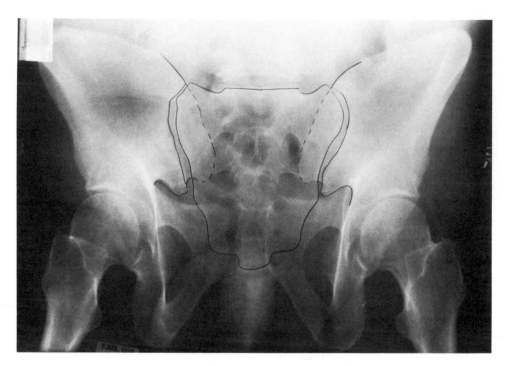

Figure 13–9.   Outlet view. Any cephalad-caudad migration of the sacrum would be evident on this view.

a diastasis of greater than 0.5 cm, or a vertical shear fracture with cephalad/caudad migration of greater than 0.5 cm[6,11,33] (Fig. 13–11A–C, Table 13–1). If the tell-tale avulsion fractures indicative of ligamentous failure are present, lesser displacements are considered unstable as the avulsion fractures indicate that greater displacement than what is evident on the x-ray occurred at the time of injury. Soft tissue recoil then allowed relaxation of the pelvis into its current position. This instability can be documented with stress films.

If there is still a question of instability based on the physical examination, CT, and plain films, stress films under anesthesia can be obtained. When stressing the pelvis, the mechanism of injury and the fracture pattern will direct the appropriate application of the stress. Fractures which fail in vertical shear can be assessed with push-pull films. An AP pelvis or outlet view is obtained with an assistant maximally pushing on the foot of the injured side with an axially directed force while pulling the foot on the uninjured side for counter-resistance. A second film is obtained by reversing the maneuver and pulling on the injured foot and pushing on the uninjured side. The hemipelvis is then evaluated for cephalad-caudad movement by comparing the two films (Fig. 13–12A–C).

"Open book" type pelvis fractures generally are already maximally opened in the supine position by the forces of gravity, but may be accentuated by frogging the leg into the figure-4 position and applying an additional vertically directed force on the bent knee to externally rotate the hip. An AP film will document the amount of opening produced. The corresponding reduction film can be obtained by an AP film taken with the patient in the

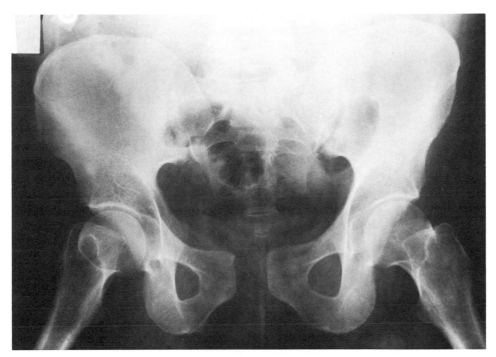

Figure 13–10. Ligamentous disruption of symphysis pubis leading to an unstable diastasis.

lateral decubitus position. The force of gravity then acts to reduce the fracture. Significant shifting as already described is indicative of an unstable pattern.

A CT scan will probably best demonstrate the pattern of difficult fractures not well characterized by routine films in the complex three-dimensional structure of the pelvis. This is especially true of the sacrum where lateral compression ala fractures can remain hidden on plain films (Fig. 13–13). If necessary for selected fractures, reconstruction in the sagittal plane or three-dimensional reconstructions can be helpful as well.

MINOR FRACTURES

Minor pelvic fractures include those fractures of the bony pelvis which do not affect the stability or integrity of the pelvic ring and the tendon avulsion fractures. The minor fractures are usually seen as isolated low-energy injuries, but can also occur in the polytrauma patient.

Isolated rami fractures (Fig. 13–14) are often the result of a fall in the elderly, and can be treated symptomatically with bed rest and progressive assisted ambulation as tolerated. Rami fractures routinely heal without further sequelae.

When the injury is the result of high energy, it is important to make sure that the rami fractures are not associated with a major pelvic ring disruption. In the cooperative patient, physical exam will suffice to rule out a major pelvic fracture by localizing other areas of pain toward which to direct the radiographic exam, or by demonstrating instability. If an

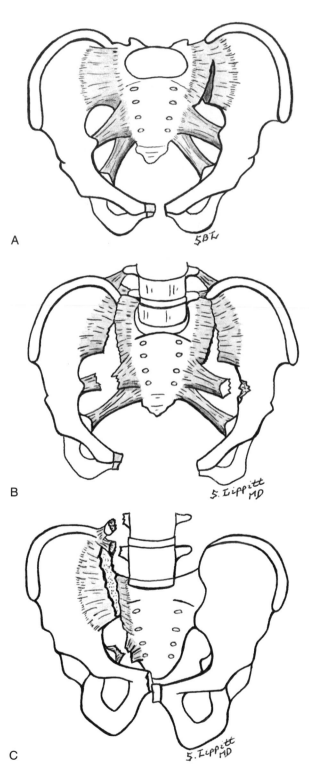

Figure 13–11. **A:** A stable anterior compression pelvis injury resulting from tearing of the anterior sacroiliac ligament and demonstrating mild widening of the pubis. **B:** An unstable anterior compression injury (the "Open Book" injury). More significant tearing of the anterior sacroiliac and sacrospinous ligaments with gross widening at the pubis. Note avulsion fracture of left ischial spine proving failure of sacrospinous ligament. **C:** Vertically unstable pelvis injury. Failure of iliolumbar and sacrotuberous ligaments. Note avulsion of lumbar transverse processes.

Table 13–1 Pelvic Instability

SI joint widening	1.0 cm
Pubic diastasis	2.5 cm
Iliac or sacral fracture widening	0.5 cm
Vertical displacement (Malgaigne)	0.5 cm

adequate physical exam cannot be obtained, further radiologic studies such as stress films or a CT may be required.

The second type of minor pelvic fracture is tendon avulsion fractures, which are to be distinguished from the destabilizing ligamentous avulsions already described. Although usually found in adolescent athletes, tendon avulsions can be seen in accident victims secondary to forceful muscle contractures which occur at the time of injury in an attempt to avoid or protect one's self from impact. The three types are hamstring avulsions off the ischial tuberosity, sartorius avulsion off the anterior superior iliac spine, and rectus femoris avulsions from the anterior inferior iliac spine (Fig. 13–15).

The isolated tendon avulsion fracture presents with symptoms consistent with a muscle pull or strain. Localized pain, swelling, and spasm of the involved muscles may be found. Passive stretching or attempted active contraction of the attached muscle will exacerbate the symptoms.

The majority of these avulsions are small and treatment for these injuries is sympto-

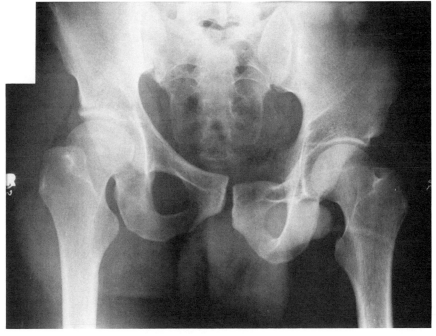

A

Figure 13–12. Push-pull views to demonstrate pelvic instability. **A:** Push view showing significant vertical displacement of right hemipelvis through SI joint and pubis of 0.8 cm. (Figure continued on next page)

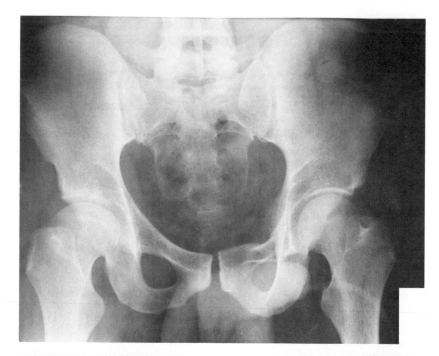

B

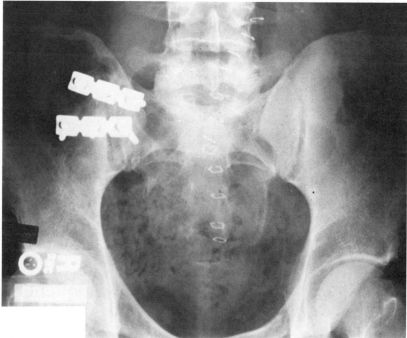

C

Figure 13–12, cont.   B: Pull view results in anatomic reduction. **C:** Surgical stabilization by anterior plates across SI joint in reduced position. (Surgical staples are from an exploratory laparotomy, not the surgical approach to the SI joint.)

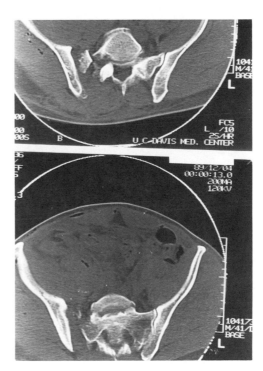

Figure 13–13. CT scan of lateral compression injury. The right sacral ala has been compressed.

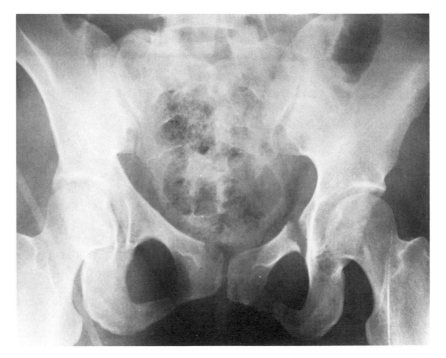

Figure 13–14. Isolated left superior and inferior pubic rami fractures, the result of a lateral compression injury.

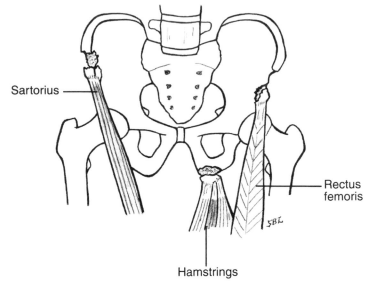

Figure 13–15.   Minor avulsion fractures from tendinous pull-offs of the rectus femoris, sartorius, and hamstring muscles.

matic. Crutch ambulation with weight bearing as tolerated, anti-inflammatories, and analgesics are helpful. Once these injuries have healed, either with bony or fibrous union, a period of muscle strengthening and stretching will help in the rehabilitative process. The athlete, especially, should be instructed in a muscle stretching routine prior to activity to prevent recurrent injury. Internal fixation may be considered for large avulsion fractures to hasten healing and recovery. These larger avulsions are rare.

Isolated fractures of the iliac wing (Duverney's fracture), although painful, are usually well stabilized by the surrounding muscles (Fig. 13–16). These require only symptomatic treatment until healed unless they are large or significantly displaced.

MAJOR PELVIC FRACTURES

A major pelvic fracture is one that disrupts the integrity of the pelvic ring such that the pelvis cannot continue to function in its capacity of transferring the forces from the trunk and upper body into the lower limbs to allow locomotion. Due to its weight bearing function, the integrity of the pelvis is ideally restored to prevent alteration of the biomechanical forces into the lower extremity. If either the direction or the magnitude of these forces are altered, the abnormal stresses can lead to chronic pain or posttraumatic arthritis.

Major pelvic fractures are the result of high energy trauma and are usually seen due to automobile or motorcycle accidents, falls from heights, or as a result of crushing from machinery. Due to the high energy associated with each of these mechanisms, major pelvic fractures are associated with an 85% incidence of other musculoskeletal injury as well as a significant incidence (Table 13–2) of injury to other body systems.

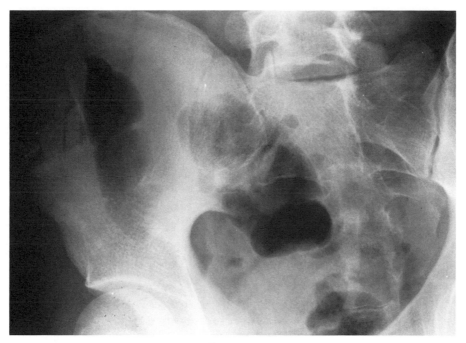

Figure 13–16.   Isolated iliac wing fracture (Duverney's fracture) of upper outer quadrant of right iliac crest.

TYPES OF FRACTURE

A complete description of the various types of fractures is beyond the scope of this chapter, but a brief mention of the classification systems will permit familiarization with the various possibilities for fracture. Fractures can be described either by their anatomic location or by their mechanism of occurrence.

Anatomically, fractures may involve the iliac wing, sacrum, the anterior or posterior columns of the innominate bone, or the pubic rami. Ligamentous injuries can lead to diastasis, subluxation, or dislocation of the sacroiliac joints or pubic symphysis.

Mechanistically, fractures occur from lateral compression, anterior-posterior compression, or from vertical shear forces across the pelvic ring. Combination and rotational injuries are also seen. The lateral compression injury is essentially an internal rotation injury causing the pelvic ring to collapse inwardly upon itself. Lateral compression injuries

Table 13–2   Associated Injuries with Major Pelvic Fractures[8]

Musculoskeletal	85%
Respiratory	60%
CNS	40%
Abdominal	30%
Genitourinary	12%
Cardiovascular	6%

(Fig. 13–21, page 234) are characterized by pubic rami fractures and anterior compression of the iliac wing, sacroiliac joint, or sacral ala (Figs. 13–13, 13–17). These injuries are often stable due to bony impaction and interdigitation of the fracture fragments.

External rotation characterizes the anterior compression injury causing the pelvic ring to spring open. This is the familiar "open book" type of injury where there is a pubic symphysis diastasis associated with a failure of the anterior sacroiliac ligaments in tension (Fig. 13–11B).

The Malgaigne fracture is a result of vertical shear. Malgaigne[22] noted that in these injuries, one hemipelvis has been disrupted from the other by a vertically directed force (Figure 13–11C). In his series, this occurred most commonly due to a fall from a height where the patient landed more on one foot than the other. The failure can be ligamentous through the pubic symphasis and sacroiliac joints, bony through the rami and sacral ala or iliac wing, or as a result of a combination of bony and ligamentous injuries. The injury pattern may be ipsilateral (Fig. 13–18), or the superior and inferior injury may be on contralateral sides.

PRINCIPLES OF EVALUATION AND MANAGMENT

Patients with major pelvic fractures must be entered into the algorithm used for polytrauma victims. Due to the high incidence of other system trauma already mentioned, an overall mortality rate of 10% is found in pelvic fractures.[33] Thus, injuries in other areas must be

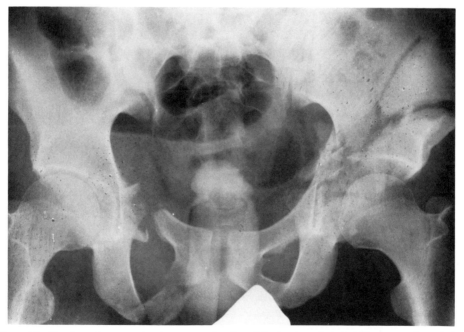

Figure 13–17. Lateral compression fracture entering the pelvic ring through the left iliac crest and acetabulum, and exiting through the right pubic and ischial rami.

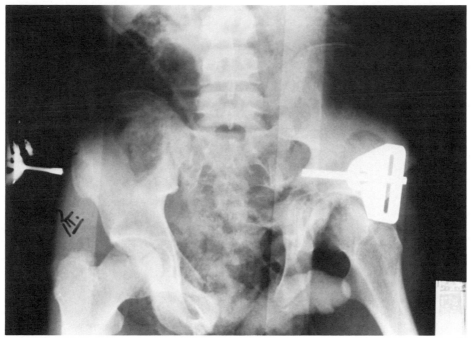

Figure 13–18. Vertically unstable Malgaigne injuries. Ligamentous instability through left SI joint and pubis. The left iliac crest has been shifted from its normal position at the L-4/5 disc space to the L-3/4 disc space. This injury was Grade III open. The patient also suffered testicular avulsions, a left traumatic above knee amputation as well as multiple chest and abdominal injuries from a high speed motorcycle injury. He expired due to massive hemorrhage from his injuries.

actively sought for and ruled out. Simultaneously with the resuscitation of the patient and assessment and management of other system trauma, the orthopaedist can begin the assessment of the "personality" of the pelvic fracture. That is, is it a stable or unstable configuration? Does the pelvis need immediate stabilization or should it be managed on a delayed basis? Is the fracture pattern conducive to internal or external fixation?

Insert a Foley catheter initially to help in fluid management and also to decompress the bladder for any anterior approach to the pelvis. As there is a high incidence of genitourinary damage found in pelvis fractures, standard protocols are followed for bladder and urethral evaluation.[1]

Often, these patients will require laparotomy for internal injuries. If so, a retroperitoneal pelvic hematoma may be found. The hematoma is be left undisturbed to allow retroperitoneal tamponade. Violating the retroperitoneum may allow venous decompression and possible uncontrollable bleeding into the abdomen. The pelvic retroperitoneal space is entered through the abdomen only if the pelvis needs exploration and ligation of vessels for uncontrollable arterial bleeding, as will be outlined below.

When a laparotomy is being performed it is important to coordinate the general and orthopaedic surgeries so that the placement of the incisions, drains, suprapubic catheters, or colostomies do not compromise the operative approach to the pelvis or application of an external fixator.

Volume loss from hemorrhage into the pelvis can be phenomenal. Blood loss of 2 to 10 units is common, and up to 20 units loss may occur, resulting in up to 40% of patients requiring transfusion.[28] The size of the hematoma can easily be appreciated on CT scan or by displacement of the bladder on plain films. Bleeding occurs primarily from the exposed cancellous bone of the fracture surfaces, as well as from torn or lacerated veins. Arterial sources are less commonly present.

Low pressure bleeding from venous and bone sources will generally tamponade itself from the accumulating hematoma. Because of the vast venous plexuses in the pelvis, it is difficult to find and control the source of the bleeding.

Minor arterial bleeders, unless a coagulapathy is present, will tamponade or usually stop spontaneously. If significant bleeding continues and does not tamponade due to a peritoneal laceration, arteriography can locate the source and moderately sized vessels such as the gluteals can be embolized to control the hemorrhage. Laceration of the larger iliac or femoral vessels will require exploration and repair. If critical arterial branches are ligated, embolized, or lost through the injury itself, the operative approach must be carefully planned to ensure that adequate blood supply to the skin flaps remain to prevent slough.[3,26]

Cancellous bone oozing is the major contributor to blood loss from pelvic fractures. Large volume losses from bleeding at the fracture site are generally found in the unstable fracture patterns. For this reason, early reduction and stabilization of the fracture can significantly contribute to hemostasis and hemodynamic stability. A three-inch pelvic diastasis will double the volume of the pelvis. Reducing the pelvic fracture will decrease the pelvic volume available for hematoma, and will contribute to the tamponade effect. Reduction also keeps the blood within the intraosseous venous plexuses, "closing the door" on the escape of the blood out of the vascular system.

Following fluid resuscitation and the removal of a MAST suit, should one have been used for initial stabilization, the application of a pelvic external fixator is the next step for uncontrollable pelvic blood loss.[29] For the patient who is exsanguinating, rapid reduction and stabilization of the pelvis can be performed through the application of an anterior pelvic external fixator as a life-saving measure. Although it will biomechanically stabilize only the anterior compression injuries or "sprung pelvis," the "ex fix" will provisionally stabilize any fracture sufficiently well to help control hemorrhage. It can then be replaced if necessary with more definitive stabilization procedures once the patient can tolerate such surgery. The ex fix has the advantage of rapid, simple application, and can even be inserted in the well-equipped emergency department for the patient in extremis.

With this approach, the majority of pelvic bleeding problems can be controlled. Only when these methods fail will embolization or exploration of vessels be necessary.

OPEN PELVIC FRACTURES

Open pelvic fractures are devastating injuries (Fig. 13–19). The mortality for open fractures remains high. Traditionally, mortality has been reported in the range of 50%,[27,28] due primarily to massive hemorrhage and late sepsis.[18] Recent reports are suggesting that with modern aggressive resuscitation and fracture management techniques, this rate may be decreasing to around 35%.[13,14] The mortality for near amputation injuries where avulsion of the sciatic nerve, lumbosacral plexus, and iliac vessels with significant muscle tearing

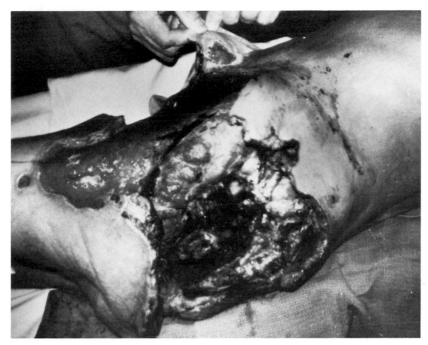

Figure 13–19. Massive open pelvis fracture with Grade IIIb wound of left buttock, sacrum, and perineum.

and a grossly unstable fracture occurs, is much higher, approaching 100%. In such cases, an immediate hemipelvectomy may be required as a life-saving measure.[20]

Open fractures of the pelvis may be obvious or occult. There is no difficulty in diagnosing the obvious open fracture with a perineal or pelvic wound that is grossly hemorrhaging. It is the occult open fracture that must be ruled out through careful examination of the genitourinary system and rectum so that it is not missed and treated as a closed fracture.

When either an obvious or occult open fracture is present, the patient is entered into the open fracture protocol with intravenous antibiotics and aggressive irrigation and debridement (see Chapter 7). Rectal and vaginal lacerations are classified and treated as Grade III injuries regardless of the size of the laceration due to the bacterial contamination in these areas. Open fractures involving the perineum, vagina, or rectum require a diverting colostomy to prevent further contamination of the wounds. Following irrigation and debridement, the pelvis can be temporarily stabilized by an external fixator (Fig. 13–20) or skeletal traction with a tibial pin for grossly contaminated wounds in which immediate internal fixation is not appropriate (Fig. 13–22).

Depending on the type of wound and fracture pattern, some provisional internal stabilization may be done in noncontaminated areas. Definitive internal fixation can be completed at a later date once the wounds are closed and clean if the patient survives, although the fracture may be healed by the time these often large wounds are closed. In addition to dressing changes, betadine whirlpools are helpful in cleaning the wounds if the patient can tolerate them.

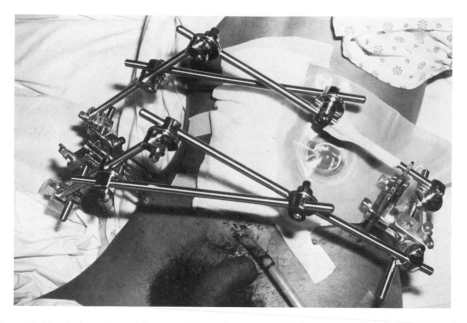

Figure 13–20. Patient with a pelvic external fixator for an open pelvic fracture not permitting internal fixation. Note colostomy to divert fecal flow from open wound, and suprapubic catheter for bladder injury.

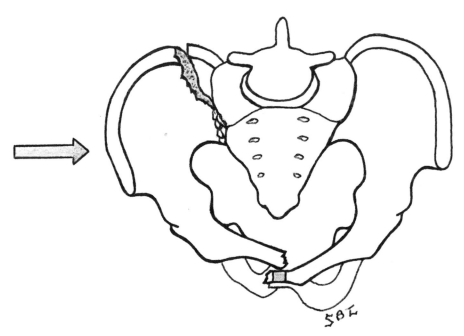

Figure 13–21. Fracture resulting from lateral compression injury of the pelvis.

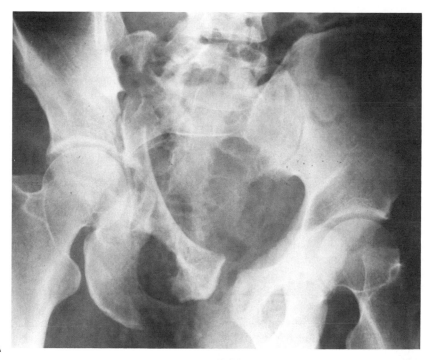

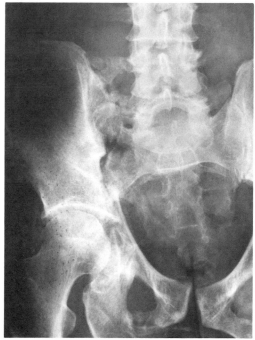

Figure 13–22.   A: Patient with vertically unstable open right Malgaigne injury. The injury passes through the SI joint, and exits through a transverse acetabular fracture and fracture through the ischial ramus. The L-4 and L-5 transverse processes were also avulsed. **B:** Following 12 weeks in skeletal traction, the hemipelvis has healed in a reduced position. Note bony bridging from the iliac wing to the avulsed transverse processes.

A

B

Specific Fracture Treatment

Stable fracture patterns may be treated with a short period of bedrest followed by rapid mobilization to a chair and ambulation as comfort allows. Unstable fractures require stabilization for two reasons. By being able to mobilize the patient with a stabilized fracture, morbidity and mortality during the recovery period are minimized. Treatment of pelvic fractures by bedrest and traction produced a mortality rate of nearly 90% in the 1890s. Surgical stabilization techniques being used today allow rapid mobilization of the patient so that "fracture disease" complications like venous thrombosis, pulmonary embolus, and respiratory distress syndrome are avoided. With this type of treatment, mortality following pelvic fractures has fallen to the rate of 5% to 20% which is being reported today.[28]

Unstable fractures which are not operatively stabilized will have a high rate of complications at long term follow-up as well, with almost one third complaining of posterior pain.[10] More severe unstable fractures can have up to a 50% incidence of chronic pain, 32% incidence of limp, and 21% incidence of motor weakness.[14] An additional benefit from stabilization of the fracture is that the patient's pain during recovery is rapidly and significantly decreased.

As the techniques for internal fixation improve, external fixation is being used less and less for fracture fixation with the exceptions of emergency provisional stabilization for the patient who is actively hemorrhaging and for open fractures. With the understanding of the mechanism of pelvic fractures, only those patients with anteriorly unstable injuries can be treated definitively with an external fixator. Posteriorly unstable injuries are not adequately controlled, and may indeed be further displaced by an external fixator.

The philosophy of internal fixation of pelvic fractures has also changed. More and more fracture patterns are being successfully fixed internally. Until recently, it was recommended that operation be carried out 5 to 7 days following injury to allow the hematoma to stabilize.[28,29] At the University of California, Davis Medical Center, early internal plate and screw fixation of unstable pelvic fractures is standard care, and in our hands this treatment gives the best overall results (Fig. 13–23).

Fractures in multiple trauma victims who are hemodynamically stable are operatively stabilized upon presentation—within the first 12 hours in most cases. The cell saver is used to cut down on transfusion needs. Entering the pelvic hematoma via the pelvis has not caused the difficulties associated with entering it through the abdomen. Rarely are major bleeding vessels encountered, and if they are, they can be addressed. Bleeding is primarily from the raw fracture surfaces, and reduction of the fracture cuts down on blood loss to such an extent that these patients will suffer less blood loss in the long run.

By early operative intervention, a much easier reduction can be obtained. Even the delay of a few days will allow the hematoma to begin organizing, and soft tissue contractures and swelling will occur making a reduction more difficult and traumatic. If the patient is not able to withstand an early surgery or the operating room is not equipped to do such procedures on an immediate basis, the fractures can be fixed within the first week. For the delayed treatment of unstable pelvic vertical shear fractures, it is helpful to place a traction pin for pain control and to prevent shortening of the hemipelvis which will complicate a late reduction.

If an external fixator is to be applied, pay attention to the technique of application (see Chapter 18). The pins may be inserted either through small incisions, or percutaneously with a stab wound. Using either technique, there must be no tension on the skin, or else skin

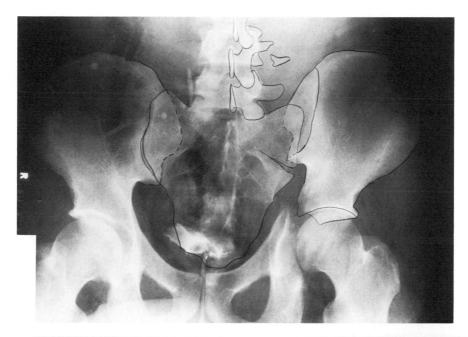

A

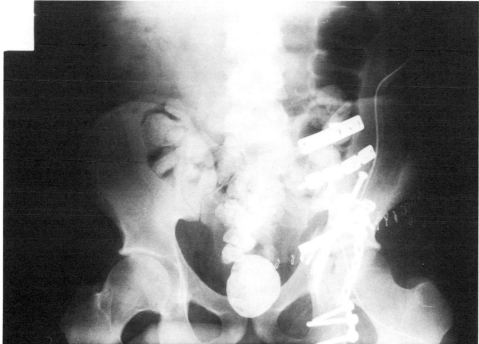

B

Figure 13–23.   **A:** Patient with unstable pelvic fracture with a widened SI joint, cephalad migration of the left iliac wing, and L-4 transverse process fracture. There is also a fracture through the left sacral ala, and a left transverse acetabular fracture involving both anterior and posterior columns. **B:** This fracture was treated acutely with open reduction and internal fixation, allowing mobilization to the chair on the first day after surgery, and the initiation of crutch ambulation (touch-down weight bearing on the stabilized side) the following day.

necrosis and superficial infection manifested by "soupy pins" will result. Soupy pins may then lead to deeper infection along the pin tract, loosening, and subsequent loss of the pin. In order to properly place the entrance points, the pelvis is reduced as much as possible first as this will change the position of the bony pelvis underneath the skin. Reduction can be done through an assistant applying manual pressure on the iliac crests to "close the book," or the patient may be placed in the lateral position in which case the pelvis will "self reduce."

After choosing the site of entrance, drill only just to penetrate through the outer cortex of the crest. Two pins are generally placed in the anterior crest, with the first at a distance of 1 to 2 cm cephalad from the superior spine to avoid the lateral femoral cutaneous nerve to the thigh. Place the pins in line with the crest, allowing them to find their own way between the inner and outer tables for a tight fit. It is crucial to be familiar with the anatomy in order to avoid the acetabulum and hip joint, to prevent exiting out of the iliac cortex, and to place the pins into optimal bone stock. Two smooth, thin wires may be slid down the inner and outer surfaces of the pelvis to act as a sighting guide if needed[23] (Fig. 13–24). Drilling between the tables is to be avoided as the pins will not fit as tightly, and the drill will sometimes unknowingly pass out of the pelvis.

Once the pins are placed and the cross bars assembled, the pins can be used as levers for any final manipulation needed for reduction before tightening the cross bar connectors to the pins. Ample room between the cross bars and the abdomen is allowed for any subsequent abdominal swelling, and to permit enough clearance for the patient to sit upright. If any skin tension is present at the pin sites, make relaxing incisions.

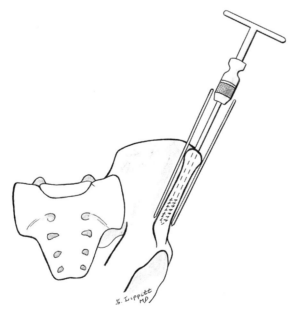

Figure 13–24. Proper method for insertion of pins for external fixator. See text for description.

REFERENCES

1. Blaisdell FW, Trunkey DD, eds. *Trauma Management, II: Urogenital Trauma.* New York, NY: Thieme-Stratton; 1985.
2. Böhler L. *The Treatment of Fractures.* 4th ed. Bristol, England: John Wright & Sons; 1935.
3. Bosse MJ, et al. Preoperative angiographic assessment of the superior gluteal artery in acetabular fractures requiring extensile surgical exposures. *J Orthop Trauma.* 1989;2:303–307.
4. Braunstein PW, et al. Concealed hemorrhage due to pelvic fractures. *J Trauma.* 1964;4:832.
5. Bucholz RW. The pathologic anatomy of Malgaigne fracture dislocations of the pelvis. *J Bone Joint Surg.* 1981;63-A:400–404.
6. Bucholz RW. Pathomechanics of pelvic ring disruptions. *Adv Orthop Surg.* 1987;10:167.
7. Carabalona P, et al. Apports du fixateur externe dans les disjonctions du pubis et de l'articulation sacro-iliaque. *Montpell Chir.* 1973;19:62.
8. Chapman M, ed. *Operative Orthopaedics.* Philadelphia, Pa: JB Lippincott; 1988.
9. Cooper A. *A Treatise on Fractures and Dislocations of the Joints.* London, England: Churchill; 1842.
10. Dickinson D, et al. Disruptions of the pelvic ring. *J Bone Joint Surg.* 1982;64-B:635.
11. Edeiken-Monroe BS, et al. The role of standard roentgenograms in the evaluation of instability of pelvic ring disruption. *Clin Orthop.* 1989;240:63–76.
12. Gertzbein SD, Chenoweth DR. Occult injuries of the pelvic ring. *Clin Orthop.* 1977;128:202–207.
13. Hanson PB, Milne JC, Chapman MW. Open pelvis fracture: a critical analysis. Presented at the Orthopaedic Trauma Association Annual Meeting; October 1989.
14. Henderson RC. The long term results of nonoperatively treated major pelvic disruptions. *J Orthop Trauma.* 1989;3:41–47.
15. Holdsworth FW. Dislocation and fracture dislocation of the pelvis. *J Bone Joint Surg.* 1948;30-B:461–466.
16. Holm CL. Treatment of pelvic fractures and dislocations. *Clin Orthop.* 1973;97:97–107.
17. Judet R, Judet L, Letournel E. Fractures of the acetabulum. Classification and surgical approaches for open reduction. *J Bone Joint Surg.* 1964;46-A:1615–1636.
18. Kellam J, Powell J, Dust W, McCormick R. The open pelvic fracture. Presented at the Orthopaedic Trauma Association Annual Meeting; October 1989.
19. Levine MA. A treatment of central fractures of the acetabulum. *J Bone Joint Surg.* 1943;23:902–906.
20. Lipkowitz G, et al. Hemipelvectomy: a lifesaving operation in severe open pelvic injury in childhood. *J Trauma.* 1982;25:823–827.
21. Mackersie RC, et al. Major skeletal injuries in the obtunded blunt trauma patient: a case for routine radiologic survey. *J Trauma.* 1988;28:1450–1454.
22. Malgaigne JF. *Treatise on Fractures.* Philadelphia, Pa: JB Lippincott; 1859.
23. Mears DC, Rubash HE. *Pelvis and Acetabular Fractures.* Thorofare, NJ: Slack Inc; 1986.
24. Peltier LF. Joseph François Malgaigne and Malgaigne's fracture. *Clin Orthop.* 1980;151:4–7.
25. Rankin LM. Fractures of the pelvis. *Ann Surg.* 1937;106:266–277.
26. Reinert CM, et al. A modified extensile exposure for the treatment of complex or malunited acetabular fractures. *J Bone Joint Surg.* 1988;70-A:329–337.
27. Richardson JD, et al. Open pelvic fractures. *J Trauma.* 1982;22:533–538.
28. Rockwood CA Jr, Green DP. *Fractures in Adults.* 2nd ed. Philadelphia, Pa: JB Lippincott; 1984.
29. Schatzker J, Tile M. *The Rationale of Operative Fracture Care.* Berlin, Germany: Springer-Verlag; 1987.
30. Sevitt S. Fatal road accidents. Injuries, complications, and causes of death in 250 subjects. *Br J Surg.* 1968; 55:481.
31. Shaftan GW. The initial evaluation of the multiple trauma patient. *World J Surg.* 1983;7:19–25.
32. Slätis P, Karaharju EO. External fixation of unstable pelvic fractures. *Clin Orthop.* 1980;151:73–80.
33. Tile M. *Fractures of the Pelvis and Acetabulum.* Baltimore, Md: Williams & Wilkins; 1984.
34. Watson-Jones R. *Fractures and Joint Injuries.* 3rd ed. Edinburgh, Scotland: Churchill Livingstone; 1943.
35. Weil GC, et al. The diagnosis and treatment of fractures of the pelvis and their complications. *Am J Surg.* 1939;44:108–116.
36. Westerborn A. Beitrage zur Kenntnisse der Beckenbrüche und Beckenluxationen. *Acta Chir Scand Suppl.* 1928:8.

14

Acetabulum Fractures and Hip Dislocation

JAMES P. KENNEDY, M.D.

HISTORY: Until the 1950s, acetabular and pelvic fractures were routinely treated with long periods of traction and bedrest until the patient was mobilized. The results of this type of treatment were so disappointing,[6,20,40] that in 1922 Cottalorda stated that "while modern industrial life gives us the means to inflict serious fractures of the acetabulum, despite sporadic attempts, the results of treatment have stayed as they were at the time of Ambroise Paré"—ie, the 1500s.[9] The surgical treatment of acetabular fractures was pioneered in the late 1950s and early 1960s by Robert and Jean Judet along with Emile Letournel[18,19,21] who proved that these fractures could be successfully surgically reduced and internally stabilized allowing good results and rapid mobilization of the patient followed by early discharge from the hospital.

Hippocrates described how to build a "scamnum," or fracture table, which was used to reduce all sorts of fractures and dislocations, including hip dislocations.[1] Illustrated in a woodcut in 1544,[16] it is very similar to the fracture tables used today. An adjustable perineal post was used for countertraction, and the extremity was attached to an axle which was cranked to supply the traction. Although Hippocrates wrote that, "by means of such machines and of such powers, it appears to me that we need never fail in reducing any dislocation at a joint,"[1] fracture tables are rarely if ever used for traumatic hip dislocations today. This method has given way to manipulative techniques which are more forgiving to articular cartilage.

INTRODUCTION

These two injuries are grouped together because of their common mechanism. They are usually seen in automobile accident victims, often as a result of a dashboard injury (a blow directed down the axis of the femur with the hip and knee flexed). The telltale sign of a knee soft-tissue injury in an auto accident victim suggests the possibility of hip injury as well[11]

240

(Fig. 14–1). The converse is also true, for as many as 25% of patients with posterior hip dislocations will have significant knee injuries.[15]

Dislocated hips are an orthopaedic emergency. The dislocation must be reduced to relieve any neurologic compression, restore joint congruency, and reduce any compromise on femoral head vasculature.[7]

In the treatment of these injuries, the initial management is the most important factor which will ultimately determine outcome. In the older patient with a poor result, a bad hip can be salvaged nicely by a total hip replacement with expectation for excellent results. Unfortunately, the majority of these joint injuries occur in the physiologically young, active population. A poor result in this group dooms the patient to either years of suffering before reaching the age where a total hip can safely be undertaken, or accepting the alternative hip fusion with its disadvantage of a stiff hip in exchange for the benefit of pain relief.

ACETABULAR FRACTURES

Acetabular fractures can be of two types. The first is the fracture associated with a hip dislocation resulting from an indirect force directed up the femoral shaft and through the femoral head into the joint. Often there is associated cartilage compression or shearing damage with these injuries. The second type of acetabular fracture results from a direct force against the pelvis and is actually a pelvic fracture which happens to be intra-articular. These injuries are discussed in Chapter 13 and will not be further addressed here.

The goals of treatment are to obtain an anatomic reduction of the articular surface and

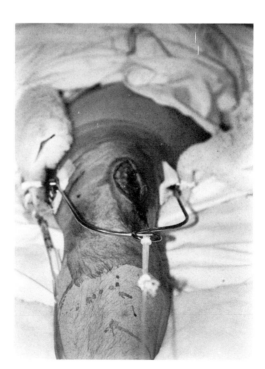

Figure 14–1. Patient with knee laceration from dashboard injury in tibial pin skeletal traction for acetabular fracture.

a concentric stable hip joint, to remove intra-articular loose bodies, and to achieve early motion to optimize cartilaginous healing.[29]

Assessment

The type of fracture is dependent upon the direction of force applied to the acetabulum which in turn is related to the position of the hip.[19,24] Most commonly due to the high incidence of automobile accidents as a cause for these fractures, the hip is in a flexed position at the time of injury. Motor vehicle accidents account for up to 80% of acetabular fractures.[19] Hip flexion, adduction, or internal rotation will direct the forces posteriorly causing a posterior acetabular wall fracture and often a posterior hip dislocation. With the hip more extended, abducted, or externally rotated, an anterior fracture or dislocation occurs. A direct blow to the greater trochanter—the source of injury in 14% of cases[19]—will result in a medially directed force which can cause a transverse acetabular fracture and "central" or intrapelvic hip dislocation.[21,25,30,35] In characterizing these fractures to determine treatment, it is also important to localize the position of the fracture in relation to the weight bearing surface, or dome, of the acetabulum.

In assessing the acetabular fracture, the most important steps are the neurovascular exam and determination of the fracture personality. Although sciatic nerve lacerations are possible, a sciatic nerve palsy is most commonly secondary to contusion and stretch of the nerve associated with the displacement of the fracture and the head of the femur posteriorly (Fig. 14–2). It is not uncommon to find the nerve entrapped within the sharp edges of the fracture site or draped over the displaced fracture under great tension. The presence of a

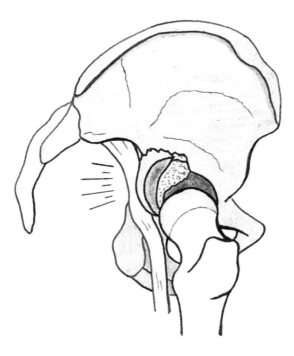

Figure 14–2. Compression and contusion of sciatic nerve from displaced posterior wall acetabular fracture. The nerve may also be lacerated by or entrapped within the sharp fracture fragments.

palsy demands rapid reduction and stabilization of the fracture to improve chances for neurologic return. The shorter the length of time that pressure is present on the nerve, the greater the chance of full return of function to the nerve.[34]

Just as one chooses one's friends by their personality, one chooses which fractures to operate upon by their personality. The personality of the acetabular fracture consists of its location, size of the fragments, degree of comminution, residual stability of the hip, degree of involvement in the weight bearing dome, displacement (congruence of the joint), and whether loose fragments are present in the joint.

Upon examining the patient, unless there is an associated hip dislocation, no deformity will be noted. The patient will complain of deep-seated hip or groin pain. An AP pelvis film will document the presence of a fracture (Fig. 14–3). Judet oblique views (Fig. 14–4) or a CT scan will further localize the fragments if necessary, and contribute to the decisions of whether the joint is congruent and the fracture is stable. Three-dimensional reconstructions of the CT scan[31] will give additional information concerning the fracture pattern.

Treatment

Some acetabular fractures can be treated with benign neglect. These are primarily small peripheral rim chip fractures that have no significant articular component and that do not

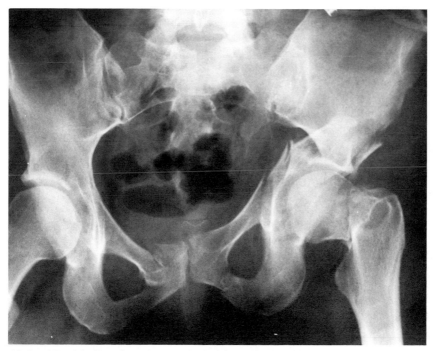

Figure 14–3. AP pelvis film of a patient who jumped from a bridge and landed on her left side in a suicide attempt. In addition to the left acetabular fracture, there are fractures of the pubic rami bilaterally and of the left femoral neck.

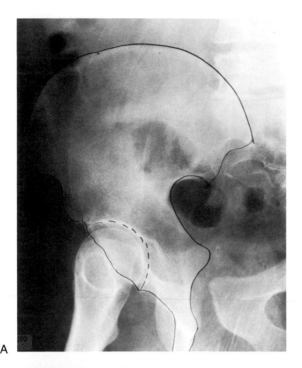

A

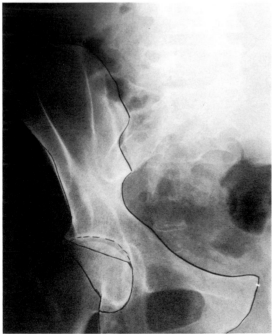

B

Figure 14–4. Judet views of acetabular fracture. **A:** Iliac oblique demonstrating posterior column of the pelvis and anterior acetabular wall. **B:** Obturator oblique showing anterior pelvic column and posterior acetabular wall.

contribute to hip stability (Fig. 14–5). If the hip is stable, rapid mobilization and immediate weight bearing as comfort allows is the treatment of choice.

Fractures that are undisplaced may also be treated nonoperatively if the configuration is stable (Fig. 14–6). Protected weight bearing must be used after an initial period of traction to prevent displacement while motion is maintained.

Operative fixation usually is required if the fracture is displaced and involves the weight bearing dome (Fig. 14–7). Fixation may also be necessary for fractures outside the weight bearing dome if their stability is required to prevent recurrent dislocation of the hip (Fig. 14–8). The presence of an incongruently reduced joint,[22] intra-articular debris, or open fractures are also indications for operative treatment.

Congruently reduced joints which are stable and do not have fracture lines involving the weight bearing dome have a high rate of successful treatment through non-operative means.[28] This generally requires 6 to 12 weeks in traction and therefore is only applicable to the isolated acetabular fracture. There is a high rate of morbidity and mortality associated with a lengthy period of enforced bedrest in the multiple trauma patient, so treatment through traction is rarely indicated for these patients. Although clinical studies have not yet been performed with adequate long-term follow-up, it seems reasonable based on current knowledge of how intra-articular fractures heal that anatomic reduction and stabilization will lead to better joint healing for most any fracture. In addition, surgical stabilization allows for a much more rapid mobilization of the patient and discharge from the hospital.

A sometimes helpful indicator to assess the area of weight bearing dome involved is the roof arc measurement. The roof arc is the angle formed by a vertical line from the center of the acetabulum and a line intersecting the acetabular fracture (Fig. 14–9). On the AP, iliac

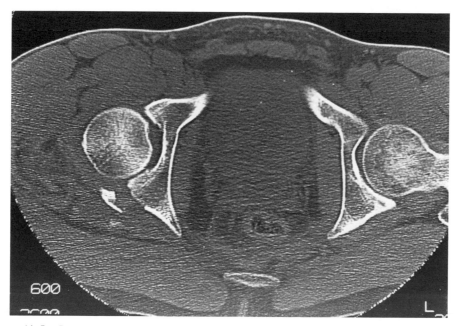

Figure 14–5. Postreduction CT scan following right hip dislocation. There is a small chip fracture off the posterior wall of the acetabulum seen only on this one cut. This small fragment is not significant for hip stability. Note concentric hip reduction.

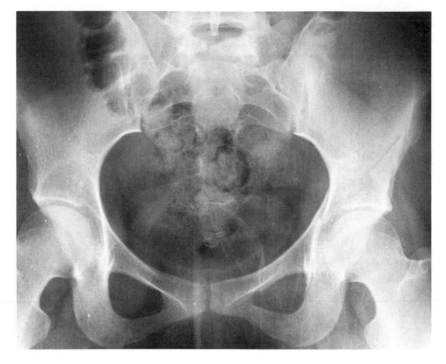

A

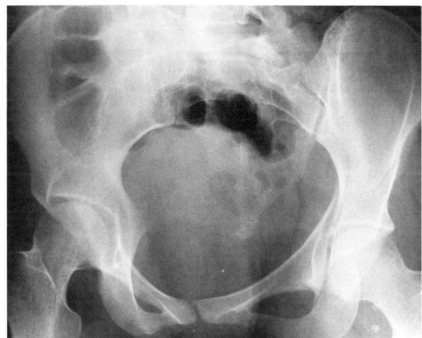

B

Figure 14–6. Nondisplaced isolated left acetabular fracture conducive to nonoperative treatment. **A:** AP view. **B:** Obturator oblique.

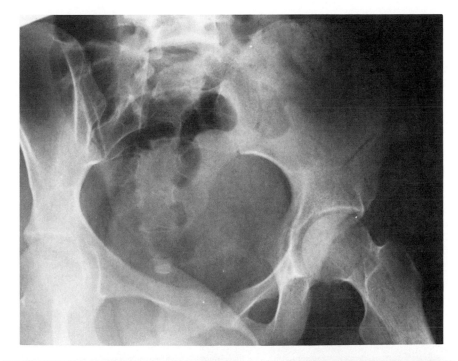

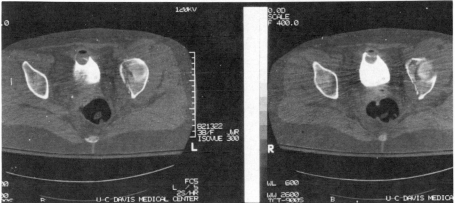

Figure 14–6, cont.   C: Iliac oblique. All three views show fracture to be nondisplaced. **D:** CT scan shows fragments of weight bearing dome (left) to be nondisplaced, and hip to be concentrically reduced (right).

oblique and obturator oblique views, any angle less than 45° would indicate insufficient intact acetabular surface for weight bearing[22] if the fracture is displaced. Fractures that are displaced but not involving significant portions of the weight bearing dome may be treated nonoperatively with traction and early motion if patient mobilization out of bed is not a concern.

The majority of acetabular fractures in the multiple trauma patient are displaced severely enough to require internal fixation, have intra-articular debris or other indications for open surgical treatment, or internal fixation is warranted to permit rapid mobilization

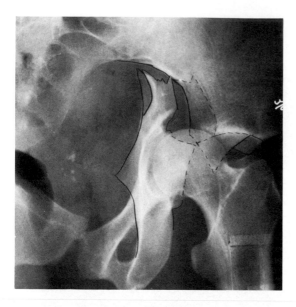

Figure 14–7. Displaced left acetabular fracture requiring surgical reduction and stabilization. Weight bearing dome of the acetabulum is disrupted, the femoral head is displaced centrally into the fracture, and the joint is incongruent and unstable.

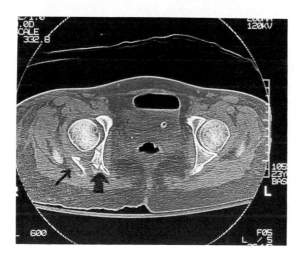

Figure 14–8. CT scan following reduction of right hip dislocation. Combination of moderately sized posterior wall fracture (small arrow) and impacted posterior wall (large arrow) leaves hip without any posterior support. If not reduced, the hip will chronically sublux out the back.

of the patient in cases where the fracture is less severe. A relative indication for surgery is the presence of a sciatic palsy to explore and decompress the nerve.

These high energy acetabular fractures in the accident victim can be greatly comminuted, displaced, or contain impacted compressed surfaces that are irreducible without elevation and grafting (Fig. 14–8). Some "blow-out" fractures (Fig. 14–10), are so severe as to be irreconstructable. If the patient is a candidate, primary total hip arthroplasty may be used, with screw fixation of the acetabular ring serving as a fixation device for the acetabular fracture. For young patients, a period of skeletal traction or the application of an external fixator across the hip to stabilize the joint is the only possible treatment. Following early

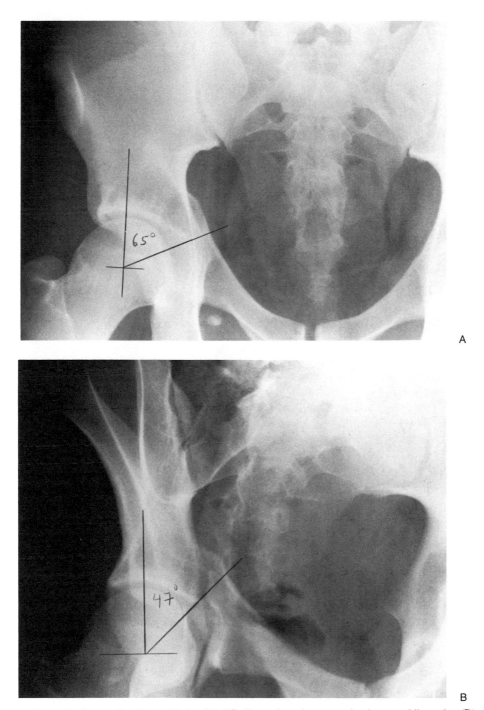

A

B

Figure 14–9.   Roof arc angles. On the AP view (**A**) 65° of intact dome is present, the obturator oblique view (**B**) shows 47° intact, and the iliac oblique (**C**) reveals an entirely intact posterior acetabular margin. (Figure continued on next page)

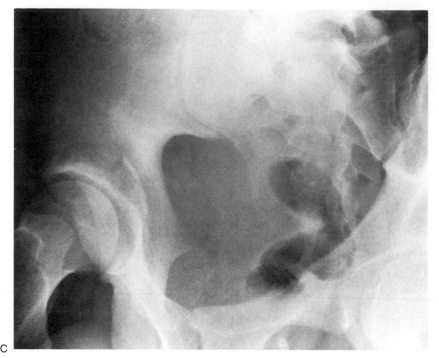

C

Figure 14–9, cont.

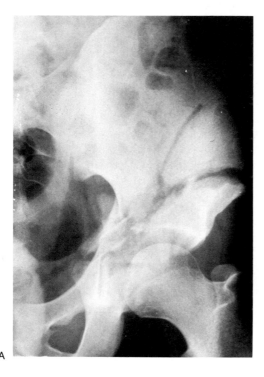

A

Figure 14–10. A: "Blow-out" fracture of left acetabulum. Marked comminution renders the hip totally unstable and unable to remain in a reduced position.

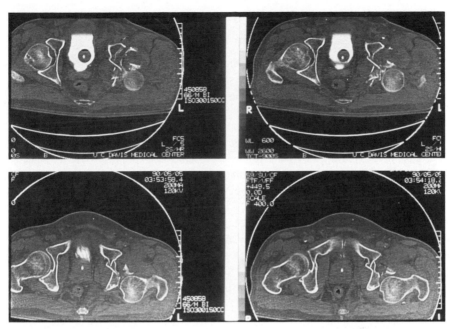

Figure 14–10, cont. **B:** CT scan showing extensive comminution and intra-articular debris blocking a reduction. This fracture cannot be surgically reconstructed.

motion, if a poor result ensues, the patient may need delayed hip fusion or a resection arthroplasty.

The operative treatment and complex reconstruction of acetabular fractures is best handled by a surgeon familiar with and experienced in their treatment. As Schatzker[30] espouses, the failure from a poorly done internal fixation is worse than the poor result from a severe injury treated by closed means, but a good result from a well done internal fixation is better than the best result possible from closed treatment.

It is now becoming evident that, as in most situations in which there has been polytrauma, the best time to fix these injuries is at presentation, both in terms of the overall condition and management of the patient, and in terms of ease of operative fixation. If a patient is too systemically unstable to allow immediate fixation, operative treatment is best done within 5 to 7 days before fibrosis and healing begin, as this will make mobilization and reduction of the fragments more difficult. Delayed surgical treatment will also lead to an increased incidence of heterotopic ossification.[14]

With unstable displaced fractures, a tibial or femoral traction pin should be inserted if the patient is not able to be operated at presentation, or if it is necessary to stabilize the patient medically prior to transfer to a facility equipped to operate on such injuries. It is remarkable how good a reduction can sometimes be obtained utilizing twenty or thirty pounds of skeletal traction. Patients with inadequate bone stock for internal fixation of acetabular fractures, or fractures that are deemed irreparable through surgical methods can be maintained for several weeks in traction allowing hip range of motion until the fracture stabilizes enough for ambulation. This is not the preferred treatment for the polytrauma patient and is generally reserved for patients with isolated injuries who are not candidates for surgery. One must be prepared for the relatively high incidence of complications that can occur with enforced bedrest. It is generally necessary to anticoagulate such patients.

After unstable fractures have been operatively stabilized, or immediately as soon as comfort allows for stable fractures and those being treated with skeletal traction, gentle range of motion should be started to help mold the cartilage and facilitate cartilage healing.[29] If the patient, due to other injuries cannot cooperate with this, continuous passive motion (CPM) can be instituted through a mechanical device with electric motor.

When an extensile surgical approach with soft tissue stripping or osteotomy is required for exposure, or if extensive soft tissue injury is present, the patient is at risk for heterotopic ossification.[3,25] This is compounded if there is an associated head injury[13] or other predisposing factor is present (see Chapter two). The overall incidence of heterotopic ossification in acetabular fractures is 55%,[12] but this can rise to more than 80% following open reduction and internal fixation.[14] Luckily, the majority of heterotopic ossification is lower grade and asymptomatic leading only to minor decreased range of motion of the hip. If severe, however, heterotopic ossification can compromise an otherwise excellent operative reduction and stabilization and lead to a poor result. Patients at risk should be considered for prophylaxis[3,23] as described in Chapter 2.

HIP DISLOCATION

Dislocations of the hip were unusual injuries prior to the mechanization of society and the high energy injuries that accompanied it. Stimson wrote in 1889 that, "the injury so rarely comes under the observation of the practitioner, even of the hospital surgeons of large cities, that our knowledge of it is, as a rule, rather theoretical than practical and personal.[33] Today, the injury is common.

Hip dislocations are classified according to their position which in turn is related to the mechanism of injury, the direction of the applied force, and the position of the hip at the time of injury. The patient with a dislocated hip has pain localized to the hip and pelvic region, has a mechanical block to hip range of motion, and holds the leg in a characteristic position. X-rays easily confirm that a dislocation is present and which direction the hip has come out.

Assessment

Anterior dislocations constitute 10% to 15% of all hip dislocations.[27] These can be further divided into superior, inferior, obturator, or perineal dislocations based on their location (Fig. 14–11). The extremity is held in a shortened, extended, externally rotated, and abducted position. Often, a fullness from the femoral head is palpable in the groin. Attempted range of motion is painful and mechanically blocked. Although neurovascular compromise is rare, the neurovascular exam should be directed toward the femoral vessels and nerve which can be compressed by the femoral head.[8,26]

Posterior dislocations (Fig. 14–12) are by far the most common type encountered. The leg is held in a position of adduction, internal rotation, flexion, and shortening (Fig. 14–13). There is a 10% to 14% incidence of sciatic nerve injury[27] from direct trauma from the femoral head[17] (Fig. 14–14). Most commonly, only the common peroneal division is

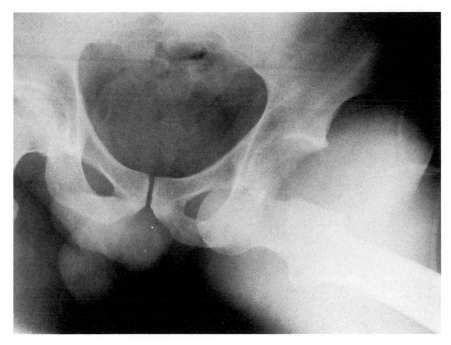

Figure 14–11.   Anterior obturator dislocation of left hip. Note abducted position of leg. The leg is also in external rotation as evident by the prominant lesser trochanter.

involved.[32] As already discussed, a posterior wall acetabular fracture, and less often a femoral head fracture, is found in association with the dislocation.

Central or intrapelvic dislocations are essentially an acetabular fracture with displacement of the femoral head into the fracture site, and not a true hip dislocation. Their treatment is directed primarily toward the acetabular fracture.

Treatment

The goals of treatment are rapid gentle reduction to obtain a stable hip. These are not as dangerous as femoral head or subcapital fractures, but the tension on the capsule and ligamentum teres can compromise circulation to the femoral head,[39] and if prompt reduction is not performed, avascular necrosis may result.[10] Avascular necrosis of the hip has been found in 8% of cases following anterior dislocation[4,27] and in anywhere from 6% to over 40% of posterior dislocations.[27,36,38]

Reductions of the hip should be performed under general or spinal anesthesia if at all possible. It would be an unusual circumstance in which hip reduction would be necessary without the help of anesthesia.

There are several reasons for a reduction under anesthesia other than, and more important than, patient comfort—although this is certainly a valid consideration. The reduction must be gentle with good muscle relaxation to prevent further articular damage from scraping the femoral head over the acetabular rim or rough fracture fragments during

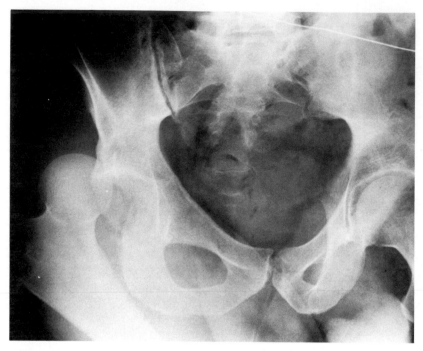

Figure 14–12.   AP pelvis of posterior right hip dislocation. Note the apparently smaller femoral head on the right. Due to the divergent x-ray beam, objects closer to the plate appear smaller and those farther from the plate appear larger. This, coupled with the physical exam, confirms the posterior location of the dislocation.

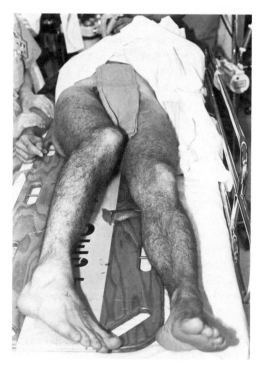

Figure 14–13.   Clinical photo of patient in Figure 14–12 with posterior right hip dislocation. The leg is held in a position of shortening, flexion, adduction, and internal rotation.

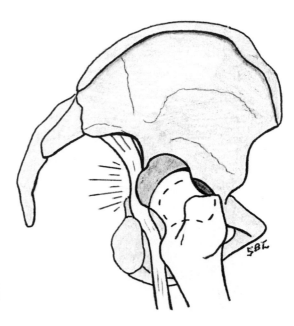

Figure 14–14. Pressure on sciatic nerve resulting in palsy from posteriorly dislocated femoral head.

the reduction maneuver. As a great deal of force can be required to reduce a hip, muscle relaxation or paralysis not only makes it easier on the surgeon, but will also help prevent precipitating an acetabular wall or femoral neck fracture from a forced reduction. Finally, examination under anesthesia permits assessment of the postreduction stability of the hip, which in turn determines the subsequent postreduction treatment.

A multitude of maneuvers have been described to reduce a hip.[27] The two most common techniques are the Stimson and Allis maneuvers. The Stimson technique[33] is most useful for posterior dislocations. Stimson devised this technique due to the amount of exertion necessary for the surgeon to reduce a hip in the supine position. He stated, "it was after having become hot and tired in thus reducing a dislocation, one summer day, that the thought occurred to me of making the patient himself do this work."[33] The patient is placed prone with the knee and hip flexed to 90°. An assistant stabilizes the pelvis by downward pressure on the sacrum. The surgeon applies gentle downward pressure to the leg just distal to the knee and gently rotates the leg to obtain reduction (Fig. 14–15). Sometimes, after maintaining this position for several minutes, the weight of the leg will effect a reduction without manipulation.

The Allis technique[2] utilizes the supine position. An assistant stabilizes the pelvis and can additionally help by applying pressure on the greater trochanter. The knee is flexed to relax the hamstrings and the surgeon applies traction in line with the femur with the hip slightly flexed. Additional flexion is sometimes helpful to allow the weight of the body to supply countertraction. The hip is then gently rotated back and forth to manipulate the femoral head back into the acetabulum (Fig. 14–16).

If one good attempt at a gentle reduction fails, one should not continue with the "death grip on a loser" philosophy. A different technique should be attempted. Alternatively, the image intensifier can be helpful in showing the surgeon a specific maneuver which might be required. If closed reduction fails, an open reduction is needed. Bony fragments can become interposed in the joint (Fig. 14–17) blocking a successful reduction as can soft

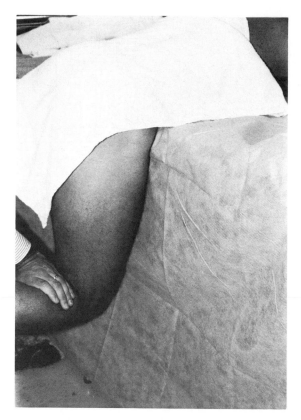

Figure 14–15.   Stimson maneuver for hip reduction.

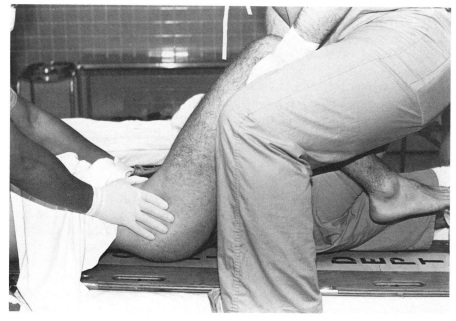

Figure 14–16.   Allis maneuver to reduce posterior hip dislocation.

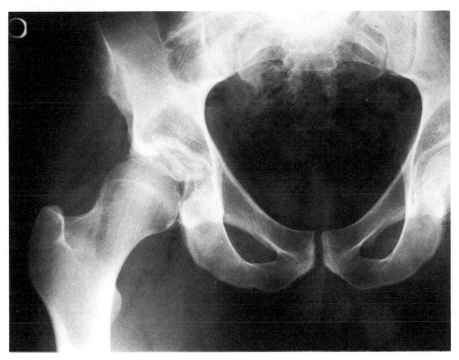

Figure 14–17.   Posterior hip dislocation following attempted closed reduction. Debris in joint blocks concentric reduction.

tissues such as capsule, muscle, or tendon.[5] The capsule may also prevent reduction if the femoral head buttonholes through it. Compounded by swelling and tension on the capsule, the capsular tear may not be large enough to allow the head to pass back through the rent into the joint.

In cases where open reduction is required, the rule of thumb is that posterior dislocations are approached via a posterior approach, and anterior dislocations are operated through an anterior approach. This allows the surgeon to directly visualize and address whatever is preventing the reduction (Fig. 14–18). Surgical insult to intact structures that will further destabilize the hip is prevented, and further devascularization of an already compromised femoral head is avoided by this technique as well.[37]

The final indication to operatively treat a hip dislocation is to stabilize significant acetabular fractures which require operative fixation on their own merit, in which case the hip dislocation is incidental (Fig. 14–19). If the patient requires surgical intervention for other orthopaedic or internal injuries, the closed reduction of the hip should be carried out first to re-establish congruency and relieve pressure on neurovascular structures. This can usually be accomplished within a few minutes once anesthesia is induced. Then, after the other injuries are addressed, the hip can be opened for internal fixation, even on a delayed basis if necessary.

Following the reduction, the hip should be examined for stability. In the absence of a fracture repair that needs protection, the following treatment protocol is advocated.

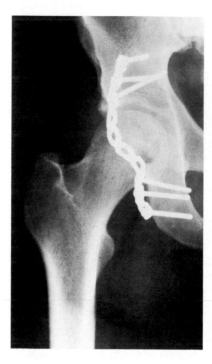

Figure 14–18. The patient in Figure 13–23 following posterior surgical approach and internal fixation of posterior wall fracture fragments displaced into joint.

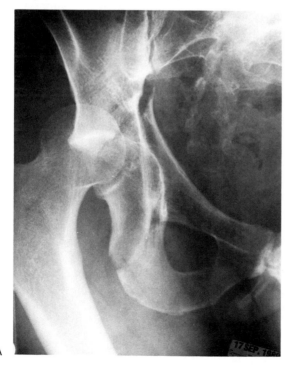

A

Figure 14–19. A: Fracture dislocation of right hip.

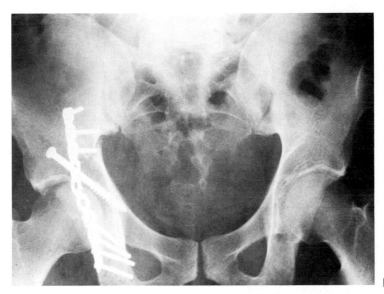

B

Figure 14–19, cont. **B:** This displaced acetabular fracture through the weight bearing dome requires reduction and fixation regardless of the presence of a hip dislocation.

1. If the hip is stable at 90° of flexion or greater, the patient can weight bear without restriction.
2. Hips that are stable up to 45° of flexion are protected either with a knee immobilizer or hip orthosis to allow flexion within the stable range. These patients may also weight bear as tolerated with crutches.
3. Hips that dislocate at less than 45° of flexion require a variable period of skeletal traction to maintain the reduction after which the patient can be mobilized in an orthosis.

For patients who have had intra-articular damage, early motion either through the use of a knee sling or CPM is helpful.[29] Hips with associated chip fractures that are closed reduced without opening the joint for inspection and debridement should have a post-reduction CT scan to determine whether intra-articular debris is present which requires removal.

REFERENCES

1. Adams F, trans. *The Genuine Works of Hippocrates*. New York, NY: Williams & Wilkins; 1939.
2. Allis OH. *The Hip*. Philadelphia, Pa: Dornan Printer; 1895.
3. Bosse MJ, et al. Heterotopic ossification as a complication of acetabular fracture. *J Bone Joint Surg*. 1988; 70-A:1231–1237.
4. Brav EA. Traumatic dislocation of the hip. *J Bone Joint Surg*. 1962;44-A:1115–1134.
5. Canale ST, Manugian AJ. Irreducible traumatic dislocations of the hip. *J Bone Joint Surg*. 1979;61-A:7–14.
6. Cauchoix J, Truchet P. Les fractures articulaires de la hanche (col du fémur excepté). *Chir Orthop*. 1951; 37:266–332.
7. Chapman M, ed. *Operative Orthopaedics*. Philadelphia, Pa: JB Lippincott; 1988.

8. Chervu A, Quinones-Baldrich WJ. Vascular complications in orthopedic surgery. *Clin Orthop.* 1988; 235:275–288.
9. Cottalorda. Les fractures par enfoncement de la cavité cotyloïde. Thesis, Montpellier, 1922.
10. Duncan CP, Shim SS. Blood supply of the head of the femur in traumatic hip dislocation. *Surg Gynecol Obstet.* 1977;144:185–191.
11. Epstein HC, et al. Posterior fracture dislocation of the hip with fractures of the femoral head. *Clin Orthop.* 1985;201:9–17.
12. Garland DE, Miller G. Fractures and dislocations about the hip in head-injured adults. *Clin Orthop.* 1984; 186:154.
13. Garland DE, et al. Resection of heterotopic ossification in the adult with head trauma. *J Bone Joint Surg.* 1985;67-A:1261–1269.
14. Garland DE. Clinical observations on fractures and heterotopic ossification in the spinal cord and traumatic brain injured populations. *Clin Orthop.* 1988;233:86–101.
15. Gillespie WJ. The incidence and pattern of knee injury associated with dislocation of the hip. *J Bone Joint Surg.* 1975;57-B:376–378.
16. Guidi G. *Chirurgie è Graeco in Latinum Conversa.* Paris, France: Petrus Galterius; 1544.
17. Hirasawa Y, et al. Sciatic nerve paralysis in posterior dislocation of the hip. *Clin Orthop.* 1977;126:172–175.
18. Judet R, Letournel E. *Traitement Chirurgical des Fractures Récentes du Cotyle. Mémoires de l'Academie de Chirurgie.* 1962;369–377.
19. Judet R, et al. Fractures of the acetabulum: classification and surgical approaches for open reduction. *J Bone Joint Surg.* 1964;46-A:1615–1646.
20. Knight RA, Smith H. Central fractures of the acetabulum. *J Bone Joint Surg.* 1958;40-A:1–16.
21. Letournel E, Judet R. *Fractures of the Acetabulum.* Berlin, Germany: Springer-Verlag; 1981.
22. Matta JM, Merritt PO. Displaced acetabular fractures. *Clin Orthop.* 1988;230:83–97.
23. McLaren AC. Prophylaxis with indomethacin for heterotopic bone. *J Bone Joint Surg.* 1990;72-A:245–247.
24. McCoy GF, et al. Biomechanical aspects of pelvic and hip injuries in road traffic accidents. *J Orthop Trauma.* 1989;3:118–123.
25. Mears DC, Rubash HE. *Pelvic and Acetabular Fractures.* Thorofare, NJ: Slack Inc; 1986.
26. Nerubay J. Traumatic anterior dislocation of the hip joint with vascular damage. *Clin Orthop.* 1976;116: 129–132.
27. Rockwood CA Jr, Green DP. *Fractures in Adults.* 2nd ed. Philadelphia, Pa: JB Lippincott; 1984.
28. Rowe CR, Lowell JD. Prognosis of fractures of the acetabulum. *J Bone Joint Surg.* 1961;43-A:30–59.
29. Salter, RB. The biologic concept of continuous passive motion of synovial joints. *Clin Orthop.* 1989;242: 12–25.
30. Schatzker J, Tile M. *The Rationale of Operative Fracture Care.* Berlin, Germany: Springer-Verlag; 1987.
31. Scott WW Jr, et al. Three-dimensional imaging of acetabular trauma. *J Orthop Trauma.* 1987;1:227–238.
32. Stewart MJ, et al. Fracture-dislocation of the hip. *Acta Orthop Scand.* 1975;46:507–525.
33. Stimson, LA. Five cases of dislocation of the hip. *NY Med J.* 1889;1:118.
34. Sunderland S. *Nerves and Nerve Injuries.* Edinburgh, Scotland: Churchill Livingstone; 1978.
35. Tile M. *Fractures of the Pelvis and Acetabulum.* Baltimore, Md: Williams & Wilkins; 1984.
36. Tronzo RG. *Surgery of the Hip Joint.* Philadelphia, Pa: Lea & Febiger; 1973.
37. Trueta J. *Studies of the Development and Decay of the Human Frame.* Philadelphia, Pa: WB Saunders; 1968.
38. Upadhyay SS, Moulton A. The long-term results of traumatic posterior dislocation of the hip. *J Bone Joint Surg.* 1981;63-B:548–551.
39. Urist MR. Fracture-dislocation of the hip joint: the nature of the traumatic lesion, treatment, late complications and end results. *J Bone Joint Surg.* 1948;30-A:699–727.
40. Waller Å. Dorsal acetabular fractures of the hip (dashboard fractures). *Acta Chir Scand Suppl.* 1955:205.

15

Hip Fractures

JAMES P. KENNEDY, M.D.

HISTORY: Ambroise Paré first noted the importance that blood supply plays in the healing of hip fractures in 1575 when he wrote, "More important than the fracture alone is that near the joints; the parts are bloodless and more difficult to treat and harder to cure. . . ."[15]

By the mid-1800s, a variety of traction methods[23,27] had been devised in an attempt to correct deformity and promote healing. In spite of this, complications remained high. Although surgeons knew that intertrochanteric fractures routinely healed, intracapsular fractures usually did not, and there was no means of clinically distinguishing the two. Although Wilhelm Röntgen discovered the process of radiography in 1895, it was not until the 1930s that adequate lateral x-rays of the hip allowing the accurate distinction between subcapital and intertrochanteric hip fractures were possible.[26]

In addition to the possible difficulties in obtaining union, there is a high rate of mortality with nonoperative treatment of femoral neck fractures, leading one author to state, "We come into the world under the brim of the pelvis and go out through the neck of the femur."[8] Mortality from nonoperative treatment was seen in one half to one third of the patients, with some reporting mortality as high as 75%.[7,24,44]

Due to the problems of nonunion and risk of death, an alternative treatment was sought. At the meeting of the American Surgical Association in 1882, Nicholas Senn presented a specimen of an impacted intracapsular fracture which had healed.[26] He was met with such ridicule that he returned the following year with documentation of 54 such cases, as well as the results of animal experiments.[37] Senn produced fractures in 23 dogs and cats and observed no cases of healing in those treated in spica casts. In eight cats treated by internal fixation with bone, ivory, or iron pegs, two became infected but the other six healed. Senn therefore concluded that fractures which were already impacted should be treated by spica casts; those that were not should be treated by immediate reduction and permanent fixation, "so as to place the fragments in the same favorable condition during the process of repair as in impacted fractures." Senn received such severe criticism over this that he never attempted the procedure in humans.[26]

Various forms of internal fixation had been attempted by the early 1900s, but required open reduction for accurate placement of the fixation devices,[26] which increased the risk for further damage to the vascular structures. With the improvement of x-ray techniques and the introduction of fluoroscopy, closed reduction and internal fixation became possible. By 1938 this method of fixation had become the standard,[28] with union rates of 70%

and a decrease in mortality to 25%.[7] The remaining years have seen further technical improvements in the various fixation devices leading to a predictably high rate of successful union and low morbidity.

INTRODUCTION

Fractures of the hip are one of the most common entities seen by orthopaedists. A substantial force is required to fracture a hip in the young, healthy accident victim,[7,40] in contrast to the commonly seen hip fracture in the elderly osteoporotic female which has occurred secondary to a minor trauma or fall.

Often the result of a dashboard injury, or from a direct lateral blow against the greater trochanter, the hip fracture in the young multiple trauma victim is usually significantly displaced or comminuted. For the young patient, rapid anatomic reduction with atraumatic techniques and stable internal fixation are crucial for good results.[7]

Hip fractures are classified according to anatomic site: 1) femoral head ("capital"); 2) the intracapsular subcapital and transcervical (or femoral neck) fractures; 3) intertrochanteric; and 4) subtrochanteric (Fig. 15–1A–E). Treatment for the various types differ slightly, with the prime influence on the type of treatment being the presence or disruption of the all important blood supply to the femoral head.

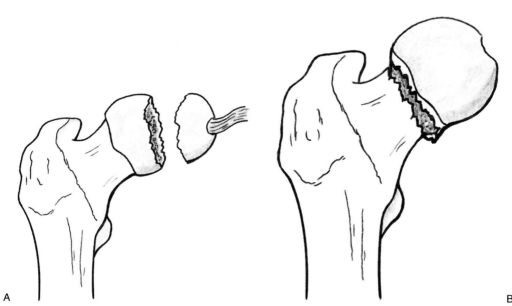

A   B

Figure 15–1. **A:** Femoral head fracture. The fracture fragment is entirely articular. **B:** Subcapital fracture. This intracapsular fracture occurs just below the articular surface at the level of the physeal scar.

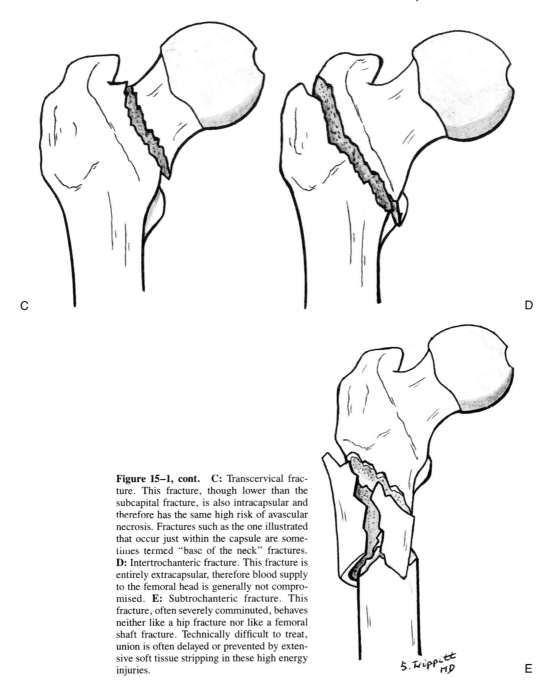

Figure 15–1, cont. **C:** Transcervical fracture. This fracture, though lower than the subcapital fracture, is also intracapsular and therefore has the same high risk of avascular necrosis. Fractures such as the one illustrated that occur just within the capsule are sometimes termed "base of the neck" fractures. **D:** Intertrochanteric fracture. This fracture is entirely extracapsular, therefore blood supply to the femoral head is generally not compromised. **E:** Subtrochanteric fracture. This fracture, often severely comminuted, behaves neither like a hip fracture nor like a femoral shaft fracture. Technically difficult to treat, union is often delayed or prevented by extensive soft tissue stripping in these high energy injuries.

ANATOMY

The hip is plagued by the same vascularity problem faced in treating fractures of the radial and humeral heads. Fractures in these areas that are intracapsular are at risk for disrupting a tenuous blood supply to the joint involved, leading to nonunion or avascular necrosis which can be compounded in the hip by collapse of the femoral head.

Three routes are available to supply blood to the femoral head (Fig. 15–2). The ligamentum teres carries a branch from the obturator artery and enters the head via the fovea centralis. Although this is a significant vascular channel in the child (and the only blood supply to the head prior to physeal closure), it is variably patent in the adult. Intramedullary vessels and the vascular sinuses present in cancellous bone serve to supply blood to the endosteal and intramedullary bone. The third and final blood source is the transcapsular branches. These derive from branches of the medial and lateral femoral circumflex arteries forming the ascending extracapsular cervical arteries. The ascending cervical branches pierce the capsule and travel up the femoral neck to enter into the head. If a fracture is intracapsular, it will often disrupt the only blood supply to the femoral head, and need emergent attention if aseptic necrosis is to be prevented.

FEMORAL HEAD FRACTURES

Fractures of the femoral head are among the most devastating of hip injuries, and must be handled as surgical emergencies.[13] A uniformly poor result can be expected with closed treatment of these injuries.[31] Operative treatment is usually necessary to provide the best chances for recovery, but often the initial trauma is so great as to preclude a good result.[41] Good results can be expected in less than 50% of cases.[13] Luckily, these injuries are rare, being seen in only 10% of posterior hip fracture dislocations with which they are almost always associated.[7] Many of these injuries may be prevented by seat belt use[14] as 85% of femoral head fractures are the result of dashboard injuries.[13] A result of severe trauma from a combination of shearing and impaction injuries, femoral head fractures are often seen in combination with other injuries to the pelvis and lower extremities.

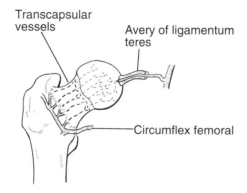

Transcapsular
vessels

Avery of ligamentum
teres

Circumflex femoral

Figure 15–2. The three sources of blood supply to the femoral head: The variably present artery of the ligamentum teres; the transcapsular vessels branching off the circumflex femoral vessels; the intraosseous vascular channels (not shown).

Assessment

These injuries are assessed in the same manner as the hip dislocation, of which they are a variant (see Chapter 14). After the examination and stabilization of the patient, and diagnosis of a fracture by x-ray (Fig. 15–3), the patient should be taken to the operating room with all possible haste,[13] for best results will be obtained only with operative treatment carried out within 24 hours of the injury.[12]

The emergency in reducing and fixing these fractures is that old nemesis about the hip, compromise of blood supply. At the level of the femoral head, the subsynovial vessels travelling up the femoral neck have all entered the bone, so unless the fracture fragment remains attached to the ligamentum teres, it will be avascular. These fragments are entirely articular and have no other soft tissue attachments as a blood supply source, and even if the ligamentum is intact, in the adult it often does not contain a patent vessel.

Treatment

The treatment of these injuries is controversial due to the poor results with the various forms of treatment. Some have advocated closed treatment,[11] others recommend reduction with excision of the head fragments,[32] while others advocate screw fixation of the fragment.[4] All of these forms of treatment probably have their place, depending upon the circumstances of the fracture present.

Impaction fractures of the head—especially if not involving the major weight-bearing

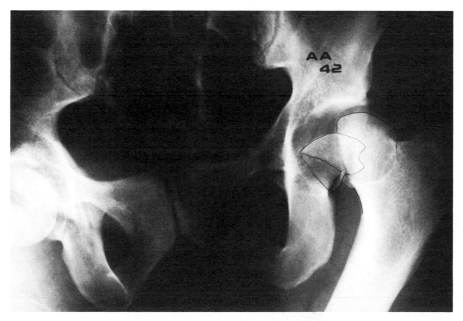

Figure 15–3.   Femoral head fracture.

surfaces, may be treated in closed fashion with early range of motion. Anatomic closed reduction of the displaced fracture dislocation probably rarely if ever[13] can be achieved due to intra-articular debris and inability to control the fracture fragment within the joint.

The surgery for the internal fixation of these injuries is technically very difficult.[7,31] A posterior surgical approach is used for associated posterior dislocations so as not to interfere with the intact anterior vascularity.[13]

In the young or active patient it is certainly worth an attempt to surgically address significant fractures. Small fragments in the non–weight-bearing inferior portion of the head are probably best excised, with the possible exception of large fragments consisting of more than one third of the diameter of the femoral head.[13]

Large fragments, or those involving the significant weight bearing dome are best treated with operative fixation, yet at the present time, no one form of treatment yields consistently good results.[13] Due to the fact that these fracture fragments are entirely articular, any fixation device must be placed through and buried below articular cartilage (Fig. 15–4). Alternatively, the fixation device may be placed laterally up the femoral neck. It can be very challenging to place screws in this fashion. Also, the fragment may be too thin to allow good purchase in this manner. In the physiologically older patient greater than 65 to 70 years old who has a significant fracture, it may be best to insert a hip prosthesis primarily.

Postoperatively, the patient should again be mobilized or placed in a continuous passive motion (CPM) device. Weight bearing must be protected until healing and revascularization of the fragment has occurred. This can take six months or longer.[7]

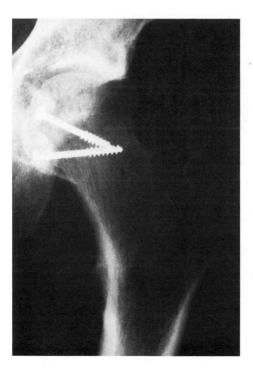

Figure 15–4. Internal fixation of femoral head articular fracture with screws countersunk below the articular surface following open reduction.

INTRACAPSULAR NECK FRACTURES

The two types of intracapsular fractures, subcapital (Fig. 15–5) and transcervical, are at great risk to develop non-union or avascular necrosis[40] and should be treated on an emergent basis, with operative fixation within 12 hours of injury.[7] Even with early optimal surgical treatment, the rate of avascular necrosis is 20%, and if near anatomic reduction is not obtained, this rate approaches 50%.[7]

In the early 1800s, Sir Astley Cooper studied 43 museum specimens and the patients in his practice with intracapsular fractures. He stated that although healing might be possible, he had never seen a case of intracapsular hip fracture which had healed.[9] As late as 1935, the intracapsular neck fractures were still termed the "unsolved fracture."[38]

This fracture should be thought of as a vascular injury to the bone's blood supply.[20] The risk of avascular necrosis is related to the amount of displacement at the time of injury (leading to tearing of blood vessels) and to the delay in reduction and stabilization.

Findings

The typical hip fracture patient presents with a shortened, externally rotated, and abducted lower extremity.[31] Intracapsular fractures do not exhibit as great a deformity as the extracapsular (or intertrochanteric) fractures. Buck's traction with a foam boot will decrease pain, but more importantly may allow increased blood flow across the neck by decreasing

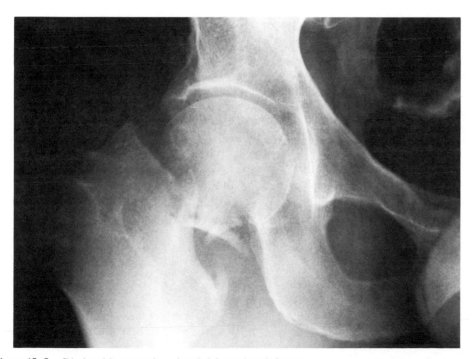

Figure 15–5.   Displaced intracapsular subcapital femoral neck fracture.

external rotation and relieving vascular occlusion due to compression from a tight, twisted capsule.[7,31]

If multiple injuries are present, the patient should be worked up for these injuries, and treatment instituted on the basis of injury priority as rapidly as possible, with the hip fracture treated on an emergent basis.[40]

Treatment

Early anatomic reduction and fixation is mandatory for badly displaced fractures to prevent the early complication of avascular necrosis and the late complication of degenerative arthritis which may result from altered joint mechanics. Fixation is also indicated for the undisplaced fracture to eliminate the risk of displacement and to permit the rapid mobilization of the patient. The incidence of avascular necrosis or nonunion with these fractures in the multiple trauma victim is higher than that occurring with an isolated fracture.[40] This is probably because there is a lesser chance of a vascular insult from the low energy trauma seen in the isolated fracture,[18,29,45] and a greater chance of a displaced fracture in the high energy multiple trauma victim.[7]

Although intracapsular fractures are not common in young patients, the fractures that are seen are most often the result of high-velocity trauma and are therefore often associated with multiple injuries.[40] The consequences of avascular necrosis are so devastating for the young multiple trauma victim, that the sooner fixed, the better. Unlike the elderly patient who can do quiet nicely with a prosthetic hip, the young active patient with a bad hip is not a candidate for such reconstruction[6,40] and must either accommodate to living with his disability, or accept a hip fusion[39]—neither choice being very appealing.

Once under general anesthetic, a closed reduction of displaced fractures is attempted. This must be gentle to prevent further vascular damage. If the closed reduction is not anatomic, an open reduction is required, being careful not to further disrupt vascularity[7] by minimizing soft tissue stripping and preserving blood vessels encountered in the approach. Following a perfect reduction, several types of fixation devices are possible. Acceptable techniques include sliding hip screw devices, blade plates, or multiple pins or screws.[7,31] The multiple pin or screw technique is probably preferable[7,40] (Fig. 15–6). These may be inserted percutaneously or through a short 3 to 5 cm incision over the greater trochanter.

For the patient physiologically over 70 years of age who is at risk for avascular necrosis due to a displaced fracture or delay in treatment, as well as those patients with pre-existing arthritic symptoms, a primary hip prosthesis is often indicated instead of internal fixation.[3] The usual multiple trauma patient who is young is not a candidate for prosthetic replacement, but rather should have immediate reduction and internal fixation even if the fracture is severely displaced.

INTERTROCHANTERIC FRACTURES

The intertrochanteric fracture, as it is extracapsular, does not threaten the blood supply to the femoral head as does its counterpart higher up the neck.[7] These fractures are below the extracapsular ring of vessels formed by the medial and lateral circumflex arteries, therefore the blood supply to the femoral head is not disrupted. However, these generally have better

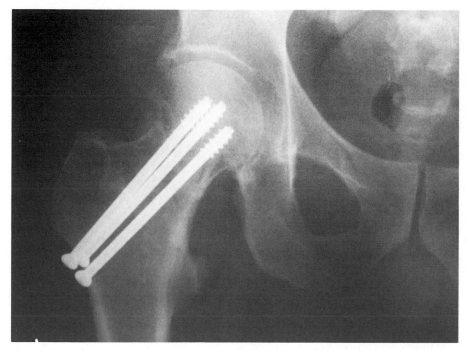

Figure 15–6. Internal fixation of subcapital fracture with percutaneous screws following anatomic closed reduction.

functional results if operatively fixed within 24 hours, and this permits rapid mobilization of the patient to help prevent systemic complications as well.

Findings

The leg is found in a markedly shortened and externally rotated (often as much as 90°) position.[19] X-ray evaluation will reveal the fracture (Fig. 15–7) which is often deformed by muscle forces into varus and external rotation. Buck's traction is used until operation unless a delay more than 12 hours is expected. Then, skeletal traction is used as it reduces the fracture better since heavier weights can be applied to counteract muscle spasm.

Treatment

Most all patients with intertrochanteric fractures are candidates for internal fixation with the exception of elderly patients suffering from significant arthritis of the hip prior to their fractures. A hip prosthesis may be considered for these patients.

A sliding hip screw device is most commonly utilized for fixation[7,31] (Fig. 15–8). Following a closed reduction on the fracture table, a lateral approach is made. The screw device is inserted under image intensifier control. After stable fixation, these patients can be immediately ambulatory, the same as subcapital femoral neck fractures,[1] with partial weight

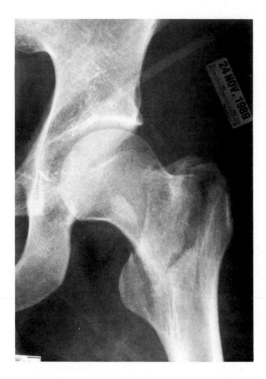

Figure 15–7. Intertrochanteric fracture.

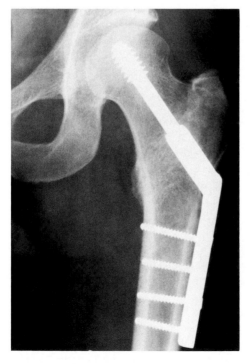

Figure 15–8. Fixation of intertrochanteric hip fracture with sliding hip screw device to allow compression at fracture site with weight bearing.

bearing. In victims of multiple trauma, open reduction through an anterior Watson-Jones exposure on a regular operating table is rapid and requires minimal fluoroscopic visualization if a fracture table is not appropriate for the patient's other injuries.

SUBTROCHANTERIC FRACTURES

The subtrochanteric fracture is a transition fracture located between the lesser trochanter and a point 5 cm distally.[42] These can be very difficult operative fixation challenges.[7,22,35] High bending forces in the region due to the angular shape of the proximal femur often lead to implant failure before union. Although newly developed devices are promising,[34] the subtrochanteric fracture can still represent an unsolved fixation problem if there is comminution in the trochanteric area.

Findings

Unlike the more proximal hip fractures, subtrochanteric fractures commonly occur in young patients, with as many as 25% being the result of multiple trauma. The remainder are pathologic fractures at the site of tumors, or low energy fractures in osteoporotic bone.[2]

The patient will present much the same as a femoral shaft fracture with pain and swelling localized at the fracture site. Shortening of the femur will be noted. Angular deformity occurs secondary to muscular forces, and without stable fixation a severe varus deformity will develop due to the high stresses of up to 1200 lb/in^2 of compression on the medial cortex.[33]

X-rays will reveal the nature of the fracture and the degree of comminution which may often be quite severe (Fig. 15–9).

Treatment

The guidelines for all fractures in the patient with multiple system injuries should be followed. Early operative stabilization allows mobilization of the patient and quicker recovery. If the fracture is not to be operated on an immediate basis, the hip should be immobilized in balanced suspension tibial pin traction[7] (Fig. 15–10).

These fractures often require bone grafting[7,22] due to delayed union of the cortical bone in this area. If comminution is present at the fracture, primary bone grafting is indicated if fixation is done open with a hip screw or plate. Bone grafting is not necessary with closed techniques using interlocking intramedullary nail devices. Due to the high biomechanical stresses in this region and sometimes slow healing, fixation devices often fail before healing occurs. For this reason, indirect reduction techniques[22]—that is using the fixation device to distract the fragments into gross alignment through ligamentotaxis without the devascularizing effect of stripping soft tissues for an anatomic reduction—may be helpful.

The search for the ideal fixation device for subtrochanteric fractures continues (Fig. 15–11). Various side-plate devices[16,34,36] as well as intramedullary implants[10,17,25,46] have been used with varying results. Many of these devices remain technically difficult to use and

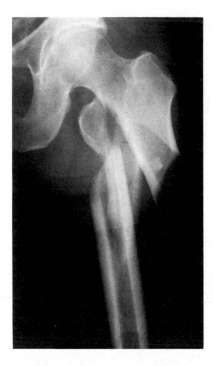

Figure 15–9. Comminuted subtrochanteric hip fracture.

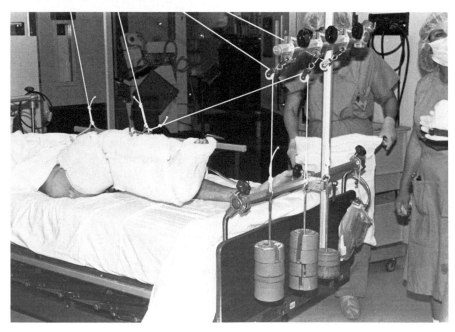

Figure 15–10. Patient with subtrochanteric fracture in tibial pin traction prior to surgery. (Short-leg Robert Jones is present for ipsilateral ankle fracture.)

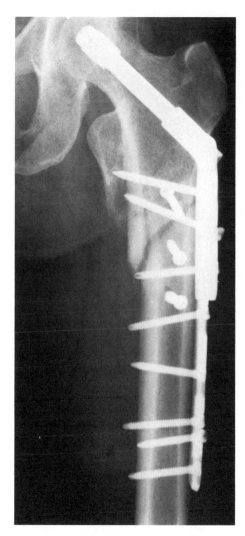

Figure 15–11. Fixation of subtrochanteric fracture with multiple interfragmentary lag screws and sliding hip bolt with side plate extension.

have a high rate of complications. Cross-locking intramedullary nails avoid soft tissue stripping, are not technically as difficult to insert, can allow earlier weight bearing, and rarely biomechanically fail as opposed to the various side plate devices.

For plates, a direct lateral approach to the greater trochanter is made similar to that used for intertrochanteric fractures. The approach must often be extended up the neck to expose the joint. Unlike femoral shaft fractures where closed nailings are routine, many of the intramedullary devices are easier to use if an open reduction and nailing is performed. For these devices a lateral position on a regular operating table is preferred to using the fracture table.

PEDIATRIC HIP FRACTURES

Fortunately, displaced intracapsular hip fractures in the child are rare, but when they do occur, are an absolute operative emergency.[43] Due to the sensitivity of the femoral head and growth plate to ischemia, immediate reduction is mandatory. Even with immediate accurate reduction, there is still a significant incidence of poor results. This is also one fracture where the "rule" of not violating the growth plate with fixation devices is broken—but only out of necessity. Smooth pins, or preferably a single screw, are passed across the plate in order to stabilize the fracture[30] but causing as little damage to the growth plate as possible. The device is removed early once healing has occurred to hopefully allow the resumption of growth.

REFERENCES

1. Arnold WD. The effect of early weight-bearing on the stability of femoral neck fractures treated with Knowles pins. *J Bone Joint Surg*. 1984;66-A:847–852.
2. Bergman GD, et al. Subtrochanteric fracture of the femur. *J Bone Joint Surg*. 1987;69-A:1032–1040.
3. Bochner RM, et al. Bipolar hemiarthroplasty for fracture of the femoral neck. *J Bone Joint Surg*. 1988;70-A:1001–1010.
4. Butler JE. Pipkin type II fractures of the femoral head. *J Bone Joint Surg*. 1981;63-A:1292.
5. Chakraborti S, Mitler IM. Dislocation of the hip associated with fracture of the femoral head. *Injury*. 1975; 7:134.
6. Chandler HP, et al. Total hip replacement in patients younger than thirty years old. *J Bone Joint Surg*. 1981; 63-A:1426–1434.
7. Chapman MW, ed. *Operative Orthopaedics*. Philadelphia, Pa: JB Lippincott; 1988.
8. Cleveland M, Fielding JW. Intracapsular fracture of the neck of the femur. In: *A.A.O.S. Instructional Course Lectures*. 1955;12:35–43.
9. Cooper AP. *A Treatise on Dislocations and Fractures of the Joints*. Hurst Reese Orme and Brown; 1822.
10. Cuthbert H, Howat TW. The use of the Küntscher Y nail in the treatment of intertrochanteric and subtrochanteric fractures of the femur. *Injury*. 1976;8:135–142.
11. Dowd GSE, Johnson R. Successful conservative treatment of a fracture dislocation of the femoral head. *J Bone Joint Surg*. 1979;61-A:1244.
12. Epstein HC. *Traumatic Dislocation of the Hip*. Baltimore, Md: Williams & Wilkins; 1980.
13. Epstein HC, et al. Posterior fracture dislocation of the hip with fractures of the femoral head. *Clin Orthop*. 1985;201:9–17.
14. Funston RV, et al. Dashboard dislocation of the hip: a report of twenty cases of traumatic dislocation of the hip. *J Bone Joint Surg*. 1938;20:124.
15. Hamby WB, comp-ed. *The Case Reports and Autopsy Records of Ambroise Paré*. Springfield, Ill: Charles C Thomas; 1960.
16. Hanson GW, Tullos HS. Subtrochanteric fractures of the femur treated with nail-plate devices. *Clin Orthop*. 1978;131:191–194.
17. Harris LJ. Closed retrograde intramedullary nailing of peritrochanteric fractures of the femur with a new nail. *J Bone Joint Surg*. 1980;62-A:1185–1193.
18. Kofoed H. Femoral neck fractures in young adults. *Injury*. 1984;14:146–150.
19. Lowell JD. Fractures of the hip. *N Engl J Med*. 1966;274:1480–1490.
20. Lucie RS, et al. Early prediction of avascular necrosis of the femoral head following femoral neck fractures. *Clin Orthop*. 1981;161:207–214.
21. Massie WK. Treatment of femoral neck fractures emphasizing long term follow-up observations on aseptic necrosis. *Clin Orthop*. 1973;92:16–62.
22. Mast J, et al. *Planning and Reduction Technique in Fracture Surgery*. Berlin, Germany: Springer-Verlag; 1989.
23. Maxwell TJ. Intra-Capsular Fracture of the Neck of the Femur. *Chicago Med J Examiner*. 1876;33:401–404.
24. Murray RC, Frew JFM. Trochanteric fractures of the femur. *J Bone Joint Surg*. 1949;31-B:204–219.
25. Pankovich AM, Tarabishy IE. Ender nailing of intertrochanteric and subtrochanteric fractures of the femur. Complications, failures, and errors. *J Bone Joint Surg*. 1980;62-A:635–645.
26. Peltier LH. *Fractures*. San Francisco, Calif: Norman Publishing; 1990.

27. Phillips GW. Fracture of the neck of the femur. *Am J Med Sci*. 1869;58:398–400.
28. Plummer WW. Comments on lateral fixation in fresh fractures of the neck of the femur. *J Bone Joint Surg*. 1938;20:97–107.
29. Protzman RR, Burkhalter WE. Femoral-neck fractures in young adults. *J Bone Joint Surg*. 1976;58-A: 689–695.
30. Rang M. *Children's Fractures*. 2nd ed. Philadelphia, Pa: JB Lippincott; 1983.
31. Rockwood CA Jr, Green DP, eds. *Fractures in Adults*. 2nd ed. Philadelphia, Pa: JB Lippincott; 1984.
32. Roeder LF, De Lee JC. Femoral head fractures associated with posterior hip dislocations. *Clin Orthop*. 1980;147:121.
33. Rybicki EF, et al. On the mathematical analysis of stress in the human femur. *J Biomech*. 1972;5:203.
34. Sanders R, Regazzoni P. Treatment of subtrochanteric femur fractures using the dynamic condylar screw. *J Orthop Trauma*. 1989;3:206–212.
35. Schatzker J, Tile M. *The Rationale of Operative Fracture Care*. Berlin, Germany: Springer-Verlag; 1987.
36. Schatzker J, Waddell JP. Subtrochanteric fractures of the femur. *Orthop Clin North Am*. 1980;11:539–554.
37. Senn N. The treatment of fractures of the neck of the femur by immediate reduction and permanent fixation. *JAMA*. 1889;13:150–159.
38. Speed K. The unsolved fracture. *Surg Gynecol Obstet*. 1935;60:341–352.
39. Sponseller PD, et al. Hip arthrodesis in young patients. *J Bone Joint Surg*. 1984;66-A:837–846.
40. Swiontkowski MF, et al. Fracture of the femoral neck in patients between the ages of twelve and forty-nine years. *J Bone Joint Surg*. 1984;66-A:837–846.
41. Urist MR. Fracture-dislocation of the hip joint: the nature of the traumatic lesion, treatment, late complications and end results. *J Bone Joint Surg*. 1948;30-A:699–727.
42. Watson HK, et al. Classification, treatment and complications of the adult subtrochanteric fracture. *J Trauma*. 1964;4:457–480.
43. Weber BG, Brunner CH, Freuler F, eds. *Treatment of Fractures in Children and Adolescents*. Berlin, Germany: Springer-Verlag; 1980.
44. White BL, et al. Rate of mortality for elderly patients after fracture of the hip in the 1980s. *J Bone Joint Surg*. 1987;69-A:1335–1340.
45. Zetterberg CH, et al. Femoral neck fractures in young adults. *Acta Orthop Scand*. 1982;53:427–435.
46. Zickel RE. An intramedullary fixation device for the proximal part of the femur. Nine years' experience. *J Bone Joint Surg*. 1976;58-A:866–872.

16

Femur Fractures

JAMES P. KENNEDY, M.D.

HISTORY: Since the time of Hippocrates, femoral fractures had been treated with various bindings, splints, and casts, but always with the limb held in extension.[19] Albucasis (936–1013) was the first to state that the knee should be maintained in flexion during the healing of the femur,[1] but his advice was ignored and subsequently forgotten.

It was not until the 1700s that the concept of deforming muscle forces was developed. Percival Pott, in his book, Some Few General Remarks on Fractures and Dislocations,[20] *stated that limbs should be positioned so that their muscles are in the greatest state of relaxation, thus minimizing the deforming forces on the fracture in order to obtain a reduction.*

Pott treated fractured femurs by lying the patients on their sides with the flexed leg resting on pillows. This was rather impractical for nursing care until Robert Chessher began using the supine position with the leg maintained in the proper position by a frame.[21] Various frames with or without skin traction were used until the advent of skeletal traction.

At about the same time, experimentation with intramedullary fixation had begun. Although the Conquistadores observed the Aztecs and Incas treating long bone non-unions with resinous intramedullary wooden pegs in the 16th century,[12] this type of fixation was not seen in traditional medical circles until Bircher began using short ivory pegs in femoral fractures in 1886.[3] Due to the problems with maintaining fixation with these short pegs, Hey-Groves began using long metal nails during World War I which closely resembled the nails of today.[13] Using the open technique of inserting the nail into the femur at the fracture site for these open war injuries without the benefit of antibiotics, he had significant problems with infection,[6] and therefore abandoned the technique.

The era of modern intramedullary nailing was introduced by Gerhard Küntscher.[17] Utilizing large intramedullary nails, he was able to obtain good results by pioneering the closed technique of inserting the nail under fluoroscopic control at the greater trochanter, without exposing the fracture site. His first report was published in Germany in the early days of World War II, so was not available to much of the rest of the world. His results were so good, that with the help of abundant fractures from the war, this technique spread across Europe. Following World War II, Küntscher's technique was discovered in the United States when American prisoners of war were noted to have intramedullary nails in healed femora, and eventually the technique became standard in America. Due to high radiation exposures from the fluoroscopes at that time, and once antibiotics became generally available,

276

closed nailing was abandoned in this country for the relative ease of open nailing.[6] As radiation safety improved, and with the development of the image intensifier, closed nailing is now again standard.

INTRODUCTION

No other fracture has been so much revolutionized in its treatment as has the fractured femur. This has been primarily through the development of intramedullary nailing techniques.[5] In the past, the patient was relegated to three months in traction with more likelihood than not of developing a complication from "fracture disease," not to mention the significant risk of mortality. Today, following intramedullary nailing, the patient can be discharged ambulatory a few days postoperatively, and can often be full weight bearing without crutches (depending on the fracture pattern) within two to four weeks.

INITIAL EVALUATION

The patient with a femoral shaft fracture should be checked for proximal and distal injuries of the ipsilateral extremity such as tibial or pelvic fractures. Knee ligamentous injuries are also common. Unfortunately, it is difficult to determine clinical knee stability in the presence of a fractured femur. Although it is possible to get some indication through palpation that the knee has been injured, the knee must always be examined under anesthesia after the femur has been stabilized to specifically assess ligamentous integrity.

A not uncommon injury pattern is ipsilateral femoral shaft and neck fractures from a dashboard injury mechanism. As the treatment for this condition requires a different device than the usual intramedullary nail used for shaft fractures alone, good x-ray views of the hip are necessary. This may require an internally rotated view to get a clear visualization of the femoral neck.

Neurovascular injuries are fairly uncommon with femoral shaft fractures except for a couple of specific instances. Femoral artery injuries must always be ruled out with shaft fractures of the distal third of the femur.[10,11] The femoral artery is tethered at the adductor canal of Hunter as it passes from the anterior compartment of the thigh into the posterior compartment, and can easily be torn by the wide displacement of the bone ends that occur at the time of fracture (Fig. 16–1).

"Floating knee" injuries (femoral shaft and ipsilateral tibial shaft fractures) are associated with a significant incidence of injuries to the structures in the popliteal fossa—the popliteal artery, and tibial and peroneal nerves. The floating knee should be treated with the knee dislocation protocol including arteriography (see Chapter 17) to rule out vascular injury. Following the arteriogram, both the femur and tibia do best with operative stabilization.

In the past, compartment syndrome of the thigh has been thought to be rare and therefore was not generally looked for. Today, compartment syndromes of the thigh are being reported more commonly, indicating that they probably were often missed in the past.[24] For this reason it is necessary to be aware of it, look for it, check pressures if indicated, and be prepared to do thigh fasciotomies when warranted.

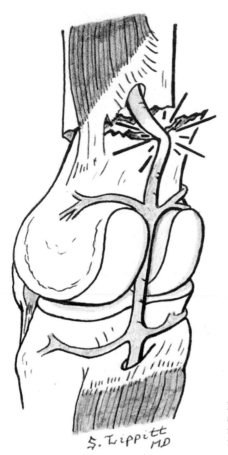

S. Lippitt
MD

Figure 16–1. Distal third femoral fracture at level of Hunter's adductor canal. Displacement can cause laceration or impingement on femoral artery.

The most popular method of immobilizing the femur fracture for transport is with a Hare or Thomas splint. These convenient devices consist of a frame buttressed up against the ischial tuberosity that uses a Spanish windlass and strap about the foot to apply traction (Fig. 16–2). This effectively immobilizes the extremity and makes the patient more comfortable. Radiographs can be easily obtained without removing the splint. The patient may be transferred back and forth to the x-ray table or CT scanner while maintaining traction sufficient to prevent shortening at the fracture site without difficulty.

In addition to holding the fracture out to length, the immobilization afforded by the splint helps prevent further soft tissue damage from the movement of sharp bone ends. Additional soft tissue trauma can lead to excessive bleeding at the injury site, as one to two units of blood can easily be lost into the thigh just due to the fracture itself. Bringing the fracture out to length through traction not only helps with the final reduction, but will result in an earlier tamponade of the hemorrhage through decreasing the volume of the thigh. Keeping surface area constant, a spherical container provides the greatest volume of any geometric shape. With muscle spasm, fracture shortening, and hemorrhage into the thigh, the thigh begins to assume a spherical contour. Lengthening the thigh changes it from a

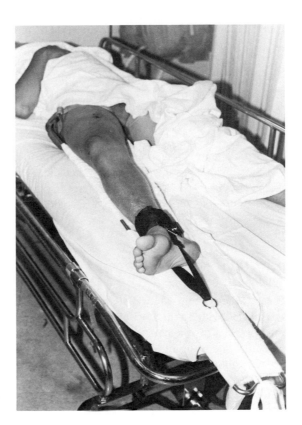

Figure 16–2. Hare splint for temporary immobilization of femur fracture.

more spherical configuration to a more cylindrical one and thereby lessens the volume available to bleed into.

Although the Hare splint is a very functional device, it cannot be left on indefinitely due to pressure from the strap about the foot. As soon as possible, the patient should be placed in skeletal traction, maintaining all of the benefits listed above. If the patient is being taken to the operating room expeditiously, there is no need to set up balanced suspension traction. The weight can simply be hung off the bottom of the bed, positioning the leg on pillows for comfort. However, if there is to be any delay in nailing the femur, balanced suspension will make the patient more comfortable and facilitate nursing care (Fig. 15–10).

The skeletal traction pin should be placed with the requirements of intramedullary nailing in mind. A tibial pin is generally placed for femur fractures so that the femur is not potentially contaminated from the insertion of the pin (see Chapter 3 for pin insertion technique). Ipsilateral proximal tibial fractures or knee ligamentous injuries may preclude skeletal traction through the tibia or across the knee joint. If this is the case, a distal femoral pin must be used. Scrupulous sterile technique should be adhered to and the pin must be placed far enough anteriorly or distally so as not to interfere with the placement of an intramedullary nail or any potential interlocking screws, but also avoiding the knee joint. If a tibial pin can be used, it should be placed distal to the anterior tubercle so that the complete femur including the knee joint can be prepped out for surgery without including the pin site.

The type of pin used will depend somewhat on the type of fracture table available and surgeon preference, but generally the largest pin possible is best. Strong traction is often necessary to reduce the fracture, especially if the nailing is delayed for any reason. A heavy pin will neither bend nor cut out under the influence of these heavy forces. A large straight pin is much easier and more atraumatic to remove than a smaller pin that has been bent from traction.

If the femur is to be immediately nailed, either a threaded or smooth pin can be used. The threaded pin has the advantage of not sliding back and forth as a smooth pin does (see Chapter 3). The best choice for long-term traction is the newer pins that are threaded in the middle intraosseous portion to prevent sliding, but smooth on the ends that protrude through soft tissue and skin.

INDICATION FOR NAILING

There are few things so absolute in orthopaedics as the fact that adult femur fractures are best treated with an intramedullary nail. It is generally felt that the indication for nailing a femoral shaft is the presence of a fracture.[6] Obviously there are some exceptions to this generalization, but not many.

Certainly, every femur fracture in the polytrauma patient that is amenable to nailing should be so treated.[4,5] This facilitates nursing care, and allows the patient to be rapidly mobilized. Nailing decreases the incidence of ARDS, blood loss, and narcotic requirement. Early IM nailing and mobilization will also prevent the problems associated with fracture disease (atelectasis, adult respiratory distress syndrome, urinary tract infection, decubiti, deep venous thrombosis, and pulmonary embolus).[4–6] Using closed nailing techniques, fracture disease is prevented, and a 99% union rate with a less than 1% incidence of infection[25] can be expected.

With the advent of today's interlocking nails, even fractures with significant comminution or other unstable configurations can be maintained in their proper alignment[15] with a much lower rate of complication than with previously available techniques.[14]

TIMING OF SURGERY

The best time for nailing the polytraumatized patient with a fractured femur is immediately.[4] Immediate stabilization will serve to help control hemorrhage at the fracture site and help stabilize the patient hemodynamically. After the initial resuscitation and stabilization, the patient generally is in the best medical condition that he will be in for the next several days. If it all possible, this small golden period of time should be taken advantage of. Otherwise, there is a high probability that medical complications will occur increasing morbidity to the patient and resulting in postponement of the surgery. Polytrauma patients with an Injury Severity Score of 18 or more who were nailed more than 48 hours after their injury were found to have a four times greater incidence of pulmonary complications requiring an average of 7.6 days stay in the intensive care unit at a total hospital cost of almost $33,000. This is in comparison to a similar group of patients nailed within 24 hours of their injury who had an average intensive care unit stay of only 2.8 days at a total hospital cost of less than $20,000.[4]

In the nonpolytraumatized patient, timing is not as crucial,[4] but the task of nailing is easier if performed in the first 6 to 12 hours. If nailing is attempted past this time, hemorrhage and swelling will make the reduction more difficult. The additional trauma from forceful traction to obtain a satisfactory reduction as well as reaming and bleeding into an already tense thigh may precipitate a compartment syndrome. Extreme traction against the stabilizing perineal post on the fracture table in these instances can also lead to a pudendal nerve injury.

TECHNIQUE

The patient may be nailed either in the supine or lateral position. It is generally felt that the patient is easier to set up in the supine position, but harder to nail, and harder to set up but easier to nail in the lateral position. It is useful to be adept at both techniques as the patient's other injuries will sometimes dictate how they can be positioned. A spinal fracture may preclude a lateral nailing unless the spine has already been stabilized.

The patient is positioned on the fracture table making sure that the perineal post is carefully padded and being careful that the genitalia are free. Skeletal traction is applied to bring the fracture out to length and slightly overdistract it, being careful that the metal traction apparatus is not in contact with the skin, or burns from the electrocoagulator may result. The position of the legs is adjusted to allow access to the image intensifier for both AP and lateral views of the entire femur (Fig. 16–3). The ability to reduce the femur is confirmed by the image intensifier. Rotation at the fracture site is carefully corrected.

Following the surgical prep and drape, access to the piriformis fossa is made through an incision at the greater trochanter. The entrance point for the nail is palpated then opened by reaming over a short guide pin placed at this position. A long intramedullary guide pin is then passed under image control across the fracture. The femur is reamed to the chosen diameter, and the nail is inserted over the guide pin. Interlocking screws are placed if necessary based on the fracture configuration (Fig. 16–4).

Modern nails are designed with flutes (Fig. 16–5) to allow rapid endosteal revascularization. Nails are now available that are sufficiently strong to allow immediate full weight bearing with crutches in stable fracture patterns. Realistically, however, most patients require six weeks to achieve full pain-free weight bearing without crutches.

OPEN FEMUR FRACTURES

Open femur fractures are rarely as difficult to deal with as the open tibial fracture. The blood supply to the femur is inherently better due to its large soft tissue envelope, and soft tissue coverage over the bone is not difficult to achieve. The protocol for all open fractures should be followed. If adequate irrigation and debridement are performed, and the wound is left open, reamed nails can be used for all Grade I and many Grade II injuries without significant increase in infection.[6–9]

Unlike lesser grade injuries, Grade III fractures must be carefully considered. Although reamed nailing may be indicated in certain polytrauma situations[9,18] (especially

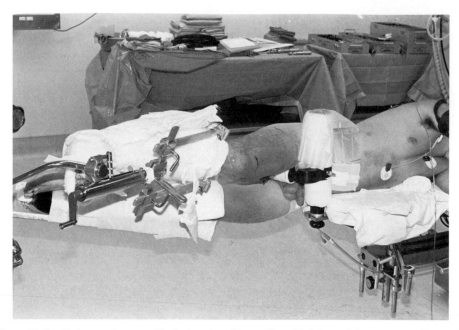

Figure 16–3. Patient on fracture table for lateral position nailing of left femoral fracture. An axillary roll is placed to prevent brachial plexus compression. The down leg is carefully padded to protect the peroneal nerve and secured. Tibial pin skeletal traction is used to bring the fracture out to length and correct rotation. Reduction is checked clinically and by biplanar image intensification. The genitalia are free to prevent a pudendal nerve palsy if strong traction is necessary.

with the Grade IIIa injury), the advantage of immediate rigid stability can be offset by an increased infection rate of 6.5%[7] from the devascularizing effects of reaming. Reamed nailing of the Grade IIIa femur must be done under ideal circumstances in which the patient has had an expeditious and thorough irrigation and debridement.

The act of reaming and nailing destroys the intramedullary blood supply, resulting in necrosis of the inner 50% to 70% of the cortex.[16] Although this bone is eventually revascularized, Grade IIIb and IIIc fractures have extensive stripping and loss of periosteal blood supply to such an extent that reaming can tip the balance over to osteonecrosis and infection. These Grade IIIb and IIIc fractures are treated better by other means, especially if they are isolated injuries.

If the patient does not have multiple injuries and can tolerate a period of bedrest, an initial period of traction can be utilized following the irrigation and debridement until the wound is closed and revascularization has begun. The femur then can be nailed on a delayed basis, once it becomes a "closed" fracture.

The standard for open fractures in other anatomic areas, the external fixator, has a higher morbidity[2] when used in the femur as opposed to locations such as the tibia, although little else may be available for the unstable IIIb and IIIc injuries. The external fixator remains the most rapid means of managing an open fracture in a patient who is medically unable to tolerate a lengthy anesthetic.

Due to the large muscle mass that the fixator pins must penetrate, pin tract problems such as drainage and infection often develop with femoral external fixators. There is also a

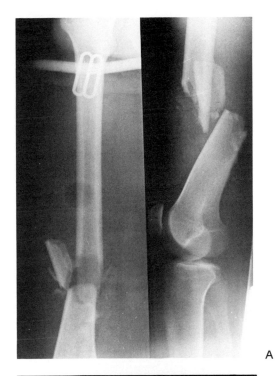

A

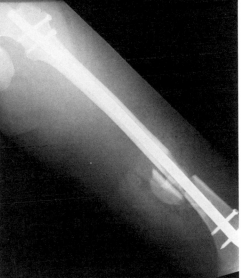

B

Figure 16–4.   Femur fracture. **A:** This fracture of the distal third is rotationally unstable as evidenced by its relatively smooth transverse nature without spikes to allow interdigitation following reduction, and is longitudinally unstable due to the large butterfly fragment preventing significant bony apposition. **B:** Anatomic nailing of the fracture with an interlocked nail. The proximal and distal interlocking screws prevent rotation and shortening at the fracture. (The displaced butterfly fragment is not significant and will serve as a vascularized bone graft.)

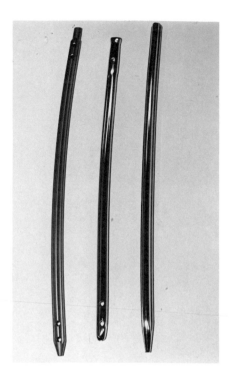

Figure 16–5. Various femoral nails. Left: Titanium interlocking Alta nail with multiple flutes, Middle: Slotted interlocking Grosse-Kempf nail, Right: Tri-flanged (or cloverleaf) Küntscher nail.

significant incidence of knee stiffness due to tethering of muscle or subsequent scarring. Fortunately, unlike the tibia, the severe open injuries of the femur that external fixation may be indicated for are relatively uncommon.

An intramedullary nail may also be inserted without reaming to preserve endosteal blood supply in these Grade IIIb and IIIc fractures. A smaller nail is used and fixation will not be as rigid as with the reamed nail. Interlocking the nail with screws will help to stabilize the fracture further if necessary. Multiple flexible nails may also be used.[8]

A way to avoid using an external fixator and its potential problems with knee stiffness and difficulty with the pins, is to plate the femur[23] (Fig. 16–6). This can be done with selected large Grade III wounds where the exposure is essentially done by the injury itself. It is necessary to be careful in applying the plate so that further soft tissue stripping and devascularization does not occur. Due to the large muscle mass of the thigh, sufficient local soft tissue is usually present to cover over the plate yet still leave the wound open. A major disadvantage to plating the femur is that unlike an intramedullary rod, weight bearing must be protected for a prolonged period until healing has progressed sufficiently so that the plate and screws are not dangerously loaded during ambulation. Bone grafting is mandatory for these open fractures which are plated once the wound is clean.

Femur fractures, although once associated with significant morbidity and mortality, are now one of the musculoskeletal injuries with the most predictable results following treatment. The vast majority of complications are secondary to technical problems at the time of nailing and therefore are preventable by paying attention to detail.

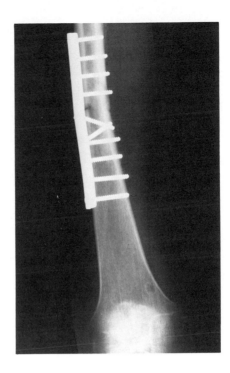

Figure 16–6. Femoral fracture stabilized by compression plate and screws.

REFERENCES

1. Albucasis, Spink MS, Lewis GL, trans-eds. *On Surgery and Instruments*. Berkeley, Calif: University of California Press; 1973.
2. Alonso J, et al. External fixation of femoral fractures: indications and limitations. *Clin Orthop*. 1989;241: 83–88.
3. Bircher H. Eine neue Methode unmittelbarer retention bei Fracturen der Rohrenknochen. *Arch Klin Chir*. 1893;34:410–422.
4. Bone LB, et al. Early versus delayed stabilization of femoral fractures. *J Bone Joint Surg*. 1989;71-A: 336–340.
5. Browner BD, Cole JD. Current status of locked intramedullary nailing: a review. *J Orthop Trauma*. 1987; 1:183–195.
6. Browner BD, Edwards CC: *The Science and Practice of Intramedullary Nailing*. Philadelphia, Pa: Lea & Febiger; 1987.
7. Brumback RJ, et al. Intramedullary nailing of open fractures of the femoral shaft. *J Bone Joint Surg*. 1989; 71-A:1324–1331.
8. Chapman MW. The role of intramedullary fixation in open fractures. *Clin Orthop*. 1986;212:26–34.
9. Chapman M, ed. *Operative Orthopaedics*. Philadelphia, Pa: JB Lippincott; 1988.
10. Chervu A, Quinones-Baldrich WJ. Vascular complications in orthopedic surgery. *Clin Orthop*. 1988; 235:275–288.
11. Cone JB, Vascular injury associated with fracture-dislocations of the lower extremity. *Clin Orthop*. 1989; 243:30–35.
12. Farill J. Orthopaedics in Mexico. *J Bone Joint Surg*. 1952;34-A:506.
13. Hey-Groves E. Ununited fractures, with special reference to gunshot injuries and the use of bone grafting. *Br J Surg*. 1918-1919;6:203–247.
14. Johnson KD, et al. Comminuted femoral-shaft fractures: treatment by roller traction, cerclage wires and intramedullary nail, or an interlocking intramedullary nail. *J Bone Joint Surg*. 1984;66-A:1222–1235.
15. Kempf I, et al. Closed locked intramedullary nailing. *J Bone Joint Surg*. 1985;67-A:709–720.

16. Kessler SB, et al. The effects of reaming and intramedullary nailing on fracture healing. *Clin Orthop*. 1986; 212:18–25.
17. Küntscher G. Die Marknagelung von Knochenbrüchen. *Arch f Klin Chir*. 1940;200:443.
18. Lhowe DW, Hansen ST. Immediate nailing of open fractures of the femoral shaft. *J Bone Joint Surg*. 1988; 70-A:812–820.
19. Peltier LF. *Fractures*. San Francisco, Calif: Norman Publishing; 1990.
20. Pott P. *Some Few General Remarks on Fractures and Dislocations*. London, England: L Hawes, W Clarke, R Collins; 1765.
21. Richter AL. *40 Lithographierte Tafeln nebst Erklarung and Erlauterung Derselben zu dem Theoretisch-Praktischen Handbuch der Lehre von den Bruchen und Verrenkungen der Knochen*. Berlin, Germany: Enslin; 1828.
22. Rockwood CA Jr, Green DP, eds. *Fractures in Adults*. 2nd ed. Philadelphia, Pa: JB Lippincott; 1984.
23. Schatzker J, Tile M. *The Rationale of Operative Fracture Care*. Berlin, Germany: Springer-Verlag; 1987.
24. Schwartz JT Jr, et al. Acute compartment syndrome of the thigh. *J Bone Joint Surg*. 1989;71-A:392–400.
25. Winquist RA, et al. Closed intramedullary nailing of femoral fractures. A report of five hundred and twenty cases. *J Bone Joint Surg*. 1984;66-A:529–539.

17

Fracture and Dislocation of the Knee and Patella

JAMES P. KENNEDY, M.D.

HISTORY: Until the late 1870s, knee injuries were treated with splinting in extension. This method when applied to patellar fractures usually resulted in a fibrous union of the distracted fragments and weakness of the knee. Sir Astley Cooper first advanced the theory of displacement of fracture fragments leading to nonunion in 1822 through his study of patellar fractures in an animal model.[8] Thus it was natural that the patella served as the impetus for the development of many surgical techniques for fracture treatment that we use today.

Malgaigne devised the first external fixator in the 1840s and used it to treat patellar fractures. A claw mechanism was employed to percutaneously gain purchase into the distracted superior and inferior pole fragments, and a screw mechanism then was used to draw the two together.[19] The actual open surgical treatment of a closed fracture was first performed in March of 1877 by Cameron, who, using Lister's recently developed aseptic techniques, successfully obtained union in an eight-week-old displaced patellar fracture which had failed closed treatment by stabilizing it with a silver cerclage wire.[4] Lister himself repeated this technique in October that same year, performing the first successful open reduction and internal fixation of an acute closed fracture using aseptic techniques.[18]

INTRODUCTION

Injury to the knee is very common in multiple trauma patients. This is in part due to the vulnerability of the knee to dashboard injuries in automobile accidents and direct trauma in motorcycle accidents—our most common causes of multiple trauma. As well, the proximity of the knee to automobile bumpers and fenders makes knee injuries common in pedestrian accidents as well.

PATELLA FRACTURES

The most common injury to the patella in the trauma victim is a stellate comminuted fracture resulting from a direct blow (Fig. 17–1). Comminuted stellate fractures comprise 30% to 35% of all patella fractures.[24] The second type of injury, avulsion fractures and ruptures of the extensor mechanism occurring secondary to tensile forces (Fig. 17–2), make up 50% to 80% of patella fractures.[24] These can occur with or without comminution, and are most often seen as isolated injuries. They may occur in the polytrauma patient due to forced flexion of the knee along with forceful muscle contracture at the time of injury as a reaction to the accident in an attempt to prevent injury.[5]

Assessment

The patient with a fractured patella usually will have both generalized soft tissue swelling about the knee as well as a hemarthrosis, which may be tense. Pain is localized to the anterior knee. Displaced fractures will often demonstrate a palpable defect. These injuries are commonly associated with a laceration over the patella (Fig. 17–3), if so, a traumatic arthrotomy must be ruled out by the techniques described in Chapter Two. If a dashboard injury has occurred, associated injuries such as cruciate ligament failure, femur fracture, hip dislocation, or posterior wall acetabular fractures may be present as well.

If the fracture itself is not of a pattern requiring surgery, the most important part of the exam is to make sure that the extensor mechanism is intact. The stellate fractures caused by direct blows are often not associated with extensor ruptures, and in fact it is the intact extensor retinaculum which may keep many of these fractures from displacing. In compari-

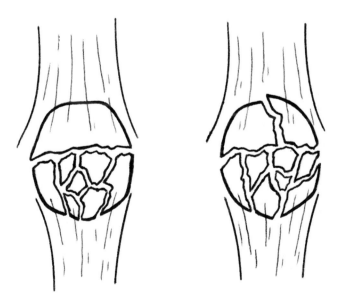

Figure 17–1. Typical stellate fractures of patella from dashboard injury or direct blow. Fragments may be maintained in proper position by intact extensor retinaculum.

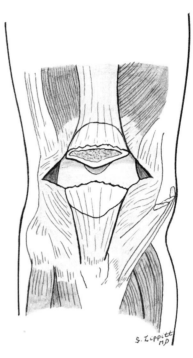

Figure 17–2. Avulsion fracture of patella resulting from tensile forces. Associated tears of extensor mechanism are often present and result in distraction of fracture fragments.

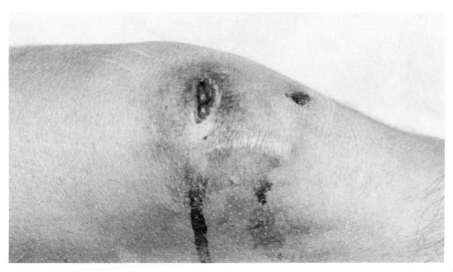

Figure 17–3. Dashboard laceration over knee. This patient needs work-up for knee injuries as well as the other injuries associated with a dashboard mechanism.

son, the avulsion fractures which fail in tension are often associated with tears of the extensor tendon which likewise has failed in tension. The patient must be able to extend the knee without a lag and perform a straight leg raise against gravity to demonstrate competence of the extensor. In most instances, pain will prevent these maneuvers even if the extensor is intact. If so, the joint should be infiltrated under sterile conditions with local anesthetic so the patient can demonstrate the maneuver.

X-rays of the knee, AP and lateral, will demonstrate the fracture pattern (Fig. 17–4). These views are generally sufficient to formulate a treatment plan. A bipartite patella can sometimes be mistaken for a fracture. The bipartite patella usually involves the supero-lateral pole, and unlike a fresh fracture its edges are sclerotic. As they are often bilateral, a comparison view of the opposite knee may be helpful in diagnosing bipartite patellae. Rarely, a CT scan or the "skyline" or "sunrise" view may be required to further evaluate the articular surfaces of a fractured patella.

Treatment

Tensile avulsion fractures usually demonstrate displacement (Fig. 17–5) and incompetence of the extensor mechanism.[5,26] If displaced, operative exploration and repair of the fracture through a direct anterior approach over the patella, as well as repair of retinacular or capsular tears to prevent resultant knee extensor weakness is necessary.[2] Nondisplaced fractures can be treated with immobilization in a knee immobilizer or cylinder cast if the patient can prove the extensor mechanism is intact by actively extending the knee.[3]

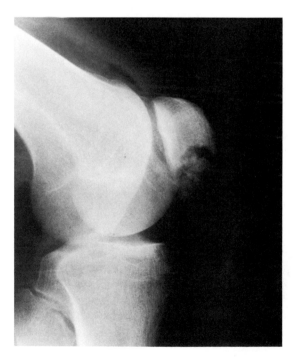

Figure 17–4. Direct blow resulting in stellate fracture of inferior pole of the patella. An intact extensor retinaculum is holding the fragments in place. (Note the air density behind the femoral condyle and above the superior pole of the patella indicating an open fracture.)

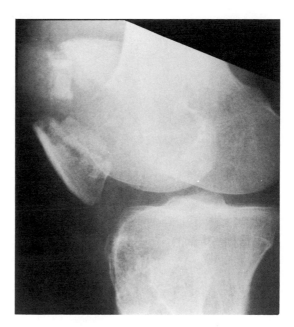

Figure 17–5. Avulsion fracture of the patella. Occurring secondary to tensile forces, the extensor retinaculum is torn as evident by weakness of knee extension and displacement of the fragments. The fracture needs to be reduced and stabilized, and the extensor repaired to restore knee function.

The stellate direct-blow fracture can be treated with simple immobilization and, later, protected motion until healed if the fractures are not displaced, there is no significant joint surface irregularity, and the extensor mechanism is intact.[5] Often, the fragments are maintained in an anatomic position by an intact extensor retinaculum which has not been damaged by the mechanism of injury. As for all joint surfaces, if the fragments are offset more than a millimeter, anatomic reduction of the joint surface is necessary to help prevent posttraumatic arthritis.[3]

Standard techniques for patellar fixation include tension band wiring or interfragmentary compression screws. The tension band serves to convert the tensile forces across the patella that occur with motion into compression forces at the patellar joint surface[23] to maintain anatomic reduction and promote healing. The tension band is used together with Kirschner wires or screws to maintain the reduction. This method is amenable to both stellate and tensile fractures.

Interfragmentary compression screws can be used only with larger fracture fragments (Fig. 17–6), and therefore usually are not suitable for stellate fractures. These screws are often protected, or "neutralized" with a tension band wire as well.

No matter what the type of fixation, if full knee flexion is permitted postoperatively, the fixation will fail. If fixation is tenuous due to poor bone stock, the surgeon may choose to totally immobilize the extremity. A better technique for appropriate candidates to promote cartilaginous healing and restore range of motion is to allow immediate motion of the knee postoperatively. After the fixation, the knee is flexed intraoperatively to see at what point the fixation device is under tension. The patient is then placed in a hinged knee orthosis or cast brace postoperatively which allows motion within a zone which will not stress the fixation.

Severely comminuted patellae may be irreparable. In these instances, a partial or total patellectomy may be required.[1] Partial patellectomy can be very functional, and it is well

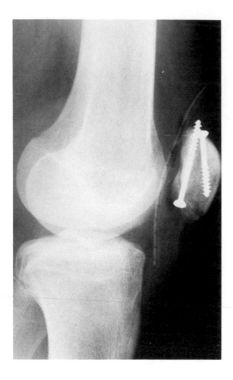

Figure 17–6. Compression screw fixation of a patellar avulsion fracture.

established that if greater than 50% of the patella can be salvaged, it is worthwhile to do so.[5] Total patellectomy can result in the loss of biomechanical advantage to the extensor mechanism afforded by the patella. For this reason, it may be worthwhile to attempt to salvage even lesser amounts of the patella.

PATELLAR DISLOCATION

Dislocation of the patella is rarely seen in the multiple trauma victim as the usual patellar dislocation is a chronic recurrent problem resulting from anatomic malalignment,[13] or a one-time occurrence following an external rotation maneuver with the knee flexed. This injury commonly occurs as a sporting injury. A valgus force or strong quadriceps contraction with the knee flexed will also produce the dislocation. Rarely, a direct traumatic blow will cause a dislocation.[5,24]

Assessment

The vast majority of patellar dislocations occur to the lateral side of the knee. The lateral femoral condyle has a lower profile than the medial, and the mechanical and anatomic axes of the lower extremity cause the patella to tend to pull toward the lateral side.

The patient with a dislocated patella will exhibit an obvious deformity. The knee is rigidly held in flexion and the patient resists any attempts to movement. Pain is localized to the anterior knee. Swelling is not normally evident when these patients are seen acutely, as it is masked by the deformity and tends to occur later following the reduction.

Treatment

The clinical picture of the dislocated patella is so classic that x-rays are not usually warranted for diagnosis prior to reduction. The anatomy is distorted so that x-rays taken in the dislocated position often are inadequate to diagnose associated injuries.

The patella is almost always easily relocated simply by extending the knee to relax the taut quadriceps. Sometimes, a gentle push on the patella is required to coax it back into the femoral groove. This can often be done expeditiously without significant pain by reassuring the patient to relax.

Once reduction is obtained, x-rays should be taken to rule out associated injuries, especially osteochondral fractures of the patella.

The more common recurrent atraumatic patellar dislocation is usually treated successfully by the nonoperative means[10,17,24] of immobilization in a cylinder cast or knee immobilizer followed by an aggressive quadriceps rehabilitation program. This mode of treatment is not always as successful in the acute traumatic dislocation.[10] For this reason, some recommend surgical repair of the torn capsular structures for better results. This is especially true if palpation of the capsule alongside the patella on the side opposite from the dislocation (ie, the medial retinaculum for lateral dislocations) reveals a defect. These capsular tears occur with the higher grade dislocations which are more unstable.

Whether treated conservatively with immobilization following reduction, or with operative repair, osteochondral fractures should be ruled out and addressed if present. Displaced fragments should be excised if small, and operatively stabilized if large.

KNEE DISLOCATION

Knee dislocations are rare, but can be potentially devastating injuries. Classified according to the direction the tibia is displaced, a dislocation may occur anteriorly, posteriorly, medially, or laterally. A mixed and rotatory pattern[24] can also be seen. Dislocation in the anterior-posterior plane is the most common. Some report that the anterior dislocation is more common,[24] while others[5] feel the posterior dislocation occurs more frequently. In the auto accident victim, posterior dislocation is more common from the dashboard injury against the flexed knee. Due to this mechanism, and the high forces involved, an open dislocation is often present. The anterior dislocation is associated with hyperextension,[15] such as when a pedestrian with the foot planted is struck from the front by an auto.

Assessment

Knee dislocations are one of the few orthopaedic surgical emergencies. The knee exhibits an obvious deformity which is characteristic. Unlike periarticular fractures about the knee, the knee is relatively immobile and rigid, without bony crepitus. A quick assessment of the neurovascular structures is mandatory due to the high number of associated nerve and vascular injuries. This injury warrants an immediate reduction upon presentation in the emergency department (even before x-rays are available) if the diagnosis is reasonably certain, and if it can be done gently. X-rays are then obtained postreduction to confirm adequate reduction and to rule out associated bony injury.

Treatment

The knee is generally easily reduced by gentle manipulation of the displaced distal leg into its normal anatomic position. Often, the knee will have been reduced in positioning the patient for transport to the hospital.[24] Gentle in-line traction followed by flexion or extension associated with manipulation of the tibia back into its normal position will usually bring about the reduction. Although the knee is ideally reduced atraumatically under general anesthesia, as the reduction must be accomplished immediately to relieve the neurovascular structures, it is rarely feasible for the multiple trauma patient to have a reduction in the operating room. Reduction maneuvers can usually be done in the emergency department with little or no analgesia, with immediate relief of the patient's complaints of knee pain. Rarely is the knee irreducible requiring open reduction. The dislocations that are irreducible are usually posterolateral dislocations where the medial femoral condyle is buttonholed through the capsule.

Urgency is required in these injuries due to the high incidence of neurovascular damage. Overall there is arterial injury in one third,[13] and neurologic compromise in one fifth.[24] If only the anterior-posterior injuries are considered, vascular injury is seen in more than 40% of cases.[5] Proximally, the femoral artery is tethered in the adductor canal of Hunter, and distally by the fibrous arch of the soleus origin (Fig. 17–7). With dislocation, the artery may be torn, stretched, go into spasm, or be occluded by pressure against the bony prominences (Fig. 17–8).

The tibial and common peroneal nerves are not as tethered as the artery, and are therefore less likely to be injured. When a nerve palsy is present, it is usually a traction injury.

Due to the high incidence of arterial injury, knee dislocations should have an arteriogram. Even if distal pulses are present, angiography is required to rule out an intimal tear or other lesion.[5,7] Some advocate repeat studies at one week postinjury to confirm that any small apparently insignificant lesion has not progressed.

If the system allows expedient studies in the radiology suite, a formal angiogram may be obtained as long as circulation to the foot is present. Often these injuries occur at night, or the patient has other injuries requiring rapid operative intervention. If this is the case, or when the distal extremity is pulseless, the radiology suite should be abandoned in favor of the operative suite. A "one shot" femoral percutaneous needle angiogram can be obtained in the operating room following the reduction to document either the location of a lesion which is then explored, or the presence of patency and flow (Fig. 17–9). A formal arteriogram can be done later when conditions are more optimal.[5] If arterial compromise is present and not repaired within eight hours, 86% of patients will go on to amputation, and two thirds of those with viable legs will suffer ischemic changes.[11] Even with repair of vascular lesions, there remains a 10% rate of amputation.[5]

Following confirmation of an intact vascular supply, the knee is splinted in a Robert Jones dressing with gentle flexion of 10° to 20°. After the swelling dissipates, a knee orthosis or cast can be applied. Some unstable knees will sublux in the Robert Jones and need

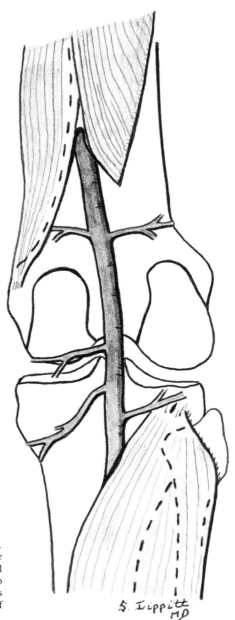

Figure 17–7. Structures in popliteal fossa. The popliteal artery is affixed to the femur proximally by fascial fibers of Hunter's canal where the artery crosses from the anterior into the posterior compartments. The artery is tethered distally at the tibia by the origin of the soleus muscle.

immediate casting, and an occasional patient is so unstable as to require an external fixator across the joint to maintain the reduced position. This is more common in the very obese in whom it is hard to apply a functional cast. If x-rays document intra-articular fractures, they are addressed as discussed below. Immobilization is continued for six weeks to allow soft tissue healing of the capsule and ligaments to occur.

Although immediate surgical reconstruction of the associated torn ligaments is

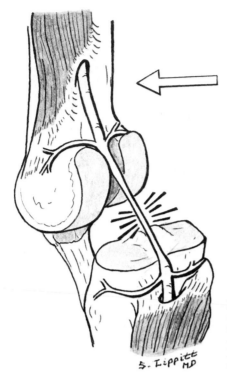

Figure 17–8. Knee dislocation. With knee dislocations, the popliteal artery which is not freely mobile may be lacerated, contused, or occluded. Arteriograms are indicated for knee dislocations to rule out popliteal artery injury.

recommended for young, athletic individuals with isolated injuries to obtain a better result,[21,27] others feel that nonoperative treatment will give results which are just as satisfactory,[5,28] especially for the more sedentary patient. The multiple trauma patient is usually not a candidate for immediate reconstruction of the ligamentous structures of the knee. Other injuries will take precedence over an elective acute ligamentous repair, and the patient with multiple system trauma often is not a candidate to undergo the lengthy postoperative immobilization and rehabilitation that such repairs require. If patients are considered to be candidates for early reconstruction, it can be done so within the first four to six weeks after they have recovered from their systemic injuries.

Open dislocations, the rare irreducible dislocation, and vascular injuries do require immediate surgical intervention,[5] and in these instances, simultaneous ligamentous repair may be acutely warranted if the knee is unstable. It is often surprising how stable these joints sometimes are following the reduction. Delayed reconstruction can be undertaken for those treated nonoperatively who develop late symptomatic instability.[24]

INTRA-ARTICULAR KNEE FRACTURES

Fractures about the knee affecting the tibial or femoral condyles (Fig. 17–10) are as much an injury to the articular surfaces of the knee joint as they are a fracture of the periarticular bone. Therefore the issues of joint alignment, stability, stiffness, and posttraumatic arthritis may compromise the clinical result even if a successful anatomic bony union is achieved.

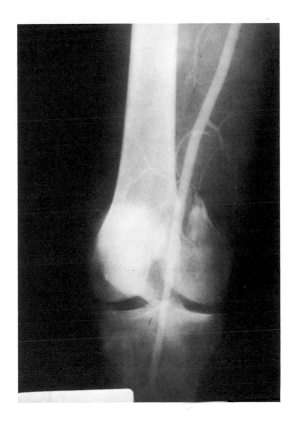

Figure 17–9. One-shot arteriogram of leg with open fracture-dislocation of the knee obtained on the operating table to determine patency of the popliteal artery.

Generally these fractures are a result of a high energy direct blow. More than half of tibial plateau fractures are the result of auto-pedestrian accidents.[12] These fractures can also result from the axial loading with rotation or varus/valgus stresses that occur with falls from a height.[24]

Assessment

Fractures about the knee are characterized by localized pain, swelling, and crepitation. A hemarthrosis forms when an intra-articular fracture is present. Bleeding into the joint will be confined within the joint only if the capsule has not been torn by the injury. If the capsule is incompetent, the hemorrhage will decompress into the surrounding soft tissue so that generalized swelling is present. Intra-articular fracture may be suspected when marrow fat globules are present in the hemarthrosis. These are easily visualized floating on top of the aspirated blood when the specimen is displayed in a shallow receptacle.

In the case of any injury about the knee, ligamentous stressing should not be performed until after x-rays confirm that no fracture is present. There is no need to test ligamentous integrity prior to x-ray. If a fracture is present but not suspected, apparent instability of the knee can be falsely diagnosed as ligamentous instability when in fact the motion is occurring due to instability at a fracture site. Not only is the wrong diagnosis

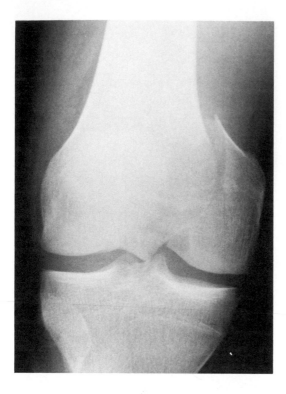

Figure 17–10. Split fracture of the medial femoral condyle which is displaced resulting in joint incongruency.

made, but further bony damage can be caused through comminution and compression from manipulation through the fracture.

An x-ray of the knee will diagnose fractures about the joint. If either a femoral supracondylar or tibial plateau fracture is discovered, x-rays of the entire length of the respective bone should be obtained to rule out other fractures.

Treatment

Unstable intra-articular fractures about the knee in appropriate candidates are best treated according to the principles for all intra-articular fractures: anatomic reduction, rigid fixation, and early motion.[5,26] Aspiration of a tense hemarthrosis is sometimes required early to decompress the joint for pain relief.

These fractures can be treated in the multiple trauma patient with the same techniques[14,22,26] used when they occur as isolated injuries. Results are almost always best when these injuries are treated by immediate stabilization through rigid internal fixation. However, delayed treatment performed at a few days' postinjury will usually give acceptable results. If delayed fixation is to be done, the extremity should be splinted or placed in balanced traction.

If for any reason it is not possible to internally fix these fractures, the patient should be placed in skeletal traction for reduction. Early range of motion is instituted to obtain the best resultant function.[25] The patient can be mobilized out of bed while maintaining reduction through the use of roller traction.

Femoral condyle fractures (even when nondisplaced initially) should be rigidly fixed[14,22] (Fig. 17–11) due to the risk of subsequent displacement[5] from muscle forces or knee motion. With rigid fixation, early motion to facilitate cartilage healing can be carried out.[25] In the obtunded patient, continuous passive motion (CPM) via mechanical devices can be utilized.

Supracondylar femoral fractures often have an intra-articular extension forming a "T" or "Y" fracture (Fig. 17–12). Like the condylar fracture, the joint surface must be anatomically restored. In order to allow motion during the healing phase, the reconstructed condyles must be rigidly fixed to the femoral shaft as well. This is usually done with a side plate device (Fig. 17–13).

Unstable or displaced tibial plateau fractures (Fig. 17–14) likewise warrant rigid fixation and early motion. There are two types of plateau fractures—splits and compressions. Plateau splits result from shearing forces and if nondisplaced are usually stable fractures unless associated with extensive soft tissue stripping. After 7 to 10 days of immobilization to allow pain and swelling to abate, these can often be treated with motion by using a hinged orthosis or cast brace molded properly to unload the injured side of the joint.

Tibial plateau compression fractures are the result of an axial load and are by definition displaced. For active individuals, anatomic reduction and fixation to allow early motion will give the best long-term results. Often, bone grafting is required due to the degree of

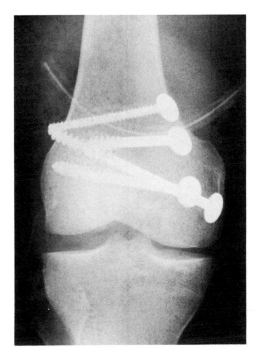

Figure 17–11. Lag screw fixation of condylar fracture in anatomic position.

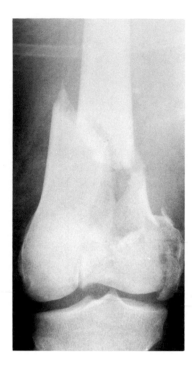

Figure 17–12. Supracondylar femoral fracture with intracondylar extension.

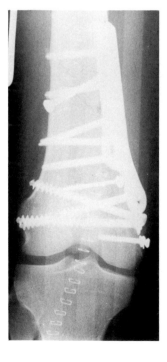

Figure 17–13. Anatomic reconstruction of femoral condyles with lag screws and stabilization of supracondylar component with buttress plate and screws.

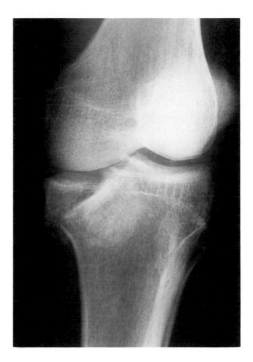

Figure 17–14. Medial tibial plateau compression fracture. Subchondral metaphyseal bone has been compressed beneath the fracture as evidenced by the increased density of the metaphysis in this region. Following elevation of the articular surface, a void will be present here requiring bone grafting.

compression of the metaphyseal bone. Once the articular surface is elevated into anatomic position, a large defect may be left underneath it needing a graft to fill the void. A buttress plate and screws are then used to protect the area until healing occurs (Fig. 17–15).

Open unstable plateau fractures which are compressed are one of the exceptions to the rule that bone grafting should not be done in the face of an open fracture. (Another exception is the unstable tibial pilon fracture—see Chapter 18.) The reason for immediate grafting at the time of fixation is that the bone graft is used not just to fill the defect and enhance healing, but is also an integral part of the fixation of these fractures. Without the graft, there would not be adequate stabilization, and the result is a risk of collapse of the articular surface. Severe open injuries such as Grade IIIb and IIIc, or those closed fractures with compromised vascularity to the skin which would be at risk for skin slough if opened (ie, the segmental amputations discussed in Chapter 21) need a period of either traction or external fixation across the joint until the wounds or skin permit definitive operative treatment.

Tibial plateau fractures which extend distally into the metaphyseal/diaphyseal area (Fig. 17–16) are at risk to develop a compartment syndrome. Often splits extend far enough to enter into the anterior compartment, but are not the result of high enough energy to cause significant soft tissue stripping. Therefore, the highly vascular proximal metaphyseal bone will bleed into a closed anterior compartment. Should there be any clinical evidence of a compartment syndrome, fasciotomy should be carried out (see Chapter 20).

Following the rigid stabilization of these fractures, the ligamentous structures about the knee should be evaluated by examination, or by stress films if warranted, as 20% to 25%

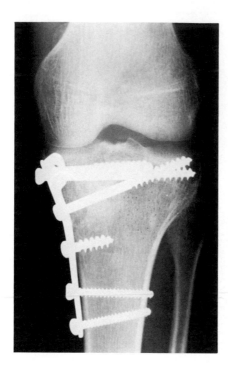

Figure 17–15. AP x-ray showing restoration of plateau after elevation, grafting, and buttress plating.

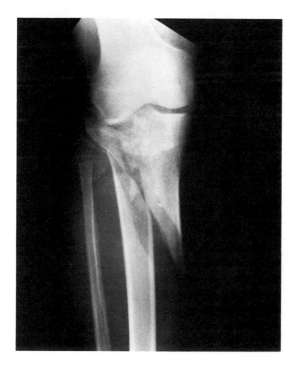

Figure 17–16. Tibial plateau fracture with metaphyseal-diaphyseal extension. Compartment syndrome may occur due to bleeding at the fracture site.

of plateau fractures are associated with ligamentous injuries.[9] Late knee instability following the treatment of tibial plateau fractures is a major cause of unacceptable results.[16]

If the ligaments themselves are not injured, restoring functional tension to the ligaments through anatomic reduction of the fracture will prevent late instability. When intraligamentous failure occurs, postoperative treatment will have to be modified to protect these ligaments as they heal. Cruciate ligament injury carries a poor prognosis when associated with these fractures, and primary operative repair at the time of fracture fixation does not significantly improve this prognosis.[9] Operative repair of collateral ligament tears may reduce the incidence of late instability. However in the multiple trauma patient, this form of treatment may be best done as a delayed reconstruction if instability becomes evident after recovery from the trauma and healing of the fracture has taken place.

REFERENCES

1. Andrews JR, Hughston JC. Treatment of patellar fractures by partial patellectomy. *South Med J*. 1977; 70:809.
2. Bostman O, et al. Comminuted displaced fractures of the patella. *Injury*. 1981;13:196.
3. Boström A. Fractures of the patella. *Acta Orthop Scand Suppl*. 1972;143:1–80.
4. Cameron HC. Transverse fracture of the patella. *Glasgow Med J*. 1878;10:289–294.
5. Chapman M, ed. *Operative Orthopaedics*. Philadelphia, Pa: JB Lippincott; 1988.
6. Cofield RH, Bryan RS. Acute dislocation of the patella. Results of conservative treatment. *J Trauma*. 1977; 17:526–531.
7. Cone JB. Vascular injury associated with fracture-dislocations of the lower extremity. *Clin Orthop*. 1989; 243:30 35.
8. Cooper AP. *A Treatise on Dislocations and Fractures of the Joints*. London, England: Hurst, Reese, Orme & Brown; 1822.
9. Delamarter RB, Hohl M, Hopp E. Ligament injuries associated with tibial plateau fractures. *Clin Orthop*. 1990;250:226–233.
10. Evarts CM, ed. *Surgery of the Musculoskeletal System*. Edinburgh, Scotland: Churchill Livingstone; 1983.
11. Green NE, Allen BL. Vascular injuries associated with dislocation of the knee. *J Bone Joint Surg*. 1977; 59-A:236–239.
12. Hohl M. Tibial condylar fractures: long term follow-up. *Tex Med*. 1974;70:46–56.
13. Hughston JC. Subluxation of the patella. *J Bone Joint Surg*. 1968;50-A:1003.
14. Johnson EE. Combined direct and indirect reduction of comminuted four-part intraarticular T-type fractures of the distal femur. *Clin Orthop*. 1988;231:154–162.
15. Kennedy JC. Complete dislocations of the knee joint. *J Bone Joint Surg*. 1963;45-A:889.
16. Lansinger G, et al. Tibial condylar fractures. *J Bone Joint Surg*. 1986;68-A:13–19.
17. Larsen E, Lauridsen F. Conservative treatment of patellar dislocation. *Clin Orthop*. 1982;171:131.
18. Lister J. An address on the treatment of fracture of the patella. *BMJ*. 1883;2:855.
19. Malgaigne JF. *Traité des Fractures et des Luxations*. Paris, France: JB Baillière; 1847.
20. McMaster PE. Fractures of the patella. *Clin Orthop*. 1954;4:24–43.
21. Meyers MH, et al. Traumatic dislocation of the knee joint. *J Bone Joint Surg*. 1975;57-A:430.
22. Mize RD, et al. Surgical treatment of displaced comminuted fractures of the distal end of the femur: an extensile approach. *J Bone Joint Surg*. 1982;64-A:871.
23. Müller ME, Allgöwer M, Schneider R, Willenegger H. *Manual of Internal Fixation*, 3rd ed. Berlin, Germany: Springer-Verlag; 1991.
24. Rockwood CA Jr, Green DP. *Fractures in Adults*. 2nd ed. Philadelphia, Pa: JB Lippincott; 1984.
25. Salter RB. The biologic concept of continuous passive motion of synovial joints. *Clin Orthop*. 1989;242: 12–25.
26. Schatzker J, Tile M. *The Rationale of Operative Fracture Care*. Berlin, Germany: Springer-Verlag; 1987.
27. Sisto DJ, Warren RF. Complete knee dislocation. *Clin Orthop*. 1985;198:94–101.
28. Taylor A, et al. Traumatic dislocation of the knee. *J Bone Joint Surg*. 1972;54-B:96.

18

Fracture of the Tibia/ Fibula Shaft and Pilon Fracture

JAMES P. KENNEDY, M.D.

HISTORY: Hippocrates stated that the average healing time for a tibial fracture was 40 days (a gross underestimation), and that it should be treated by immobilization in full extension.[1] Various splints and bandaging techniques were used as immobilization devices at that time. At the beginning of the Christian Era, Celsus noted that an intact fibula was important for the stabilization of the tibial fracture[35]—a concept that remains important even today in the closed treatment of these fractures.

Little changed in the treatment of tibial shaft fractures until the mid-1700s when Pott determined that fracture displacement was secondary to muscular forces, and that tibial fractures should therefore be immobilized with hip and knee flexion to prevent displacement.[36]

The ambulatory treatment of tibial fractures was introduced by Krause[24] with the development of the walking cast in the late 1800s. He used a tight cast with minimal padding and devised a protective cast shoe. At the turn of the century, the standard became the skin-tight cast applied with no padding for maximal control and stability of the fracture as developed by Korsch[23] and Albers.[2] Great skill was required to apply these casts so that underlying skin problems would not develop. Codavilla's pins and plaster technique was used by Böhler[8] at this same time for the additional stabilization it offered for grossly unstable tibial fractures.

In spite of these advances in the closed treatment of tibial fractures, complications remained high. As late as 1928,[42] a mortality rate of 7%, amputation rate of 4%, and a delayed or nonunion rate of 15% was reported for closed tibial fractures. In 1961, Dehne[13] reported his results from casting of tibial fractures followed by immediate weight bearing in a long leg cast. Interestingly, the Hippocratic technique of immobilization in extension is required for these casts. With this technique, results equivalent to those of internal fixation can be achieved,[41] although early mobilization may not be possible if used in the trauma patient.

Steinbach first attempted open reduction and internal fixation on the tibia in 1900 using silver plates and galvanized steel screws,[43] but open techniques did not become widely accepted until the 1960s, when experience proved their efficacy.[3] Internal fixation is especially applicable to the multiple trauma patient. Early motion can be instituted to prevent stiffness, and nursing care of the patient's other injuries is optimized.

INTRODUCTION

Fractures of the tibia are among the most difficult fractures that the orthopaedist is called upon to treat. Due to anatomical and vascular factors discussed below, the treatment of severe fractures is often fraught with complications such as compartment syndrome, nonunion, delayed union, malunion, or infection. Amputation is commonly the end-result of the severest of these injuries.

Fractures of the tibia generally occur secondary to high energy trauma, the majority being the result of automobile or pedestrian-auto accidents. The subcutaneous location of the tibia offers little protection from direct violence. Other causes include gunshot injuries, falls, and injuries during sporting activities. High energy fractures are associated with an increased healing time in 50% of cases.[19]

TIBIA SHAFT

Introduction and Anatomy

The tibia is the most common location for a shaft fracture of the long bones.[11] Even in the best of circumstances an isolated, closed, low energy, stable fracture treated in a cast may have a stormy course before healing. Contrary to Hippocrates' teachings, the more "minor" fractures take approximately 10 to 16 weeks to heal, and have a 2% delayed union rate. However, in the more severe fractures (the type usually seen in the total body traumatized patient) average time to healing is 23 weeks with a 60% delayed union rate.[39]

The blood supply to the tibia is notoriously poor. Due to its largely subcutaneous location, a good soft tissue envelope exists only posteriorly, and to a lesser extent, laterally. This means that unlike the femur, relatively few areas are available for blood vessels to enter the tibia through muscular attachments. In addition, open fractures are very common in high energy trauma as the tibia needs only to displace a moderate amount to breach the skin. In such open injuries, the bone is further devascularized by the stripping of what little soft tissues there are, increasing the chances for complications in healing.

Another common problem associated with tibial fractures is compartment syndrome. The calf is composed of four tight fascial compartments. With swelling of the soft tissues from edema or hemorrhage following a trauma, the fascia can become constrictive leading to a compartment syndrome. Vigilance must be maintained for such a development—even with open fractures, as an open fracture does not automatically decompress the compartments through an "auto-fasciotomy." In fact, 10% to 20% of open tibia fractures can develop compartment syndrome, as energy high enough to cause the open tibia fracture is also sufficient to precipitate a compartment syndrome. Compartment syndromes are discussed in further detail in Chapter 20.

Assessment

While the stabilization and assessment of the trauma victim's other injuries is taking place, the suspected tibia fracture can be quickly assessed by the orthopaedist. Most importantly, a quick feel of the compartments will help rule out compartment syndrome. If there is any question of a compartment syndrome being present, further detailed examination or pressure measurements as discussed in Chapter 20 are necessary. The distal neurovascular status is assessed. If the fracture is grossly angulated or malaligned, a gentle restoration of axial alignment will help to relieve any vascular kinking and compromise that may be present. More so for the tibia than for any other fracture, open wounds must be quickly addressed as described in Chapter 7, because the avascularity of the region places the tibia at greater risk for the development of infection. The splinted extremity is then x-rayed to assess the type of fracture present (Fig. 18–1). Following the x-rays, the tibia is tempo-

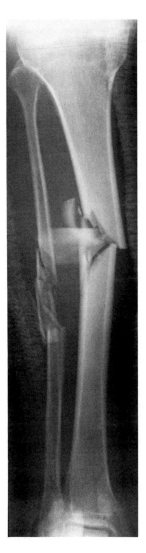

Figure 18–1. Comminuted mid-shaft tibia fracture.

rarily stabilized by a Robert Jones dressing and splint, or with skeletal traction through a calcaneal pin.

Management Considerations

Stable fractures include simple transverse or short oblique fractures without comminution or shortening, fractures with jagged ends that interdigitate with one another adding stability, or fractures with an intact fibula or a fibula fracture at a different level so that the fibula can act as an internal splint. Bony apposition of 50% or more is necessary for axial stability. Unstable fractures include long spirals, those with butterfly fragments or significant comminution, segmental fractures, tibia and fibula fractures that occur at the same level, those that lack bony apposition and are shortened, and most high energy and open fractures where the effects of soft tissue stabilization has been lost through stripping. These fractures, even when occurring as isolated injuries, are very difficult to control by casting procedures. If casted, careful and frequent exams to confirm maintenance of reduction are required, and even then the reduction may not be maintained. For this reason, operative fixation of these unstable fractures should be considered the treatment of choice.

Isolated stable tibia fractures can be treated by a long leg cast and early weight bearing with expectation of a high rate of success. However, if the patient has significant other injuries, the cast may interfere with nursing care and mobilization, and thereby contribute to fracture disease. Comatose patients are at risk for the development of pressure sores underneath the cast. For these reasons, internal fixation may be indicated in the multiple trauma patient for any tibia fracture, not so much to treat the tibia fracture, but rather to treat the overall patient. Operative fixation should also be considered for head injured patients who are agitated or uncooperative, where a cast may not control even the more stable fractures.

Treatment

The standard fixation technique for closed tibial shaft fractures is closed, reamed intramedullary nailing,[9] which has a high rate of success and low rate of complications. Closed technique helps to preserve the extraosseous blood supply as the intraosseous vasculature supplying the inner two thirds of the cortex[44] will be lost through the reaming and nailing procedure. If both intraosseous and extraosseous blood supplies were to be deleteriously affected by the operative treatment, the relatively tenuous blood supply to the tibia may be compromised enough to lead to osteonecrosis and corresponding complications in healing.

A reamed nail (Fig. 18–2) is generally chosen for closed fractures, as a larger nail that fits tightly into the prepared intramedullary canal will enhance fixation stability even though the intramedullary preparation will completely obliterate the intramedullary blood supply. If a fluted or clover-leaf nail is used, neovascular ingrowth is possible along the length of the nail in these channels. In dogs, this has been shown to occur within four weeks, with complete revascularization of the cortex by twelve weeks.[38,44] Closed fractures can tolerate this brief insult, but as will be discussed below, open fractures cannot. Therefore, nonreamed nails must be chosen for the open fractures that are to be nailed.

If the decision is made to treat the fracture by intramedullary nailing, a calcaneal traction pin is often helpful for the stabilization and maintenance of reduction during the operative procedure (Fig. 18–3). This pin should be inserted with a local anesthetic in the

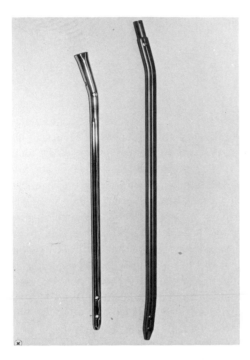

Figure 18–2. Reamed tibial nails with capability for interlocking.

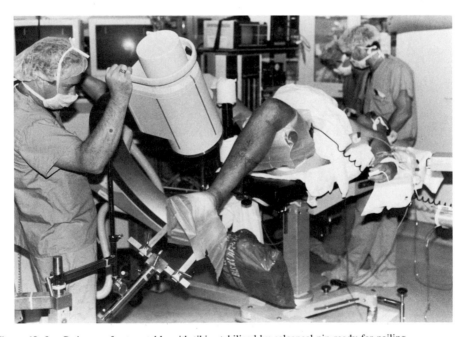

Figure 18–3. Patient on fracture table with tibia stabilized by calcaneal pin ready for nailing.

emergency department if there will be a delay before the nailing can be performed. Skeletal traction will help keep the fracture from shortening which leads to a difficult reduction resulting in further soft tissue trauma. In most cases, however, early if not immediate nailing will be performed, so the pin (if it is desired) can be inserted in the operating room. The fractures which are to be treated immediately may be stabilized for transport with a Robert Jones dressing and splint to make the patient more comfortable and decrease further soft tissue injury.

Rotationally or axially unstable fractures will require interlocking screws[9,10] (Fig. 18–4). After nailing, the knee is checked for ligamentous stability. Up to 22% of knees can exhibit significant ligamentous instability in association with tibial fractures.[45]

Plating of the tibia is usually not performed for shaft fractures due to the extensive soft tissue stripping necessary to apply these larger plates. Rarely, the fracture pattern does not permit insertion of an intramedullary rod. This is the case when the fracture extends proximally or distally into the articular areas. In these instances, plates may be the only fixation devices that can be used (Fig. 18–5). When plating tibias, a relatively high rate of nonunions can be expected.

Certainly, open fractures and fractures in the multiple system injured patient demand immediate stabilization for best results and lowest incidence of complications. However, there is some indication that delayed nailing for the patient whose only injury is an isolated tibia fracture offers some advantages. By allowing the soft tissue injury and swelling to subside, less pressure will be generated in the fascial compartments from the extravasation of blood that occurs during the reaming at the time of surgery. More importantly, by waiting 7 to 14 days, the periosteal blood supply will begin to hypertrophy. This neovascularity,

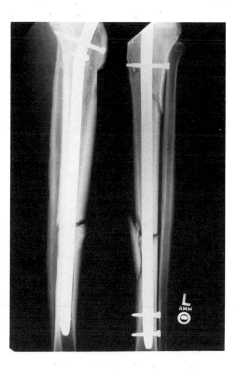

Figure 18–4.   X-ray showing reduced tibial fracture locked with reamed intramedullary nail.

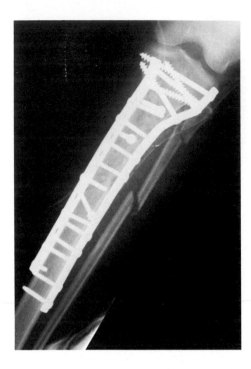

Figure 18–5.   Tibial plates for proximal tibial fracture too comminuted to be treated with
nail.

termed the extraosseous blood supply of healing bone, can form as early as 5 days postinjury,[37] and its contribution to cortical vascularity will decrease the amount of osteonecrosis from the generation of heat and destruction of blood vessels that occur from
reaming. These factors may lead to a lower incidence of complication and higher and faster
rates of healing.[10,41]

The difficulty in putting this theory into practice is maintaining the reduction while
waiting to do the nailing. The additional trauma from the difficult reduction of a shortened
fracture may outweigh any benefit gained from a delayed nailing, plus the patient is at
higher risk to develop systemic complications while waiting for the nailing.

Open Fractures

The open tibia fracture was once the unsolved problem of orthopaedics. Although the
perfect solution has still not been found, some techniques have been developed to make the
odds of a good result from treatment at least more acceptable.

In the tibia, more so than any other bone, the protocol for open fractures must be
strictly adhered to. Any slight advantage that can be obtained from antibiotics, rapid
surgical treatment, aggressive debridement, and stable fixation[33,34] may mean the difference between an uncomplicated union and non-union or infection.

The grade of the open fracture must be critically assessed, because as already
discussed in Chapter 7, Grade IIIc tibia fractures are often best treated by primary
amputation—especially in the multiple trauma victim.[25]

Prior to the era of vascular repair, these popliteal artery injuries associated with open fractures resulted in a 75% amputation rate.[14] Although vascular repairs have improved the salvage of such limbs, the severe soft tissue injury of the Grade III fracture results in a leg that eventually will require an amputation in up to 70% of patients.[25] If such extremities are able to be salvaged, they will be less functional than a prosthesis. The type of treatment that can be successfully and safely used without high risk depends on the severity of the open injury.

The well established standard for the stabilization of severe open tibial fractures is the external fixator[11,15,39,41] (Fig. 18–6). This is a simple, quick technique in the hands of those experienced with it that will stabilize the fracture, and allow access to the large open wounds, permit mobilization of the patient, and facilitate nursing care. Minimal internal fixation through the use of a single lag screw or screws across the fracture can be added[41] for the additional stability afforded by compression at the fracture site. These should be used only if their insertion does not require dissection that will further devascularize the bone. This lag screw, although giving the advantage of compression at the fracture site to facilitate primary bone healing, does not permit later stressing of the fracture to use motion as a clinical assessment of the progression of healing.

The fixator is not without problems.[17] A thorough knowledge of cross sectional anatomy is necessary to prevent damage to underlying structures from the insertion of the percutaneous pins.[6] Pin sites must be predrilled prior to pin insertion. Drilling in pins directly generates heat significant enough to cause thermal necrosis, pin loosening, and possible ring sequestrum formation.[28]

The use of half pins generally is preferable. For maximum stability of the frame the central pins are inserted as close as possible to the fracture site—the eccentric pins are

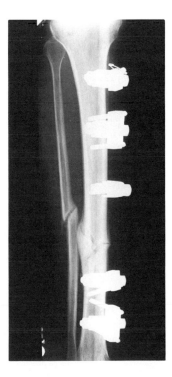

Figure 18–6. Grade II open tibial shaft fracture healing with external fixator in place. (Pins are connected with radiolucent graphite rods.)

placed as far as possible from the central ones. Pins should always be placed into cortical rather than metaphyseal bone if possible for best purchase. Pin fixation and strength will also be enhanced by using short threads on the pin so that the thicker shaft of the pin is within cortical bone. Larger diameter pins are stiffer and contribute to frame stability as well. Placing the connecting bars as close as possible to the bone will increase the stability of the entire construct,[11] as will the addition of a second bar to make a double frame (Fig. 18–7). In addition, various fixator brands[30] and frame configurations[16] differ in their rigidity. For unstable fractures, the double frame in a delta arrangement gives the best stability (Fig. 18–8).

Once a frame is applied, no good alternative fixation device for treatment exists if the frame must be removed. In severe injuries, pin tract infections occur in up to one third of cases.[29] Such infections are usually secondary to a loose pin, and therefore often require the replacement of that pin. Early removal of the fixator and application of a cast, though solving an infection problem, can lead to angulation at the fracture site.[11] Changing from

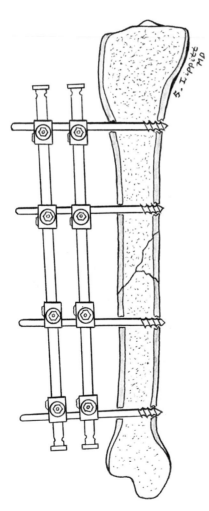

Figure 18–7. Double frame external fixator on tibia. Factors which contribute to increased frame stability are placing the central pins as close as possible to the fracture and the eccentric pins as far away as possible. Pins are placed into thick diaphyseal cortical bone and not thinner metaphyseal cortex using short threaded pins so that the thicker shaft fits tightly into the near cortex. The connecting bar is placed as close as possible to the tibia.

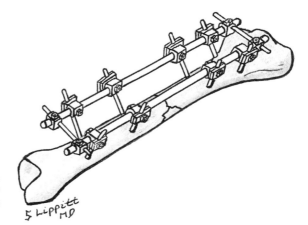

Figure 18–8. Triangulation of two frames connecting them in a delta arrangement for increased frame strength resulting from the biplanar fixation.

external fixation to an internal nailing can be risky with up to 25% incidence of subsequent deep infection. Risk is greatest (an incidence of 71%) for those with evidence of pin tract infection compared to a 6% incidence for those without pin problems.[29] It is felt that a delay between removal of the fixator and insertion of a nail as well as the use of antibiotics will help decrease the problem of delayed infection. However, the best timing for this has not yet been resolved.

So, while the external fixator can be the only or best treatment means for severe open fractures, it is not without its problems. For lesser injuries, other means of fixation may be superior, and as our experience increases and techniques improve, internal fixation means may make the external fixator obsolete for the severe injuries.

Grade I open fractures can be treated with a non-reamed intramedullary nail. Grade II fractures can likewise be handled in this manner, but only the "ideal" cases in which the traumatic wounds are rapidly and aggressively treated. A nonreamed nail is necessary in open fractures to preserve as much endosteal blood supply to the fracture site as possible. The periosteal blood supply about the fracture has been lost to a variable degree depending on the amount of soft tissue stripping. With the use of nonreamed nails (Fig. 18–9), the endosteal vasculature is lost and the cortex devascularized only in those areas of direct contact with the nail. The remaining areas rapidly regain normal vascularity within three weeks.[38]

Either multiple small nails of the flexible type or the standard single nail may be chosen. Multiple flexible nails do not maintain length well when the fracture is axially unstable secondary to comminution, but can serve as an internal splint in selected cases.[20]

With the recent development of non-reamed nails that can be interlocked, any fracture pattern that can be nailed in a closed injury can be nailed in an open injury. This allows the expansion of this form of treatment to include those fractures which are rotationally and axially unstable. As the nonreamed nail is smaller than its reamed counterpart, it is not as strong or as stable. Thus, these fractures sometimes must be casted to protect the operative fixation. Recently developed titanium nails which are much stronger than the nails made out of steel alloys may make this casting obsolete except for the non-compliant patient. An infection rate of less than 5%[18,46] can be expected through proper treatment of the lesser grade open tibia fractures and use of a nonreamed nail.

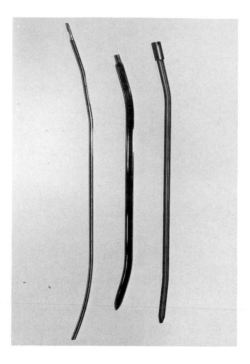

Figure 18–9.   Unreamed tibial nails. *Left:* flexible nail. *Middle and Right:* rigid nails.

An alternative favored by some for open tibia fractures is the use of plate and screw fixation,[12,41] yet others condemn it.[4,11] If plating is to be attempted, scrupulous technique in rigid fixation must be adhered to, and absolutely no further soft tissue stripping can be done. The plate must be applied only to the bone that was stripped by the injury itself to prevent further devascularization. For these reasons, this method is probably best left to the hands of experts, and the surgeon who sees an occasional open tibia fracture should probably use one of the other techniques.

Grade III fractures and Grade II fractures that are not expeditiously addressed are most safely treated by avoiding initial internal fixation. Some have reported excellent results in nonreamed nailing of Grade III open fractures.[46] A higher infection rate of 8% to 15% is seen when Grade II and III fractures are nailed acutely. The advantage and lower systemic risk of early stabilization makes this rate acceptable for the multiple trauma victim, but not for the isolated open tibia fracture. The isolated open fracture is best treated by delayed nailing after the wound problem has been resolved.

The acute nailing of severe open tibia fractures remains somewhat controversial, and as our experience with nonreamed nails increases, perhaps good results will be confirmed and this type of treatment will become standard. At the present time however, the majority of surgeons feel that external fixation techniques are safest for the severe open tibia fracture.

Bone Grafting

Many of these open fractures of all Grades, regardless of the form of treatment, can benefit from an early bone grafting procedure once the soft tissues have recovered (anywhere from

2 to 6 weeks).[5,7] Although a delayed union cannot be confirmed at this early date, many severely comminuted fractures or those with bone loss will predictably go on to delayed or nonunion. Early application of a bone graft can save several months of healing time over simply waiting for an obvious nonunion to be manifested.

Routine early grafting of Grade II and III open tibias, those with segmental bone loss, or high energy closed fractures can be done in an attempt to neutralize the high incidence of delayed or nonunion. If one does not act quickly with many of these cases, it is easy to spend upwards of two years working to get a successful union. Excellent results consisting of a 96% healing rate in a mean time of 46 weeks has been shown using posterolateral bone grafting for a population of severe tibia fractures in which 79% were Grade III injuries, 40% of which had significant bone loss.[7]

Recently described techniques of bone transport for limb lengthening[21,22] are beginning to be used in acute trauma. Circular external frames with thin wire fixation can be used initially as stabilization, then bone may be transported as necessary to stimulate union or replace areas of bony loss. Although excellent results can be obtained in the delayed reconstruction of such cases, data are not yet available to confirm the efficacy of this technique in the acute trauma case. Such frames are also complicated and time-consuming to apply.

FIBULA

Fractures of the fibular diaphysis generally are ignored and readily heal—sometimes to the point of interfering with union of an associated tibial fracture. Fibular shaft fractures usually occur along with a tibial fracture, unless they are the result of a direct blow (the "night-stick" fracture of the leg). Such isolated midshaft fibular fractures that do not involve the ankle joint can be treated purely symptomatically, and often do not even require a cast.

Usually, the concern with the fibular fracture is more how it affects the healing of the tibia than the healing of the fibula itself. The fibula is routinely stabilized in the treatment of tibial pilon fractures as discussed below. Plating the fibula fracture can also give added stability to an unstable tibial shaft fracture. However, rendering the fibula intact may diminish the cyclic compression that occurs with weight bearing at the site of the tibial fracture and which is conducive to fracture healing. Therefore, in most cases of tibia-fibula shaft fractures, the fibula is not stabilized.

Although most all fibular fractures heal readily, some will go on to a fibrous nonunion. This is not a serious problem as it usually is not symptomatic. Only in rare instances will a painful non-union occur requiring operative intervention.

Fractures at the ends of the fibula can be a more serious problem and require closer scrutiny. If the ankle joint is disrupted, anatomic reduction, usually with internal fixation, is required to prevent chronic pain or late arthritis from altered joint mechanics. The distal fibula fracture is addressed further in Chapter 19.

The proximal fibular head fracture is rarely displaced due to the surrounding soft tissues which tend to stabilize it. Fractures at this location are usually the result of a direct blow or a valgus deforming stress to the knee. Another mechanism causing proximal fibular fractures occurs with the Maissoneuve fracture. This rotational injury is significant because of its destabilizing effect on the ankle. This fracture is also discussed in Chapter 19.

The lateral collateral ligament of the knee attaches to the fibular head, so a fracture at this location may cause instability of the knee. The ligament itself is intact, so with adequate immobilization, the fracture will heal to return stability to the lateral side of the knee.

The most common problem with these proximal fibular head injuries is a peroneal nerve palsy. This is especially true with the fractures that occur due to a direct blow. The peroneal nerve is very sensitive to injury. The bleeding and swelling from the fracture will often result in pressure on the nerve, leading to a drop foot. These peroneal palsies will often resolve over several weeks, but until they do, the drop-foot must be managed with an ankle-foot orthosis (AFO) to prevent a rigid equinus deformity. For cases of permanent neurologic drop-foot, a posterior tibial tendon transfer to the dorsum of the foot can restore active ankle dorsiflexion. Return of nerve function can be quite prolonged in some cases.

PILON FRACTURES

The pilon fracture is the last important fracture of the tibia. Named so by the French (pilon = pile-driver), it can be one of the most technically challenging fractures to treat, and like the tibial shaft, is associated with a whole complement of complications. Even with the best healing of the bony injury, a poor outcome may result from the high degree of irreparable articular damage that may occur.

Mechanism

The pilon fracture occurs from an axial compression injury across the ankle joint which drives the talus up into the tibial plafond resulting in a severe intra-articular fracture (Fig. 18–10). It commonly is seen in falls from a height, or in motor vehicle accidents from the position of the foot on the brake or floorboards at the time of impact. A variant associated more with a shearing mechanism than pure compression is seen in skiing injuries. Pilon fractures make up 10% of all tibial fractures,[11] and are usually accompanied by a fracture of the distal fibular diaphysis. Some of these injuries are so comminuted and severe that it is not technically possible to surgically reconstruct them (Fig. 18–11) and a primary ankle fusion may be necessary. Open fractures are commonly present, and if severe, amputation may be required (Fig. 18–12).

Assessment and Goals

Neurovascular compromise with pilon fractures is not common. The axial loading mechanism does not normally damage the neurovascular structures, and as angular forces and deformation are not a major part of the injury mechanism, tension on the nerves and vessels from deformity does not normally occur either. Although severe swelling is the norm, compartment syndrome is not seen as the distal tibia is mainly subcutaneous at this level with only tendinous structures traversing the swollen injured area. The muscular compartments of the leg are proximal to the distal tibia, and the compartments of the foot are not yet present.

If reconstruction is to be attempted, it must be done within the first few hours of the

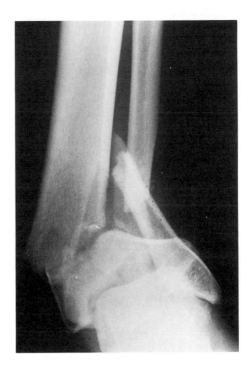

Figure 18–10.   Pilon fracture of distal tibia and fibula.

injury—the earlier the better—or on a delayed basis after the swelling has resolved. Swelling from these fractures is massive due to the soft tissue edema and bleeding from the vascular metaphyseal bone into the limited confines of the ankle region. Fracture blisters commonly occur. Even with immediate fixation, the swelling can be such that by the end of the operation, the skin may not close and must be left open. Often, these injuries must be temporized with closed or indirect reduction techniques due to the bad condition of the skin until surgery can be safely undertaken.

X-rays will reveal the type of fracture present. The degree of comminution, displacement of fracture fragments, amount of metaphyseal compression, condition of the articular surfaces, and the size and number of fracture fragments must be taken into consideration along with the condition of the enveloping soft tissues in order to determine the best treatment plan. In addition to the nature of the fracture, the "nature" and demands of the patient must be considered as well. An elderly sedentary smoker with diabetes and peripheral vascular disease is a very high risk operative candidate in comparison to the young, healthy, active individual.

The goals of treatment are the restoration of ankle joint integrity, congruency, and stability; achievement of bony union; and functional painless motion. This will be best achieved by open reduction and internal fixation in the appropriate candidate, but only if the fracture is amenable to it and the surgeon is capable of such a reconstruction. If both of these requirements are not present, a better result will be achieved in the long run through closed treatment. Using proper operative technique, an overall incidence of 74% to 84% good results can be obtained, but only 50% good results can be expected for the severest of pilon fractures.[26,32,41]

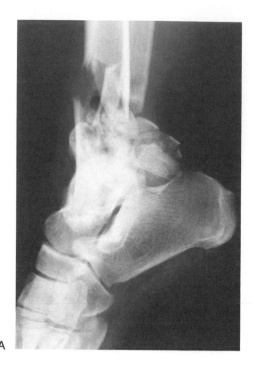

A

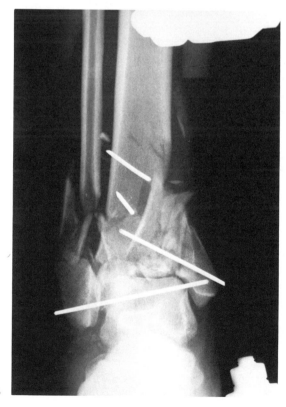

B

Figure 18–11.   A: Severe pilon fracture with extensive comminution. **B:** Treated by primary ankle fusion with compression across joint provided by external fixator (not shown) due to severe articular damage.

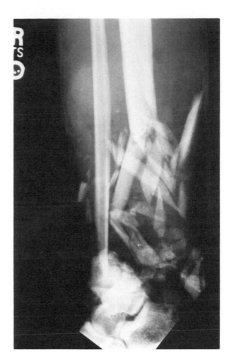

Figure 18–12.   Irreconstructable open pilon
fracture necessitating primary amputation.

Treatment

If open reduction is chosen, it must be done as early as possible using meticulous technique
and careful handling of the soft tissues. The surgeon should remind his assistants of this,
making sure they use gentle retraction techniques. Remove or relax the retractors any time
there is a "break in the action." Tourniquet time must be carefully monitored with deflation
after 90 minutes. It may be reinflated after a 5-minute period of reperfusion.[40] The fibula is
generally fixed first through a lateral approach to re-establish the proper length of the
injured area and afford additional stability to the tibial repair. The tibia is then approached
through an antero-medial incision being sure that an adequate skin bridge of 7 cm[26] is left
between the two incisions to prevent skin slough from vascular compromise. The fracture
fragments are reconstructed using meticulous "no touch technique"[31] leaving soft tissue
attachments intact to prevent devascularization of the fragments. Dissection should also be
minimized to avoid further soft tissue injury which results in additional swelling. Recently
described indirect reduction methods[27] can also be very helpful. All depressed articular
surfaces are elevated into anatomic position and voids are bone grafted. This is another
area where bone grafting in the face of an open fracture must often be done primarily if the
bone graft is necessary for the inherent stability of the construct.

Any debris is removed from the joint, including irregular cartilaginous flaps. The
fracture can be provisionally reduced and held with smooth thin wires if necessary. Once the
reduction is acceptable, the wires are sequentially replaced with interfragmentary compression screws and a buttress plate. The wound is closed only if it can be done so without
tension. If the skin cannot be closed, muscle and soft tissue is used to cover the metallic

implants, and the skin is left open. Early motion is instituted for improved cartilage healing if the fixation is stable.

When the tibial fracture is not reconstructable, plating only the fibula will help bring the tibia out to length, maintain alignment, and afford some stability. It is often surprising how well the tibial fragments will be reduced by this indirect method. The fibula alone can also be plated as a temporizing measure if swelling will not permit early fixation of the entire fracture, making delayed fixation of the tibia easier by holding the fracture out to length.

Another temporizing technique is calcaneal pin traction. This keeps the fracture out to length and allows elevation of the leg to decrease the swelling. Motion can even be instituted while in traction to help mold the articular cartilage and promote its healing. An external fixator can likewise be used, but will not allow range of motion.

If the tibia is not reconstructable, or in severe open injuries, it can be treated definitively with the calcaneal pin traction and early motion, or an external fixator to maintain length and alignment. Percutaneous pins and a cast may also be used to hold fragments in position. In these severest of injuries, a poor result is a foregone conclusion, so motion and function of the ankle is sacrificed in order to obtain union of the fracture with the foot in a plantigrade position. If posttraumatic arthritic pain is severe, a delayed fusion may be required.

REFERENCES

1. Adams F, trans. *The Genuine Works of Hippocrates*. Baltimore, Md: Williams & Wilkins; 1939.
2. Albers. Über Gehverbande bei Bruchen der unteren Gliedmaßen. Verh Dtsch Ges Chir, 23rd Congress: 1894; 75–91.
3. Allgöwer M, Perren SM. Operating on tibial shaft fractures. *Unfallheilk*. 1980;83:214–218.
4. Bach AW, Hansen ST Jr. Plate versus external fixation in severe tibial shaft fractures. *Clin Orthop*. 1989; 241:89–94.
5. Behrens F, et al. Treatment of severe open tibial fractures—prospective evaluation. *Orthop Trans*. 1983; 7:528. Abstract.
6. Behrens F, Searls K. External fixation of the tibia: basic concepts and prospective evaluation. *J Bone Joint Surg*. 1985;68-B:246–254.
7. Blick SS, et al. Early prophylactic bone grafting of high-energy tibial fractures. *Clin Orthop*. 1989;240: 21–41.
8. Böhler L. Apparate zum Einrichten von Knochenbruchen unter Schraubenzug. *Münch med Wschr*. 1928; 75:2047.
9. Bone LB, Johnson KD. Treatment of tibial fractures by reaming and intramedullary nailing. *J Bone Joint Surg*. 1986;68-A:877.
10. Browner BD, Edwards CC. *The Science and Practice of Intramedullary Nailing*. Philadelphia, Pa: Lea & Febiger; 1987.
11. Chapman MW, ed. *Operative Orthopaedics*. Philadelphia, Pa: JB Lippincott; 1988.
12. Clifford RP, et al. Plate fixation of open fractures of the tibia. *J Bone Joint Surg*. 1988;70-B:644–648.
13. DeBakey ME, Simeone FA. Battle injuries of the arteries in World War II: an analysis of 2471 cases. *Ann Surg*. 1946;123:534–579.
14. Dehne E, et al. Nonoperative treatment of the fractured tibia by immediate weight bearing. *J Trauma*. 1961; 1:514–535.
15. Edwards CC, et al. Severe open tibial fractures. Results treating 202 injuries with external fixation. *Clin Orthop*. 1988;230:98–115.
16. Finley JB, et al. Stability of ten configurations of the Hoffmann external-fixation frame. *J Bone Joint Surg*. 1987;69-A:734–744.
17. Green SA. *Complications of External Skeletal Fixation*. Springfield, Ill: Charles C Thomas; 1981.
18. Harvey FJ, et al. Intramedullary nailing in the treatment of open fractures of the tibia and fibula. *J Bone Joint Surg*. 1975;57-A:909–915.

19. Hoaglund FT, States JD. Factors influencing the rate of healing in tibial shaft fractures. *Surg Gynecol Obstet.* 1967;124:71–76.

20. Holbrook JL, et al. Treatment of open fractures of the tibial shaft: Ender nailing versus external fixation. *J Bone Joint Surg.* 1989;71-A:1231–1238.

21. Ilizarov GA. The tension-stress effect on the genesis and growth of tissues: Part I. The influence of stability of fixation and soft-tissue preservation. *Clin Orthop.* 1989;238:249–281.

22. Ilizarov GA. The tension-stress effect on the genesis and growth of tissues: Part II. The influence of the rate and frequency of distraction. *Clin Orthop.* 1989;239:263–285.

23. Korsch. Über den ambulatorischen Verband bei Knochenbruchen der Unter und Oberschenkels, sowie bei komplizierten Bruchen. *Berl klin Wschr.* 1983;30:29.

24. Krause F. Beiträge zur Behandlung der Knochenbrucke der unteren Gliedmaßen im Umhergehen. *Dtsch med Wschr.* 1891;17:457–460.

25. Lange RH, et al. Open tibial fractures with associated vascular injuries: prognosis for limb salvage. *J Trauma.* 1985;25:203–208.

26. Mast JW, et al. Fractures of the tibial pilon. *Clin Orthop.* 1988;230:68–82.

27. Mast JW, Ganz R, Jakob R. *Planning and Reduction Technique in Fracture Surgery.* Berlin, Germany: Springer-Verlag; 1989.

28. Matthews LS, et al. The thermal effects of skeletal fixation-pin insertion in bone. *J Bone Joint Surg.* 1984; 66-A:1077–1083.

29. Maurer DJ, et al. Infection after intramedullary nailing of severe open tibial fractures initially treated with external fixation. *J Bone Joint Surg.* 1989;71-A:835–838.

30. Moroz TK, Finlay JB, Rorabeck CH, Bourne RB. External skeletal fixation: choosing a system based on biomechanical stability. *J Orthop Trauma.* 1989;2:284–296.

31. Müller ME, Allgöwer M, Schneider R, Willenegger M. *Manual of Internal Fixation.* 3rd ed. Berlin, Germany: Springer-Verlag; 1991.

32. Ovadia DN, Beals RK. Fractures of the tibial plafond. *J Bone Joint Surg.* 1986;68-A:543–551.

33. Patzakis MJ, et al. Considerations in reducing the infection rate in open tibial fractures. *Clin Orthop.* 1983; 178:36–41.

34. Patzakis MJ, Wilkins J. Factors influencing infection rate in open fracture wounds. *Clin Orthop.* 1989; 243:36–40.

35. Peltier LF. *Fractures.* San Francisco, Calif: Norman Publishing; 1990.

36. Pott P. *Some Few General Remarks on Fractures and Dislocations.* London, England: L Hawes, W Clarke, R Collins; 1765.

37. Rhinelander FW, Baragry RA. Microangiography in bone healing. *J Bone Joint Surg.* 1962;44-A:1273.

38. Rhinelander FW. Tibial blood supply in relation to fracture healing. *Clin Orthop.* 1974;105:34.

39. Rockwood CA Jr, Green DP. *Fractures in Adults.* 2nd ed. Philadelphia, Pa: JB Lippincott; 1984.

40. Sapega AA, et al. Optimizing tourniquet application and release times in extremity surgery. *J Bone Joint Surg.* 1985;67-A:303–314.

41. Schatzker J, Tile M. *The Rationale of Operative Fracture Care.* Berlin, Germany: Springer-Verlag; 1987.

42. Speed K. *A Textbook of Fractures and Dislocations.* Philadelphia, Pa: Lea & Febiger; 1928.

43. Steinbach LW. On the use of fixation plates in the treatment of fractures of the leg. *Ann Surg.* 1900;31: 436–442.

44. Summer-Smith G, ed. *Bone in Clinical Orthopaedics.* Philadelphia, Pa: WB Saunders; 1982.

45. Tempelman DC, Marder RA. Injuries of the knee associated with fractures of the tibial shaft. *J Bone Joint Surg.* 1989;71-A:1392–1395.

46. Velazco A, et al. Open fractures of the tibia treated with the Lottes nail. *J Bone Joint Surg.* 1975;57-A: 909–915.

19

Fractures and Dislocations of the Ankle and Foot

JAMES P. KENNEDY, M.D.

HISTORY: The association of specific fractures with their mechanism of injury was first described by Pott (Pott's fracture of the ankle) in the mid-1700s,[19] and subsequently by others.[18] In the early 1800s, Dupuytren subjected cadaveric ankles to various forces, then dissected them to study the fracture patterns produced.[8] By the 20th century, with the advent of radiographs, ankle fractures were being treated based on the fracture pattern and the knowledge of the mechanism that produced it.[3] A closed reduction was performed to reduce the fracture using manipulative forces in a direction opposite to those traumatic forces which produced it—a technique still used today.

INTRODUCTION

Injuries about the foot are often complicated by early and severe swelling. In such cases, operative injuries must be addressed promptly before swelling occurs if complications such as skin slough and inability to close the wound are to be avoided. When the patient's other injuries or general condition precludes early definitive operative treatment, gentle closed reduction of fractures or dislocations can be performed if needed as a temporizing measure to relieve the neurovascular structures. The extremity can then be immobilized in a bulky dressing until the patient is able to be returned to the operating room for final treatment. For convenience of discussion, injuries are divided in this chapter into ankle, hindfoot, midfoot, and forefoot problems.

ANKLE INJURIES

Fractures and Sprains

Ankle fractures and sprains generally are found as isolated injuries following a twist, misstep, or athletic injury. In the multiple trauma victim, the ankle injury is usually secondary to a crushing or direct blow, or from an axial load with the type of fracture produced dependent on the position of the foot at the time of impact. These injuries are addressed with the same techniques used for the patient with an isolated ankle injury. Fractures and sprains occur from the same mechanism, the only difference being the site of failure—bone or ligament. Often, ligamentous tears will be present on one side of the joint associated with a fracture on the other side.

Ankle dislocations are associated with higher degrees of energy. Dislocations rarely occur without associated bony or ligamentous avulsion fractures. Following the failure of the ligaments, sufficient energy remains to disrupt the integrity of the joint producing the dislocation.

Ankle fractures are classified by one of two main methods. The Lauge-Hansen system describes the position of the foot and the direction of force at the time of injury—for example: supination-adduction, supination-eversion, pronation-abduction, and pronation-eversion.[13] Various stages of injury exist with a progression of structures failing as the amount of energy increases. The simpler Danis-Weber classification describes three variations—Type A, B, and C—based on the type of fibular fracture present.[17]

Type A fractures are ligamentous avulsions occurring below the level of the intact syndesmosis (the distal tibial-fibular joint) so that the tibial-fibular ligaments remain intact. A fracture at the level of the syndesmosis (Type B) disrupts the mortise, but the syndesmosis may or may not be compromised (Fig. 19–1). The mortise is reconstructed through fracture fixation, the syndesmosis through ligamentous repair if needed. A suprasyndesmotic fracture, or Type C fracture (Fig. 19–2), results in a mortise that remains incompetent even after the fracture repair due to the disrupted distal tibial-fibular ligaments

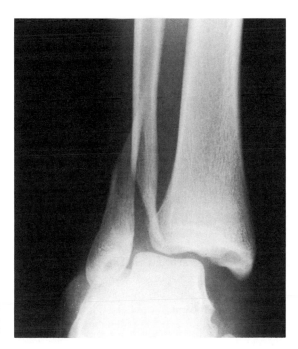

Figure 19–1. Mortise view of Weber Type B fibular fracture. The mortise is disrupted, but the syndesmosis (distal tibial-fibular joint) is intact.

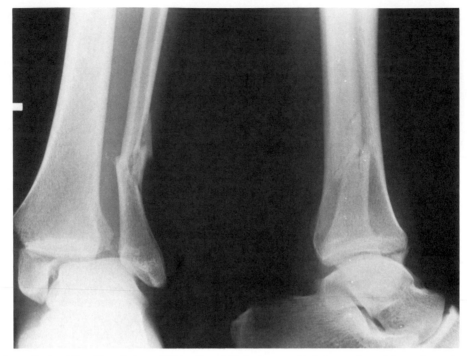

Figure 19–2. AP and lateral views of Weber Type C fibular fracture. Both the mortise and the syndesmosis are disrupted requiring internal fixation after anatomic reduction. The medial malleolus fracture is also intra-articular with a displaced joint surface.

and usually requires the addition of a transfibular-tibial syndesmosis screw for stability (Fig. 19–3).

Assessment

The physical exam consists of a complete distal neurovascular exam and search for associated injuries. Palpation of the medial and lateral malleoli and their ligamentous structures will help to localize bony and soft tissue injuries and to determine if the normal anatomic relationships have been preserved. This is especially important with fractures of a single malleolus which may be accompanied by a ligamentous injury involving the opposite malleolus. Purely ligamentous lesions require a stress exam of the ligaments to check for instability. Stress x-rays can be helpful for selected cases. The ankle can be thought of as a bony and ligamentous ring just as the pelvis is, although not as rigid (Fig. 19–4). A single bony or ligamentous disruption in the ring should lead to a search for others. More than one break in the ring increases the instability of the ankle.

Scrutinize the entire tibia and fibula. If the patient cannot be adequately examined due to altered consciousness, then the complete tibia and fibula must be x-rayed. Only in this way can a Maissoneuve injury be ruled out. The Maissoneuve injury, first described in

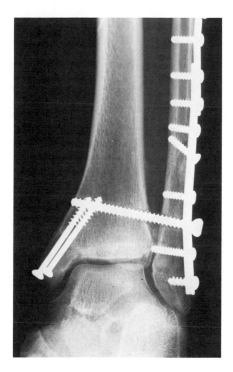

Figure 19–3. Reconstructed ankle mortise and intra-articular medial malleolus fracture of Weber C fracture seen in Figure 19–2, shown here with a mortise view. A screw between the tibia and fibula is used to stabilize the syndesmosis.

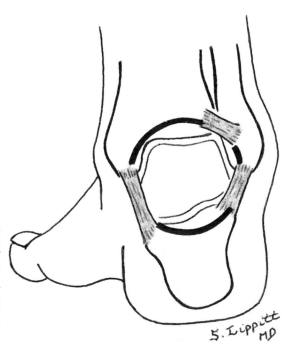

Figure 19–4. The ringlike structure of the ankle joint. The medial deltoid and the lateral ligamentous complex (anterior and posterior fibulotalar and fibulocalcaneal ligaments) are coupled with the bony mortise and the anterior and posterior syndesmotic tibiofibular ligaments. If one break occurs in the ring through fracture or ligamentous tears, failure of the other structures in the ring should be ruled out.

1840,[15] is the result of an external rotation force which produces a fracture of the medial malleolus, or a tear of the medial deltoid ligament. The force then tears the tibial-fibular syndesmotic ligaments and travels up the syndesmotic membrane, exiting at the fibular neck where a fracture is found (Fig. 19–5). This injury results in an unstable ankle mortise, and therefore cannot be thought of as a routine sprain or medial malleolar fracture.

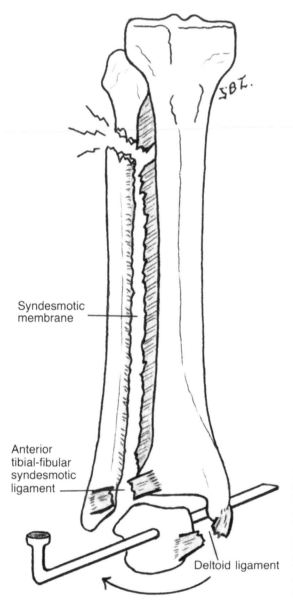

Syndesmotic membrane

Anterior tibial-fibular syndesmotic ligament

Deltoid ligament

Figure 19–5.   The Maissoneuve injury. A twisting injury results in a medial ligamentous tear (or medial malleolus fracture) and rupture of the syndesmotic ligaments. As the force travels up the syndesmotic membrane, it exits at the proximal fibula, fracturing it. Most commonly, the syndesmotic membrane remains intact; it may also tear as shown here. Whenever a fibular neck fracture is found with a medial ankle injury, the Maissoneuve injury has rendered the mortise unstable.

Radiology

The radiologic exam consists of AP, lateral and mortise views (taken in 15° of internal rotation) to diagnose the injury and assess the integrity of the ankle joint. The entire lower leg is x-rayed if a reliable exam cannot be performed based on the cooperativity of the patient, or if any areas of tenderness or signs of injury such as bruising or lacerations are noted.

In selected cases, stress films may be required to confirm or refute the ligamentous stability of the joint. This would rarely be required early in the evaluation of a multiple trauma victim as more serious issues are usually present and take priority.

Principles of Management

Sprains are immobilized with devices based on their grade of severity (see Chapter 2) for comfort and to allow healing of the ligaments without stress on these structures. Mild Grade I sprains may require only an elastic bandage or a removable varus-valgus brace. Severe Grade III sprains often warrant cast immobilization and crutches. Although the repair of torn ligaments in Grade III sprains may be indicated for active individuals with isolated injuries, repairs should not generally be done acutely in the multiple trauma victim unless a surgical approach to these areas is already being made for other reasons—such as to repair a fracture or irrigate and debride an open wound. In such cases, the additional ligamentous repair adds no further time or morbidity to the operative procedure.

Stable nondisplaced fractures that do not disrupt the stability, integrity, or alignment of the ankle joint can often be treated with a well molded cast—especially if the patient is not an operative candidate. A Robert Jones dressing and splint is used initially if the swelling is too great to allow the safe immediate application of a cast. Most multiple trauma victims will not have the care of their other injuries compromised by a short-leg cast, and they can still be adequately mobilized in the cast for their systemic well-being.

Fractures with a step-off of the articular surface of more than 1 to 2 mm need to be surgically treated. If there is any disruption of the ankle mortise (Fig. 19–2), open reduction and internal fixation is also warranted.[23] As little as 1 mm of shifting of the talus can cause a decrease of 42% in the tibial-talar contact area.[20] With the increased stresses generated due to the decreased joint surface area, compounded by any instability, early degeneration of the joint may occur. The threshold for fixing ankle fractures is becoming smaller and smaller. Indeed, many fractures may benefit from operative fixation through debridement of any articular cartilage damage, irrigation of the hemarthrosis, and the institution of early motion, even if the fractures are minimally displaced. This is true especially for young, active patients.

Treatment

The goals of operative fixation are the same as that of all intra-articular fractures: restoration of joint anatomy and stability, early range of motion permitted by stable fixation, and bony healing.

If operative fixation is to be performed, the earlier the better. This is both from the standpoint of the patient's overall medical condition, and from that of the ankle injury. Depending on the severity of the injury, a delay of 24 hours can result in a degree of swelling that will make the surgery more difficult, and can precipitate post-operative problems with wound healing.

During the surgical procedure, the skin and soft tissues must be handled with care. The fracture fragments are reduced and held in their anatomic position, usually with plates and screws. An arthrotomy is performed to irrigate out the hemarthrosis, and debride any articular damage. Associated ligamentous tears found at the operative site are repaired. A deltoid ligament tear associated with a fibular fracture does not need surgical repair unless the ligament flips into the joint, blocking the reduction of the mortise.

If surgery cannot be performed early due to the degree of swelling or the severity of the patient's other injuries, the extremity is placed in a Robert Jones dressing, and operated upon when the swelling abates in three to five days, or when the patient is stable. The patient can be mobilized out of bed in the Robert Jones dressing prior to fracture fixation, and good results can still be obtained with delayed fixation even at 7 to 10 days.

Treat open ankle fractures according to the open fracture protocol (Chapter 7). They then can be internally fixed, being sure to leave the traumatic wound open. Due to the good blood supply found about the ankle and foot,[5] open fractures in this location can be treated with immediate internal fixation without significant increased risk for infection.[4,9]

Ankle Dislocation

Dislocation of the tibial-talar joint is a ligamentous injury of the medial deltoid ligament and the lateral ligamentous complex with an associated disruption of the joint capsule. Pure dislocations can only occur anteriorly and posteriorly due to the restraints of the malleoli. More commonly, a fracture of one or both of the malleoli will occur, permitting a medial or lateral component to the dislocation (Fig. 19–6A). Dislocations about the hindfoot and ankle are frequently open injuries as the bony structures lie just under the enveloping skin.

Assessment.   Dislocations of the ankle are a true limb-threatening emergency. Due to the close confines of the region, the neurovascular bundles to the foot are generally compromised, and a careful exam is required. As the skin in the foot has very little subcutaneous tissue, pressure from the talus can rapidly cause necrosis of skin that is tented over it under tension.[14] It is possible to literally watch the progression of necrosis as it occurs over the course of a few hours. For this reason, gently reduce ankle dislocations immediately upon their presentation—even before x-rays are obtained—if the foot is dysvascular, if skin changes (blanching or discoloration) are present, or if any delay in obtaining films is anticipated.

Following the reduction, reassess the status of the neurovascular bundles. X-rays are then obtained to characterize any fractures that are present and confirm an adequate reduction. Search for talonavicular and subtalar dislocations as well as talar fractures as these injuries commonly occur with ankle dislocations.

Treatment.   Due to swelling of soft tissues or button-holing of bones through the capsule, pure dislocations of the ankle and dislocations and fracture-dislocations of the subtalar joint are frequently irreducible by closed methods even under a general anesthetic. It is not uncommon for the posterior tibial, flexor digitorum, or flexor hallucis longus tendons on

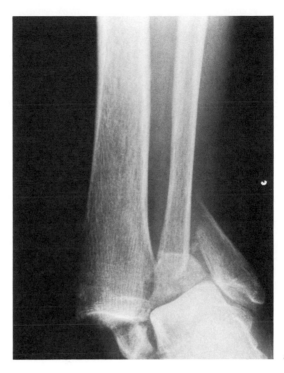

Figure 19–6. **A:** Fracture dislocation of the ankle. (Figure continued on next page)

A

the medial side, and the peroneal tendons on the lateral side to block the reduction as well. The neurovascular bundles may also become entrapped blocking reduction.

If one good try at a closed reduction in the emergency room fails, an emergent open reduction in the operating room is necessary. The reduction maneuver is longitudinal traction, increasing the deformity to unlock any impinging structures, then finally, correction of the deformity. These injuries tend to either reduce easily or with great difficulty; there is no middle road.

Irrigate and debride open injuries as for any open joint and leave the wounds open. Close the capsule over a drain to prevent articular cartilage dessication and necrosis.

Following the reduction, fractures are addressed. With the exception of ligamentous avulsion chip fractures, fractures associated with an ankle dislocation are operatively stabilized because they are by definition unstable (Fig. 19–6B).

Dislocations generally are fairly stable following their reduction and fixation of any fractures that are present. They can then be treated with a bulky dressing followed by casting to immobilize the ankle during ligamentous and soft tissue healing. Severely injured joints with more significant soft tissue disruption may be unstable and require pinning of the joints to maintain the reduction during healing. Many open dislocations fall into this category. An external fixator can also be used for immobilization.

Most ankles treated in this fashion will do well following rehabilitation therapy. Delayed ligamentous reconstruction can be done for the few cases of late instability that occur.

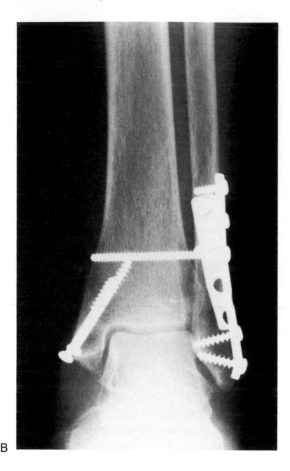

Figure 19–6, cont. B: Internal fixation of fracture to stabilize dislocation of mortise and unstable syndesmosis.

B

HINDFOOT INJURIES

Talus Fractures

The talus fracture is a high energy dorsiflexion injury. It was known as "aviator's astragalus" (astragalus = talus) in the early 1900s as it was often seen in airplane crashes from the dorsiflexion forces that were transmitted through the rudder controls into the pilot's feet.[1] Today, the fractured talus is usually seen secondary to motor vehicle accidents through the related mechanism of forces applied to the patient's foot on the brake pedal or floorboards at the time of an accident. This injury may also be seen following a fall from a height. In these latter instances, other axial load injuries such as tibial plateau and lumbar compression fractures may be present also.

Assessment

Fractures can involve the body, neck, or head of the talus with neck fractures being the most common if the minor chip avulsion fractures are excluded.[12] Talar fractures are initially approached in the same manner as the ankle dislocation. Due to the high energy involved and the lack of abundant soft tissue covering, these injuries are also often open (Fig. 19–7). The open talus fracture occurs not from sharp bone fragments cutting through the skin, but rather a tearing of the skin due to its failure in tension from the deformity produced at the time of injury.

The greatest management problem with this injury occurs when it is significantly displaced. When the head or body fragment is displaced (resulting in a subtalar or ankle dislocation in association with the fractured talus), it can cause the same skin and neurovascular compromise as the ankle dislocation. The incidence of late complications is also related to the initial fracture displacement.

The surface of the talus is 60% articular,[21] and it has no attachments of muscle or tendon. Therefore its blood supply, through only three nutrient vessels[10,11] and minimal synovial attachments, is easily threatened by displaced fractures or dislocations.[16] The risk of avascular necrosis (AVN) of the talus increases with the amount of displacement of the fracture. Nondisplaced fractures (Hawkins I) exhibit a 0% to 13% rate of AVN. Fractures where the ankle joint remains reduced, but the subtalar joint is subluxed or dislocated (Hawkins II) have a 20% to 50% rate of AVN. Avascular necrosis is seen in 83% to 100% of Hawkins III fractures where the body fragment is dislocated from both the ankle and subtalar joints, and virtually all Hawkins IV fractures go on to AVN.[10,12] The Hawkins IV fracture results when the body fragment is dislocated from the ankle and subtalar joints, and the head fragment is dislocated from the talonavicular joint.

Treatment

Anatomically reduced fractures can be treated through cast immobilization and protection from weight bearing. Displaced fractures require immediate reduction to relieve any neurovascular or skin compromise, followed by operative stabilization[10] to maintain the reduction. As for all intra-articular fractures, the joint anatomy must be restored if post-

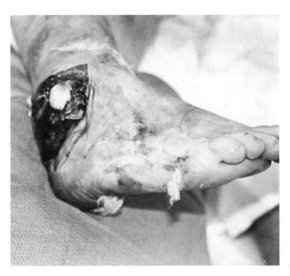

Figure 19–7.   **A:** Open Hawkins III fracture dislocation of the talus. The dome of the talus is rotated 180° and is presenting itself through the wound. (Figure continued on next page)

A

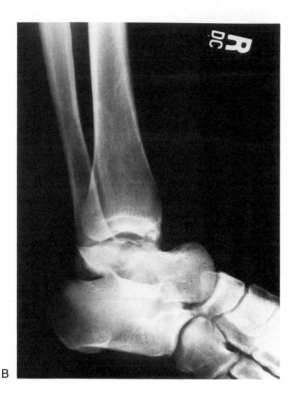

B

Figure 19–7, cont.   B: Lateral x-ray of talar fracture dislocation. Note talar dome rotated 180° facing plantarwards.

traumatic arthritis is to be minimized. Vascularity will also improve with reduction as tension on the vascular structures will be relieved.

Mildly displaced fractures can often be manipulated through closed methods, then fixed percutaneously with screws (Fig. 19–8). Pieces that are displaced out of the joint can be difficult to reduce even with open reduction. A medial malleolar osteotomy may be required to permit the talus to fit back into the mortise. If open treatment is required, it too must be done early before swelling or fracture blisters occur. If the skin condition does not permit immediate operative intervention, the joint is closed reduced as best as possible and immobilized in a Robert Jones dressing and splint. The surgery must then be delayed until the skin condition improves.

Subtalar Dislocation

Dislocations of the talo-calcaneal joint are addressed with the same philosophy as that for the ankle dislocation and talar fracture. These are all variations of the same injury with the difference being the level at which the structures fail.

The subtalar joint dislocation may be an open or near-open injury, or exhibit neurovascular compromise to the foot. If so, it is to be rapidly managed as outlined above for ankle dislocations. A good rule of thumb is that any dislocation should be reduced as quickly as possible, and certainly within the first six hours after injury. Due to the complex orientation of the three facets of the subtalar joint, most are fairly stable following reduction and can be treated in a Robert Jones dressing followed by casting. A Steinmann pin can be

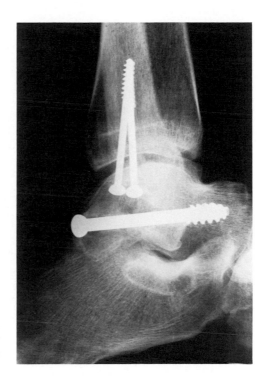

Figure 19–8. Talar fracture following anatomic reduction and fixation with a percutaneous screw from posterior. (The two smaller vertical screws are for an associated medial malleolus fracture.)

placed across the joint for a few weeks to ensure maintenance of reduction if the joint is very unstable following reduction.

Calcaneus Fracture

Fractures of the calcaneus are usually the result of falls from a height, crushing injuries, or axial loads from motor vehicle accidents. The geometry of the calcaneus is complex with three articulating facets for the talus, and articulations with the cuboid and navicular bones. The heel pad is made up of specialized chambers of fat acting as shock absorbers, and injury or scarring of these soft tissues can lead to chronic heel pain.

Assessment. Calcaneus fractures usually do not present with visible deformity. Hindfoot swelling and ecchymosis are present. Ecchymosis is characteristically seen in the plantar arch of the foot, but is only visible late after the bleeding has had time to dissect its way to the surface. Pain and swelling will easily localize the injury. Typically, pain will be present with medial-lateral compression of the calcaneus between the thumb and fingers. In addition to the routine foot films (AP and lateral), Harris axial views of the calcaneus are required to evaluate the posterior tuberosity for loss of height and widening (Fig. 19–9). Often CT scans (Fig. 19–10) and lateral or 3-dimensional reconstructions are helpful in fully assessing the injury due to the complex anatomy of the calcaneus.

There are many types of calcaneal fractures, but they all can result in the same problems. Disruption of any of the calcaneal articulations, loss of heel height, and widening of the heel can lead to chronic pain and difficulty with shoe wear if not corrected. As well,

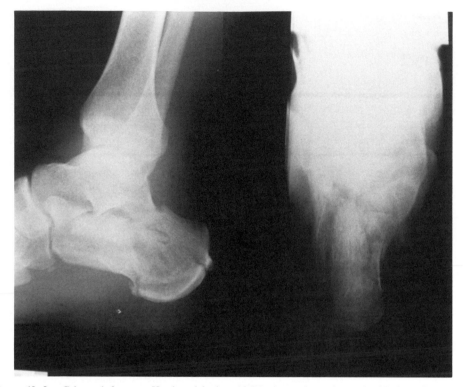

Figure 19–9. Calcaneal fracture. Harris axial view (right) shows shortening and widening of posterior tuberosity which will lead to difficulty with shoe wear if not reduced. Lateral view (left) demonstrates complete collapse of superior articular surface of calcaneus.

the heel fat pad injury and peroneal tendinitis or tendon entrapment in nonreduced fractures will add to the patient's complaints.

Treatment. A wide variety of treatments have been described for calcaneal fractures ranging from preserving the status quo and not intervening to operative restorations. Casting and/or protective weight bearing should only be used for stable nondisplaced fractures for the reasons outlined above. Unfortunately, due to the high energy imparted to the trauma patient, this type of fracture is rarely seen in this setting. Most calcaneal fractures in the high-energy trauma victim are severely comminuted and collapsed. Healing is not a problem, due to the vascularity and abundance of cancellous bony surfaces found in the calcaneus. The difficulty in treating these injuries is in maintaining reduction and preventing late disability.

Closed reduction has been performed for displaced fractures. In the past, such devices as padded mallets and clamps to pound and squeeze the calcaneus back into shape were used. Closed reduction generally is unsuccessful as the calcaneus is primarily cancellous bone. This cancellous bone is compressed during the act of fracturing. Even if the fragments can be reduced through closed means, voids are present from the compressed bone leaving nothing to hold the pieces in their reduced position. This results in the tendency for them to recollapse.

The Essex-Lopresti maneuver and its modifications[7,21] are a slight improvement as they use a percutaneous pin to manipulate the fragments then stabilize them. However, the

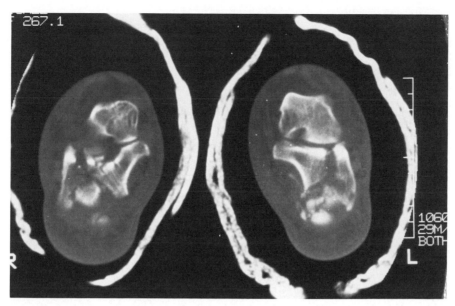

Figure 19–10.   CT scan of calcanei showing bilateral comminuted fractures in a roofer who fell 20 feet, landing on both heels.

voids in the bone are not corrected and if there are several fracture lines, they cannot all be stabilized by this one pin. Therefore, many patients treated in this fashion will also go on to late collapse.

Although more technically challenging, open reduction and internal fixation or a combination of internal and external fixation is probably the best treatment for fractures which are amenable to it, if the surgeon is comfortable with the technique. All articulating surfaces can be elevated back into anatomic position, fracture lines can be stabilized, but most importantly, the compressed areas can be generously bone grafted for additional stability.

MIDFOOT INJURIES

The midfoot is made up of the navicular, cuboid, and three cuneiform bones. Injuries here consist of ligamentous sprains and chip avulsions, dislocations, fractures, and the Lisfranc injury to the metatarsal-tarsal joints. As elsewhere in the foot, massive swelling can occur. At this level, compartments are again found, and swelling within these closed compartments can result in compartment syndromes of the foot.

Ligamentous Injury

Ligamentous midfoot sprains and chip avulsion fractures can be treated through immobilization until healing. Due to the interlocking geometric configuration of the bones, late instability generally is not a problem if bony alignment has not been disrupted.

The more minor dislocations and subluxations (the exception being the Lisfranc injury) can generally be reduced by closed manipulation then percutaneously pinned for stabilization. If closed reduction is not possible, open reduction is required to remove the offending tissue blocking the reduction.

Fractures

Fractures of the midfoot likewise can generally be treated through closed means if nondisplaced. However, due to the high energies found in patients with multiple trauma, significant disruptions can occur. If disruption of articular surfaces is present, open reduction is usually indicated to prevent late posttraumatic arthritis. More commonly, one sees crushing and collapse of these cancellous bones—such as in the "nutcracker fracture" of the cuboid. If the loss of integrity of the bone is significant, the pieces are elevated back into position and buttressed with bone graft to prevent collapse and imbalance of the foot.[22]

Lisfranc's Injury

Lisfranc's joints consist of the tarsal-metatarsal articulations, that is, the joints where the forefoot and midfoot join. Lisfranc was a surgeon in Napoleon's army, and described this injury in the cavalry who received it via forces transmitted through their mounts' stirrups. Lisfranc treated these injuries, which were often open, by amputation. Today, we see Lisfranc's injury from the axial loads, twisting, and crushing found in automobile and motorcycle accidents.

The injury consists of a combination of ligamentous avulsions and fractures in this region rendering the forefoot unstable and causing the metatarsals to displace in a variety of patterns (Fig. 19–11). This region forms the transverse and longitudinal arches of the foot (Fig. 19–12). Although flexible, the extreme tight-fitting and keystone nature of the articulations—especially the base of the second metatarsal (Fig. 19–13)—and the numerous strong ligaments across these joints (Fig. 19–14) are necessary to maintain the arch during weight bearing. It therefore takes a great deal of force to disrupt the anatomy of the midfoot. As a result, when these injuries occur, the midfoot will balloon up like a fat sausage and can result in compartment syndrome. Early operative intervention is warranted within the first 12 to 24 hours. The suspicion that a Lisfranc's injury has occurred is raised whenever there is severe swelling in the midfoot.

Closed reduction and stabilization by pinning is generally insufficient. Due to the forces, a great deal of debris is present in the area (Fig. 19–15). Upon opening these joints, sheared pieces of articular cartilage, flaps of ligaments, and pieces of bone are often present blocking anatomic reduction. Reduction can usually only be produced by an open procedure to permit debridement of the intra-articular debris.

If an anatomic reduction is not obtained, the mechanics of the foot and arch are disrupted, and chronic pain may result. Following the open reduction, stabilize the joints. Usually this can be done through stout pins (Fig. 19–16) which are later removed in the office after ligamentous healing. Some advocate the use of screws for more stable fixation,[2] however this requires a second operation for removal to free the joints, and there may be more damage to the articular surfaces through the use of the large threaded screws across

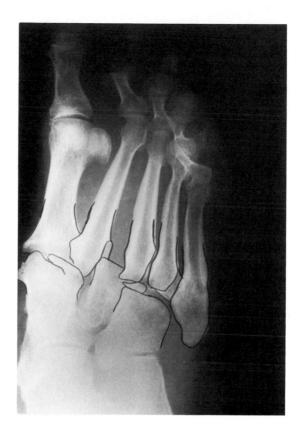

Figure 19–11. Lisfranc injury demonstrating widely displaced metatarsal bases and some bony intra-articular debris. The thick ligaments of the metatarsal-cuneiform joints are also present blocking reduction.

the joints in comparison to the smooth pins. In severe cases with significant articular cartilage damage, a primary fusion of the joints may be required.

FOREFOOT

Forefoot injuries result from the same mechanisms already discussed for the midfoot. Digital dislocations and fractures as well as metatarsal fractures can be found. Commonly occurring as a low-energy isolated injury, these injuries in the trauma patient can be treated with the same techniques used in their lower energy counterparts. If, due to the higher energy, they are displaced significantly, surgical intervention may be necessary.

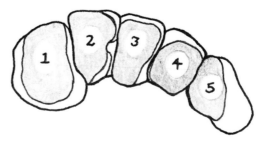

Figure 19–12. The keystone nature of the bases of the metatarsals forming the transverse arch.

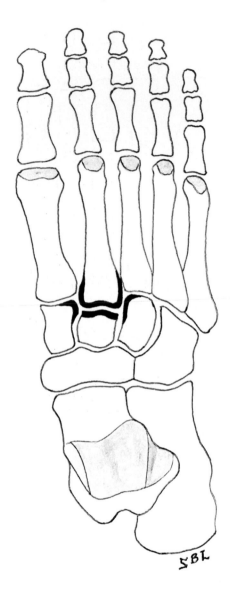

Figure 19–13. Recessed base of the second metatarsal as it tightly locks into its articulation with the cuneiforms is the key to maintaining the arch at Lisfranc's joints.

The most important aspect of these injuries is that they are commonly missed. Even if the patient is conscious and coherent, he often does not feel the pain of these injuries due to the more severe pain from other major trauma. It is always crucial to do serial exams to ferret out these minor injuries in the foot and elsewhere. The patient and family should be warned that further minor injuries may turn up later and to bring up new aches and pains to the physician's attention. Diagnosis of these injuries are in many instances made on a delayed basis.

Dislocations of the digital and metatarsal-phalangeal joints generally can be closed reduced and are stable requiring only "buddy-taping" to an adjacent intact toe. Occa-

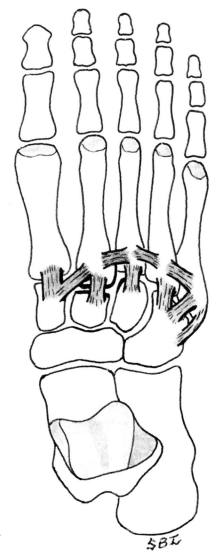

Figure 19–14. Strong ligaments maintaining the integrity of Lisfranc's joints.

sionally, the bone will buttonhole through soft tissue and become entrapped requiring open reduction. In such cases, the destabilizing nature of the surgery warrants the short use of a pin across the joint.

Minor nondisplaced fractures of the digits and metatarsals likewise can often be treated closed with protective weight bearing, but the principles of fracture treatment must not be ignored for these seemingly lesser injuries. Displaced intra-articular fractures require open reduction and internal fixation to reconstruct the joint.

Commonly, grossly displaced fractures, especially of the metatarsal heads, may be present (Fig. 19–17). If left to heal this way, the patient will walk on bony prominences

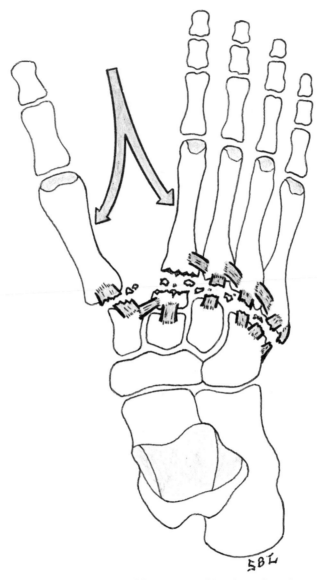

Figure 19–15. Lisfranc's injury consisting of fractures and dislocations of tarsal-metatarsal joints. Note the abundant debris in the joints blocking an anatomic closed reduction without debridement.

causing callouses and severe pain. He will describe a sensation of having a loose stone in the shoe. Such displaced injuries require reduction and stabilization with pins (Fig. 19–18). Occasionally these fractures can be reduced and pinned by closed technique, however this is difficult[6] and multiple attempts will result in prolonged surgery and cause further damage to the soft tissues leading to increased swelling. Especially in the patient with other injuries who must be operated upon expeditiously, open reduction is quick and adds no further morbidity.

These injuries to the forefoot can all be taken care of on a nonurgent basis, provided

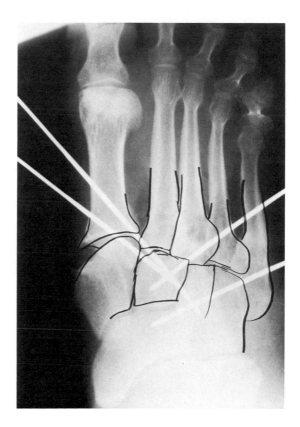

Figure 19–16. Lisfranc injury following excision of intra-articular debris, open reduction, and pinning.

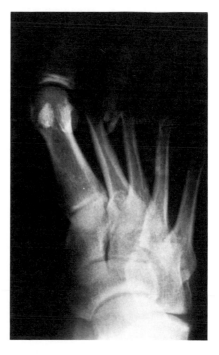

Figure 19–17. Displaced metatarsal head fractures.

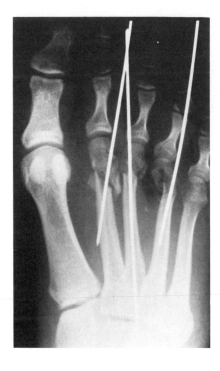

Figure 19–18.   Metatarsal head fractures after pinning.

compartment syndrome is not present. The only requirement is intervention before they start to heal (which begins quite quickly), as having to take down a partially healed injury makes reduction more difficult and will not give as good a result.

REFERENCES

1. Anderson HG. *Medical and Surgical Aspects of Aviation*. London, England: Oxford Medical Publications; 1919.
2. Arntz CT, et al. Fractures and fracture-dislocations of the tarsometatarsal joint. *J Bone Joint Surg*. 1988; 70-A:173–181.
3. Ashhurst APC, Bromer RS. Classification and mechanism of fractures of the leg bone involving the ankle. *Arch Surg*. 1922;4:51–129.
4. Bray TJ, et al. Treatment of open ankle fractures. *Clin Orthop*. 1989;240:47–52.
5. Chapman MW. The use of immediate internal fixation in open fractures. *Orthop Clin*. 1980;11:579–591.
6. Chapman MW, ed. *Operative Orthopaedics*. Philadelphia, Pa: JB Lippincott; 1988.
7. Crenshaw AH, ed. *Campbell's Operative Orthopaedics*. 7th ed. St. Louis, Mo: CV Mosby; 1987.
8. Dupuytren G. Mémoire sur la Fracture de l'Extrémité Inférieure de Pérone, les Luxations et les Accidents qui en sont la Suite. *Annuaire Méd-Chir*. Hôp. Paris. Crochard, Paris; 1819.
9. Franklin JL, et al. Immediate internal fixation of open ankle fractures. *J Bone Joint Surg*. 1984;66-A:1349–1356.
10. Grob D, et al. Operative treatment of displaced talus fractures. *Clin Orthop*. 1985;199:88–96.
11. Halliburton RA, et al. The extra-osseous and intra-osseous blood supply of the talus. *J Bone Joint Surg*. 1958;40-A:1115.
12. Hawkins LG. Fractures of the neck of the talus. *J Bone Joint Surg*. 1970;52-A:991–1002.
13. Lauge-Hansen N. Fractures of the ankle. *Arch Surg*. 1950;60:957–985.
14. McKeever F. Treatment of complications of fractures and dislocations of the talus. *Clin Orthop*. 1963;30:45–52.

15. Maisonneuve JG. Recherches sur la fracture du perone. *Arch Gen Med.* 1840;7:165– 187, 433–473.
16. Mulfinger GL, Trueta J. The blood supply of the talus. *J Bone Joint Surg.* 1970;52-B:160–167.
17. Müller ME, Allgöwer M, Schneider R, Willenegger M. *Manual of Internal Fixation.* 3rd ed. New York, NY: Springer-Verlag; 1991.
18. Peltier LF. *Fractures.* San Francisco, Calif: Norman Publishing; 1990.
19. Pott P. *Some Few General Remarks on Fractures and Dislocations.* London, England: L Hawes, W Clarke, & R Collins; 1768.
20. Ramsay PL, Hamilton W. Changes in tibiotalar area of contact caused by lateral tibia shift. *J Bone Joint Surg.* 1976;59-A:356.
21. Rockwood CA Jr, Green DP. *Fractures in Adults.* 2nd ed. Philadelphia, Pa: JB Lippincott; 1984.
22. Sangeorzan BJ, et al. Displaced intra-articular fractures of the tarsal navicular. *J Bone Joint Surg.* 1989; 71-A:1504–1510.
23. Schatzker J, Tile M. *The Rationale of Operative Fracture Care.* Berlin, Germany: Springer-Verlag; 1987.

20

Compartment Syndrome

JAMES P. KENNEDY, M.D.

HISTORY: Richard von Volkmann reported the sequelae of compartment syndrome in 1881,[27] although Malgaigne described ischemic contractures from tight bandages 34 years earlier.[21] Volkmann also felt that the contractures he observed occurred from ischemic changes in limbs that were too tightly bandaged. Later, Jepson[13] proved in 1926 that the Volkmann's contracture could be prevented in patients with compartment syndrome by prompt fascial decompression.

INTRODUCTION

Compartment syndrome due to trauma is usually the result of interstitial edema or hemorrhage into the soft tissues enclosed within a fascial space. This results in high tissue pressure within the compartment impeding perfusion of the tissue on the microvascular level with tissue necrosis being the end result. Untreated, it can lead to an extremity left functionless from a Volkmann's ischemic contracture.

Due to the severe impairment resulting from the resultant contracture of an untreated compartment syndrome, it is important to predict when it is going to occur and to be able to recognize when it exists so that it can be prevented or treated. Details about the various compartment syndromes as they relate to specific injuries are discussed in the chapters pertaining to each anatomic location.

Two types of compartment syndrome exist, the acute and the chronic, or exertional. The acute compartment syndrome occurs secondary to an acute traumatic insult to the extremity. Chronic compartment syndrome is a painful condition brought on by exertion. This is a less severe, atraumatic form of the syndrome and will not be further discussed here.

LOCATION

Most clinicians are aware of the compartment syndromes occurring in the classic locations of the forearm and lower leg, and any physician treating trauma will encounter compartment syndromes in these locations. These two anatomic locations have well defined fascial compartments that are unyielding to swelling that occurs within them. Orthopaedic subspecialists are also well aware of the compartment syndromes that occur in the hand and foot.

Compartment syndrome has also been described in less well known locations such as the shoulder, upper arm, buttock, and thigh.[2,3,22] These anatomic areas do not have as well defined tight fascial boundaries to their compartments as the lower leg and forearm, so compartment syndromes are less common, but they do occur. These perhaps are the most dangerous of compartment syndromes because they may easily be overlooked as the physician doesn't think of compartment syndrome occurring in these locations. Compartment syndrome of the thigh, especially, may be seen in the badly traumatized patient.[23]

It is widely, but incorrectly, believed that open fractures cannot develop a compartment syndrome because the open nature of the injury has already provided decompression. This is a dangerous misconception. The extensive soft tissue injury that can accompany an open fracture puts many of these cases at risk for a compartment syndrome. Up to 10% of open tibial fractures will develop a compartment syndrome.[1]

It should be realized that compartment syndrome can occur in virtually any location. The symptoms are the same regardless of the location, so if the clinical picture fits, compartment pressures are measured and fasciotomies performed when indicated. Symptomatology and physical findings, and not location, are the key to recognizing compartment syndromes.

ETIOLOGY

There are many potential causes of compartment syndrome.[3,6,18,22] Traumatic direct crush injuries are the most common. Fractured extremities can develop the syndrome through bleeding from the fracture, vessel laceration (such as following a supracondylar humerus or distal femur fracture), or bleeding from torn muscle fibers into the closed space. Dressings or casts which are too tight are another common cause or contributor to increased compartment pressures. Burns are associated with a special type of compartment syndrome when the swelling underlying a burn is encased by an unyielding enveloping skin eschar.

Ischemia from arterial insult can cause or contribute to increased compartment pressures. "The Saturday-Night Syndrome"[18,19] results from patients who in an alcoholic or drug-induced stupor remain motionless for hours in a position which cuts off the circulation to an extremity or results in direct compression of a compartment. This same mechanism occurs in patients trapped in cramped quarters in automobile accidents or during the destruction associated with natural disasters. In both of these situations, not only does the ischemia contribute to soft tissue damage, but when circulation is restored, postischemic swelling from the hyperemic response can be massive,[15] compounding the insult. After three hours of tourniquet-induced ischemia to a limb, the muscle will increase in weight by 50% once perfusion is restored[8] secondary to the development of postischemic edema. For this reason, it is possible to see a compartment syndrome precipitated following surgery for an arterial bypass, repair of an arterial laceration, or an acute embolism. Even short-term use of a tourniquet will cause swelling upon deflation. With less than an hour of tourniquet time, limbs will increase 10% by volume following tourniquet deflation.[24] For this reason, tourniquets should always be deflated prior to wound closure or casting to help prevent problems with postoperative swelling. Venous obstruction secondary to avulsion, laceration, or thrombosis is another cause which is often unsuspected.

Other less common causes of compartment syndrome include various congenital or acquired bleeding disorders in which bleeding into a compartment will occur spontaneously or following minor trauma. Massive soft tissue swelling and edema can also occur secondary to various toxins found in venomous snakes, spiders, and scorpions. A more rare cause is an iatrogenic compartment syndrome induced by the MAST garment. Several cases of compartment syndrome have been reported[25] following lengthy use of the MAST garment.

PATHOPHYSIOLOGY

There is much that is yet to be understood about the pathophysiology of compartment syndrome. The lesion occurs on the microvascular level, and seems to be related to both an increase in pressure within a closed compartment and ischemia of the tissue within the compartment.[10]

The normal fluid exchange that occurs during perfusion is related to the filtration pressure within the capillaries and the osmotic differential of the plasma proteins.[26] These are such that at the arterial end of the capillary the filtration force is greater than the osmotic pressure, so fluid will leave the capillary into the interstitial tissue. At the venous end, the osmotic force is greater than the filtration pressure, so fluid returns to the vascular space.

As the compartment syndrome develops, pressure within the compartment increases. When the pressure within the compartment exceeds that in the microcirculation, the venous end of the capillaries are functionally occluded.[26] High proximal pressures in the distally occluded capillary plus anoxic damage to the capillary endothelium results in increased transudation of fluid into the soft tissues. Since the osmotic differential has increased due to loss of colloid through the "leaky" capillary, the transudate exceeds the amount of fluid resorption by the venous system resulting in progressive edema. As fluid slowly builds up in the compartment, pressures increase further, and a vicious cycle develops. Eventually, the pressures reach such a magnitude that microvascular circulation stops and the tissues within the compartment are no longer perfused. Irreversible damage to the muscles in the involved compartment can occur within 4 hours of anoxia, and irreversible damage to nerves within 12 hours.[22] The end result of an untreated compartment syndrome is death of all the tissues within the compartment. The muscle will become fibrotic and a Volkmann's contracture with its characteristic contracted, insensate, functionless extremity will result. A spectrum of Volkmann's ischemic contracture is possible ranging from mild cases without much functional loss to the full-blown cases with useless, contracted limbs.

It is crucial to note that the compartment syndrome occurs on the microvascular level. Therefore, as will be discussed further below, distal pulses may still be present even when muscle perfusion has stopped. This is because nutritive circulation in the compartment occurs at levels roughly 50% of arterial pressure so that the differential between the large arterial and compartment pressures remains sufficient to drive the blood through a tight compartment that is not being perfused. It is therefore possible to completely necrose the forearm or leg musculature, but maintain viability to the hand or foot and their intrinsic muscles.

DIAGNOSIS

The key to diagnosis is continual assessment of those injuries that are at risk for developing a compartment syndrome. These include fractures of the tibia, forearm, and supracondylar humerus; the Lisfranc injury of the midfoot, and any comminuted fracture with severe soft tissue injury. The diagnosis of compartment syndrome is a clinical diagnosis, with the measurement of compartment pressures used for confirmatory evidence when needed, or more often, for use in those patients where an adequate examination cannot be carried out.

The hallmark of the compartment syndrome is the "Four P's"—Pressure, Pain, Paresthesias, and Pulses Intact.[18] The first of these, pressure, is the sine qua non of the compartment syndrome. The patient will have tensely swollen compartments to palpation. This finding alone may be an adequate indication for fasciotomies in patients at risk. Measurement of compartment pressures help to confirm the diagnosis in borderline cases, or are helpful in following the progression of pressures to permit recognition before a full-fledged syndrome develops.

Pain has two components in the compartment syndrome. The first is pain out of proportion to that expected for the patient's level of injury. The second is pain with passive stretch. The origin of pain is from the ischemic muscle, so passively stretching the muscle will cause severe aggravation of the pain. Active stretch will cause this pain as well, however it is difficult to get patients to perform this painful maneuver voluntarily. No matter how severe the injury might be, limited range of motion of the distal parts to gently stretch the muscle traversing the compartment in question should be able to be performed without undue discomfort if compartment syndrome is not present. When the compartment syndrome is developing, this gentle maneuver will set off severe pain from the ischemic or necrosing muscle.

Muscle is more sensitive to anoxia than nerve, so muscle pain occurs earliest and numbness or anesthesia occurs later. As the syndrome progresses, paresthesias begin, progressing to eventual anesthesia. Paresthesias will be present in the areas innervated by the nerves traversing the involved compartments. Thus, pain will be absent late in the syndrome after anesthesia sets in as the nerves become ischemic. This is a poor prognostic sign.

The final physical finding is the presence of distal circulation confirmed by capillary refill and distal pulses. The two differential diagnoses to consider are a nerve or arterial lesion. The nerve laceration or contusion presents with neither pressure increases nor pain with range of motion, so this is not often confused with the compartment syndrome. A case of primary arterial insufficiency may be more difficult to distinguish. Pain with stretch is present with arterial insufficiency due to the soft tissue ischemia, but it involves the entire extremity and is not confined just to the compartment. Also, the pain is more severe in the most distal portion of the extremity (fingers and toes), and findings such as a cold distal extremity with color changes may be present. The other distinguishing feature is that the distal circulation will be poor (Table 20–1).

ASSESSMENT

The most important factor in managing the compartment syndrome is prevention, or if this is not possible, early intervention to break the cycle before irreversible damage occurs.

Table 20–1   **Compartment Syndrome Findings**[17]

	COMPARTMENT SYNDROME	ARTERIAL INJURY	NERVE INJURY
Pressure increase	+	−	−
Pain with motion	+	+	−
Paresthesia	+	+	+
Pulses intact	+	−	+

Early, if not immediate operative fixation, when warranted for those fractures at risk, can help avert a compartment syndrome by helping maintain compartment volume by reducing and stabilizing the fracture. This decreases further damage and swelling from mobile fracture fragments, stops fracture bleeding through the reduction and surgical hemostasis, and evacuates any traumatic hematoma. Prophylactic fasciotomies may be considered after revascularization procedures for traumatic arterial lesions in which the ischemic time has been greater than 4 to 6 hours[3] to help prevent a return to the operating room to do so later if a compartment syndrome develops.[3]

When the patient first begins to complain of undue pain, and the issue of impending compartment syndrome is raised, all circumferential bandages are split down to skin to relieve any possible constriction. Likewise, casts and cast padding are split to skin. To relieve pressure, the cast is univalved and spread, or removed. If necessary, maintenance of reduction must be sacrificed.

The limb should be placed no more than 10 cm above the level of the heart. Although helpful for venous drainage, elevation can theoretically impede perfusion of the compartment. Additional arterial pressure is needed to "pump the blood uphill" to the extremity and maintain the same filtration pressure. As the arterial pressure usually remains constant with limb elevation, the additional pressure to maintain the filtration pressure is not available. The filtration pressure therefore decreases and thereby the threshold for development of the compartment syndrome decreases to a lower pressure as well.

If the above measures don't quickly alleviate the clinical findings of a compartment syndrome, decompressive fasciotomies must be performed. For borderline cases, pressure measurements can be taken for documentation purposes and to help chart the course of treatment. If fasciotomies are not immediately needed, the patient should be closely monitored with frequent examination. Indwelling catheters may be helpful to provide continuous compartment monitoring.

Compartment pressures are also measured whenever there is any question about the accuracy of the clinical exam. This would include all pediatric patients, patients who are obtunded from head injury, and patients under the influence of alcohol or drugs. In the trauma patient with multiple injuries requiring lengthy surgery, the compartment syndrome could develop while the patient is under anesthesia. Continuous pressure monitoring is very helpful in these instances as well as to evaluate those extremities at risk.

Compartment pressures can be measured through the use of a wick or slit catheter attached to an arterial line setup (Fig. 20–1), or more conveniently with a hand-held battery operated digital self-contained measuring device (Fig. 20–2). The catheter is introduced with a needle into the desired compartment. The most commonly involved areas include the calf and forearm. The calf is composed of four compartments, the anterior, lateral,

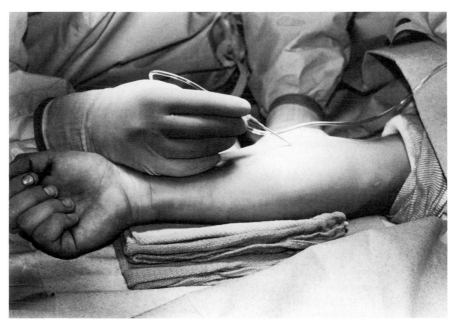

Figure 20–1. Measuring compartment pressures in volar forearm with arterial line transducer connected to a wick catheter for continual monitoring of compartment pressures. If arterial line set-up is used, be certain not to use a pressure bag or fluid will be forced into the compartment compounding the problem. The transducer should be placed at the level of the compartment being measured for zeroing.

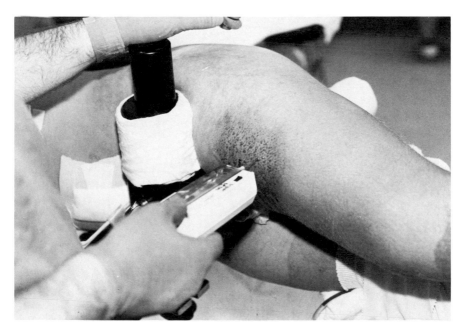

Figure 20–2. Convenient hand-held transistorized pressure monitoring device. Easily portable, it requires no additional equipment. May be used as a "one-time stick" or with an in-dwelling catheter for continual measurements.

superficial posterior, and deep posterior, which are defined by the anterior and posterior intermuscular septae, the tibia, the fibula, and the interosseous membrane (Fig. 20–3). The anterior compartment contains the tibialis anterior, extensor digitorum longus, extensor hallucis longus, and the peroneus tertius muscles as well as the anterior tibial artery and deep peroneal nerve.

The lateral compartment contains the peroneus longus and brevis muscles and the superficial peroneal nerve. The gastrocnemius and soleus muscles, and sural nerve make up the superficial posterior compartment. The tibialis posterior muscle, flexor hallucis longus, flexor digitorum longus, posterior tibial nerve, and posterior tibial artery are found in the deep posterior compartment.

The three compartments of the forearm are formed by the antebrachial fascia, the radius and ulna, and the interosseous membrane, but do not have as definite fascial divisions as the leg.[7] These compartments are the volar (flexor) and dorsal (extensor) compartments and the mobile wad proximally (Fig. 20–4). The carpal tunnel at the wrist level can also be involved. The volar compartment contains the flexors and pronators and is subdivided into deep and superficial defined by a thin intermuscular fascia. The dorsal compartment contains the extensors of the wrist and fingers. The dorsal and volar compartments are separated by the mobile wad made up of the extensor carpi radialis longus and brevis and the brachioradialis.

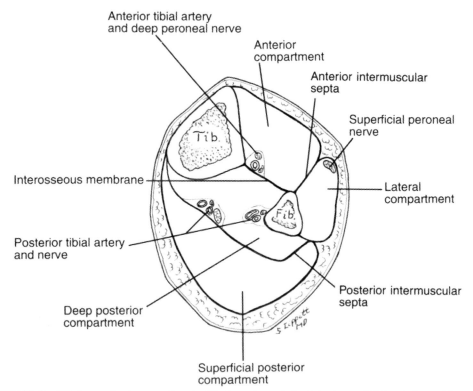

Figure 20–3.   The four anatomic compartments of the lower leg: anterior, lateral, superficial posterior, and deep posterior with their associated nerves and vessels.

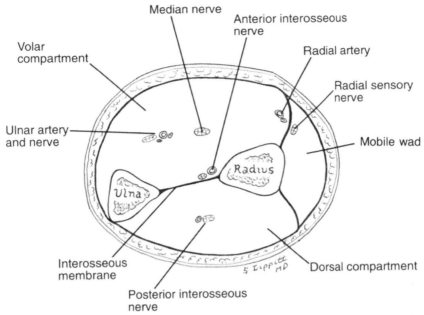

Figure 20–4. The three anatomic compartments of the forearm: the volar, dorsal, and mobile wad with the associated neurovascular structures.

Other compartmental areas include the anterior, posterior, and medial or adductor thigh compartments; the intrinsic, thenar, hypothenar, and deep palmar compartments of the hand; and the medial, lateral, central, and interosseous compartments of the foot.[9]

PRESSURE MEASUREMENTS

After prepping the skin over the chosen site, the needle is held at the planned angle of entrance and the device zeroed. The catheter should be placed into the compartment obliquely, paralleling the muscle fibers as closely as possible to prevent muscle laceration and further bleeding. This also prevents occlusion of the catheter if it abuts a muscle fiber leading to a false reading.

Normal compartment pressures in the resting individual range from zero to plus or minus 4 mm Hg.[3,18,22] Anything greater than this is abnormal. The difficulty is that there is no absolute threshold at which compartment syndrome develops, as the syndrome is both pressure- and time-related.[3,10,18] It has also become evident that as systemic blood pressure decreases, the threshold for compartment syndrome decreases as well.[3,12,16,22]

Compartment pressures of 30 mm Hg for more than 8 hours have been shown to be associated with irreversible damage.[18] For normotensive individuals, compartment pressures measuring less than 30 mm Hg can be closely observed. Pressures greater than 50 mm Hg require immediate fasciotomy. The grey zone is the 30 to 50 mm Hg range. Here, the estimated time the pressure has been present; the expectation of whether the pressure will continue, increase, or diminish; the patient's systemic blood pressure; and the overall general status will enter into the decision on whether or not to perform the fasciotomy. Generally, it is appropriate to decompress extremities in patients whose pressures fall within this grey zone when their clinical findings are suggestive of compartment syndrome, or if the injuries are such that swelling can be expected to continue. It is better to unnecessarily decompress some patients in order to be sure to decompress the ones that need it.

When the patient is hypotensive, the above pressure guidelines may not hold true. Various recommendations in these circumstances have been developed. Whitesides recommends to decompress whenever the compartment pressure rises to within 10 to 30 mm Hg of the diastolic blood pressure in symptomatic patients.[28] Perhaps a better guideline is to decompress whenever the difference between the mean arterial pressure (diastolic pressure plus 1/3 of the pulse pressure) and the compartment pressure is within 30 to 40 mm Hg.[11] This difference between the mean arterial pressure and the compartment pressure has been termed the perfusion index. Heppenstall has found cellular changes relating to impaired perfusion with a perfusion index of 30 or lower present for 6 hours, or 40 or lower present for 8 hours.[12]

TREATMENT

For acute compartment syndrome, wide decompressive fasciotomies are required. To decompress the forearm, two incisions are made, one volar and one dorsal (Fig. 20–5). The longitudinal dorsal incision allows approach to the extensor compartment and mobile wad. The fascia overlying these compartments must be widely opened. A curvilinear volar incision allows approach to the flexor compartment from proximal to the antecubital fossa

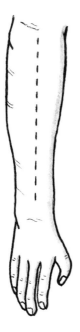
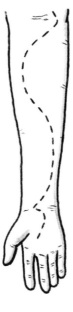

Figure 20–5. Incisions for decompression of forearm compartment syndrome.

to the midpalm. Again, the fascia is widely opened. In severe cases, the deep intermuscular fascia enveloping the flexor digitorum superficialis and profundus and the flexor pollicis longus may need to be opened as well. The thick transverse carpal ligament is divided distally to perform a carpal tunnel release.[7] The proximal end of the incision is used to release the lacertus fibrosus which must be done to decompress the median nerve at the elbow. As well, the proximal edges of the pronator teres and flexor digitorum superficialis must be inspected to make sure median nerve compression is not present from these structures.[3] Following the fascial incision, the tensely swollen muscle will bulge out through the incision and confirm the presence of compartment syndrome (Fig. 20–6).

To decompress the lower leg, three techniques have been used—the two incision decompression,[20] the single incision transfibular approach,[5] and fibulectomy.[14] Regardless of which procedure is used, the surgeon must have a good understanding of the anatomy to permit access to the compartments without surgical damage to the nerves and vessels within each compartment.

Fibulectomy should generally be avoided as it is a more lengthy and traumatic procedure, may cause resultant ankle instability or pain if not properly done, and may not adequately decompress all four compartments. It also seems somewhat ill-conceived to remove a normal anatomic structure when the condition can be easily addressed through other means.

The two incision decompression uses a lateral incision between the tibial crest and fibula for approach to the anterior and lateral compartments. A short transverse incision can be made through the leg fascia to identify the location of the intermuscular fascia (Fig. 20–7A). The superficial peroneal nerve lies just posterior to this septum in the lateral

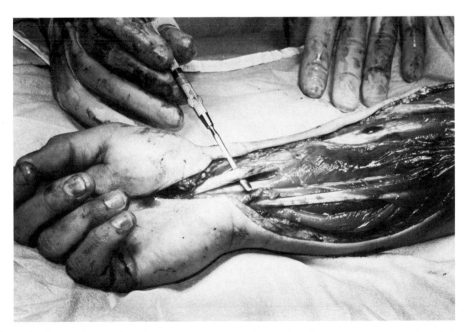

Figure 20–6. Bulging muscle of forearm following compartment release for "Saturday-Night Syndrome" due to heroin overdose. Note complete release of median nerve (elevator is under nerve) in carpal canal.

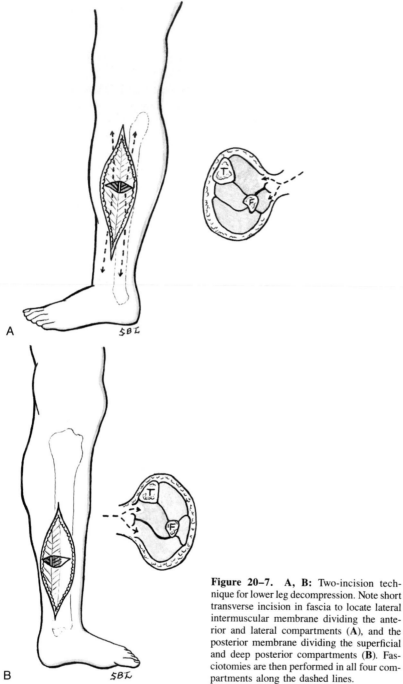

Figure 20–7. A, B: Two-incision technique for lower leg decompression. Note short transverse incision in fascia to locate lateral intermuscular membrane dividing the anterior and lateral compartments (**A**), and the posterior membrane dividing the superficial and deep posterior compartments (**B**). Fasciotomies are then performed in all four compartments along the dashed lines.

compartment and must be avoided. The fascia of the two compartments is then widely opened longitudinally with blunt scissors using a generous skin incision until the muscles are soft and all pressure is dissipated. A medial incision 2 cm posterior to the posterior crest of the tibia is used to gain access to the posterior compartments (Fig. 20–7B) and avoid the saphenous nerve and vein. Again, a short transverse incision can be used through the enveloping fascia to identify the septum between the deep and the superficial compartments.

In utilizing the single incision technique, a lateral incision is made over the fibula just distal to its head, and ending just short of the lateral malleolus (Fig. 20–8). The skin is undermined as needed anteriorly to allow approach to the anterior and lateral compartments as described above. Undermining the skin posteriorly exposes the superficial posterior compartment which is fasciotomized. Through the lateral approach, access to the deep compartment can only be made through Harmon's approach[4] to the posterior tibia. The flexor hallucis longus in the superficial posterior compartment is subperiosteally dissected off the posterior border of the fibula, and retracted with the peroneal vessels until the posterior tibialis is reached. The fascia overlying it is then released to decompress the deep compartment.

The issue of whether to use one or two incisions for the lower leg is not as important as using a technique through which a good decompression can be obtained. The two incision technique may be safer and easier for the surgeon not thoroughly familiar with the anatomy of the area or experienced in the technique of the single incision. Subcutaneous fasciotomies through small skin incisions have been advocated. These are appropriate only for the chronic exercise induced syndrome, but not for the acute compartment syndrome.

No matter what the technique used, or the anatomic area of the compartment syndrome, a complete decompression must be obtained. The skin incision should be sufficient enough to allow safe exposure of the area and equal the fasciotomy incision in length. The fascia should be incised sufficiently to ensure that the entire compartment is completely soft.

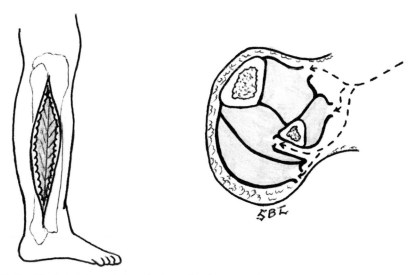

Figure 20–8. Single-incision technique for lower leg decompression.

At the time of decompression, muscle will dramatically bulge out through the fasciotomy site. With prompt diagnosis and treatment, the muscle should be pink, viable, and, most importantly, contractile. With later intervention, some necrotic muscle may be present. Noncontractile and grossly nonviable muscle can be excised at this time. All wounds are left widely open. If a skin closure is attempted, the enveloping skin can become a tight constriction and reprecipitate the loss of perfusion leading to another acute compartment syndrome. This same phenomenon can occur if a subcutaneous fasciotomy is attempted through small incisions.

After applying sterile dressings to the open wound, a Robert Jones dressing is applied. A split-thickness skin graft can then be applied to healthy muscle or granulation tissue at 5 to 7 days. Delayed primary closure can sometimes be used for part of the wound as the swelling diminishes, or for one of the incisions when the two-incision technique is used. At the time of any wound closure, the fascia should never be approximated or closed due to the risk of precipitating another compartment syndrome.

If the compartment syndrome is diagnosed late, after muscle has necrosed, no decompression is warranted. Decompression will not restore the muscle, and in fact may be detrimental by increasing the risk for infection in the exposed, dead muscle. This situation is most likely when the cause of the compartment swelling follows delay in repair of an arterial injury. When collateral flow is negligible and restoration of circulation cannot be accomplished within eight hours, death of some, if not all of the nonperfused muscle is usual.

REFERENCES

1. Blick SS, et al. Compartment syndrome in open tibial fractures. *J Bone Joint Surg.* 1986;68-A:1348–1353.
2. Brumback RJ. Traumatic rupture of the superior gluteal artery, without fracture of the pelvis, causing compartment syndrome of the buttock. *J Bone Joint Surg.* 1990;72-A:134–137.
3. Chapman MW, ed. *Operative Orthopaedics.* Philadelphia, Pa: JB Lippincott; 1988.
4. Crenshaw AH, ed. *Campbell's Operative Orthopaedics.* 7th ed. St. Louis, Mo: CV Mosby; 1987.
5. Davey JR, et al. The tibialis posterior muscle compartment: an unrecognized cause of exertional compartment syndrome. *Am J Sports Med.* 1984;12:391.
6. Evarts CM, ed. *Surgery of the Musculoskeletal System.* Edinburgh, Scotland: Churchill Livingstone; 1983.
7. Gelberman RJ, et al. Decompression of forearm compartment syndromes. *Clin Orthop.* 1978;134:225–229.
8. Harman JW, Gwinn RP. The significance of local vascular phenomena in the production of ischemic necrosis in skeletal muscle. *Am J Pathol.* 1949;24:741–755.
9. Heckman JD, Champine MJ. New techniques in the management of foot trauma. *Clin Orthop.* 1989; 240:105–114.
10. Heppenstall, RB, et al. A comparative study of the tolerance of skeletal muscle to ischemia. *J Bone Joint Surg.* 1986;68-A:820–828.
11. Heppenstall RB, et al. The compartment syndrome. An experimental and clinical study of muscular energy metabolism using phosphorus nuclear magnetic resonance spectroscopy. *Clin Orthop.* 1988;226:138–155.
12. Heppenstall RB, et al. Compartment syndrome: a quantitative study of high-energy phosphorus compounds using 31P-magnetic resonance spectroscopy. *J Trauma.* 1989;29:1113–1119.
13. Jepson PN. Ischemic contracture, experimental study. *Ann Surg.* 1926;84:785–795.
14. Kelly RP, Whitesides RE Jr. Transfibular route for fasciotomy of the leg. In: Proceedings of the American Academy of Orthopaedic Surgeons. *J Bone Joint Surg.* 1967;49-A:1022–1023.
15. Klenerman L, et al. Hyperaemia swelling of a limb upon release of a tourniquet. *Acta Orthop Scand.* 1982; 53:209.
16. Morrey BF. *The Elbow and Its Disorders.* Philadelphia, Pa: WB Saunders; 1985.
17. Mubarak SJ, Carroll N. Volkmann's contracture in children: aetiology and prevention. *J Bone Joint Surg.* 1979;61-B:290.
18. Mubarak SJ, Hargens AR. *Compartment Syndromes and Volkmann's Contracture.* Philadelphia, Pa: WB Saunders; 1981.

19. Mubarak SJ, Owen CA. Compartment syndrome and its relation to the crush syndrome. *Clin Orthop*. 1975; 113:81–89.
20. Mubarak SJ, Owen CA. Double-incision fasciotomy of the leg for decompression in compartment syndromes. *J Bone Joint Surg*. 1977;59-A:184–187.
21. Peltier LF. Joseph François Malgaigne and Malgaigne's fractures. *Clin Orthop*. 1980;151:4–7.
22. Rockwood CA Jr, Green DP. *Fractures in Adults*. 2nd ed. Philadelphia, Pa: JB Lippincott; 1984.
23. Schwartz JT Jr, et al. Acute compartment syndrome of the thigh. *J Bone Joint Surg*. 1989;71-A:392–400.
24. Silver R, et al. Limb swelling after release of a tourniquet. *Clin Orthop*. 1986;206:86–89.
25. Teeny SM, Wiss DA. Compartment syndrome: a complication of the use of the MAST suit. *J Orthop Trauma*. 1987;1:236–239.
26. Turek SL. *Orthopaedics*. 4th ed. Philadelphia, Pa: JB Lippincott; 1984.
27. von Volkmann R. Die ischaemischen Muskellähmungen und Kontrakturen. *Zentralbl Chir*. 1881;8:801.
28. Whitesides Jr, TE, et al. Tissue pressure measurements as a determinant for the need of fasciotomy. *Clin Orthop*. 1975;113:43.

21

Traumatic Amputation

JAMES P. KENNEDY, M.D.

HISTORY: Amputations are one of the earliest described operations. Characteristic signs of amputations having been performed have been found in prehistoric bones.[6] Albucasis (1013–1106) wrote about amputations for gangrene in his second volume. Brunschwig (1497), in the first detailed account of treating gunshot wounds by amputation, applied boiling oil to check the hemorrhage from the stump. Later, Gersdorff (1517) described amputations for gunshot wounds in more detail. During the amputation he applied a constricting band, then afterwards enclosed the stump in the bladder of a bull, ox, or hog to control hemorrhage. His text contained the first illustration of an amputation.[6]

Ambroise Paré, while an army surgeon in 1537, observed that amputations following gunshot wounds did better when not cauterized. He reintroduced the ligature which had been abandoned since the time of Celsus. Even by the middle of the 19th century, during the Civil War, the routine treatment for open fractures was still amputation due to the high mortality rates associated with attempts at limb salvage. Prior to World War II, the majority of amputations were performed above the knee due to the presence of good soft tissue for wound coverage and good guarantee of wound healing.[3]

Hippocrates described three indications for amputation: to remove useless limbs, to reduce invalidism, and to save the patient's life.[5] These principles still hold true today when applied to the polytrauma patient.

INTRODUCTION

Trauma is the second leading cause of amputation after peripheral vascular disease, and is the number one cause in patients less than fifty years of age.[4]

Management of the polytraumatized patient with a completely severed lower extremity presents no difficulties in deciding the course of treatment—the decision to treat the injury as an open amputation has already been made. The difficulty in the decision-making process arises when there has been a near-amputation. In such cases it is imperative to quickly decide whether to embark on an often lengthy and difficult course of limb salvage,

358

or whether to complete the amputation. Limb salvage can require multiple operations that are expensive[2] and fraught with morbidity or even mortality and yet may not be successful. Delayed amputation has been shown to be two to three times more expensive than primary amputation, and a delay often results in a more proximal level of amputation or other complications such as higher infection and mortality rates.[2] The most difficult cases to manage can require two to three years of multiple operations in an attempt to gain union. In spite of heroic measures, the severe Grade IIIc tibia fractures still have an amputation rate of 20% to 75%.[8]

INDICATIONS

Faced with a patient in extremis or with severe systemic injuries, immediate amputation of crushed limbs can be life-saving by removing the metabolic demands of the injured tissue and the breakdown products generated by such critical injuries. A severe extremity trauma may also be the source of a coagulopathy.

The stress of multiple operations required to reconstruct a severely crushed extremity may not be well tolerated in these gravely injured patients. In these instances, primary amputation may be the treatment of choice. In other cases—overwhelming infection, sepsis, or gas gangrene[5]—amputation is necessary as a life-saving measure. Another indication for immediate amputation is the technical or anatomic impossibility of sufficiently reconstructing a mangled limb so that it will be a functional extremity. This is especially true in severe injuries of the tibia which are notorious for developing infected nonunions following such open fractures.

As medical science progresses, more and more severely injured limbs are being salvaged. Skin grafting and flap techniques are such that soft tissue loss alone is rarely an indication today for amputation. Microvascular repair and vascular bypass techniques have eliminated isolated blood vessel injury as a cause for amputation, so long as warm ischemia time can be kept less than 6 hours.[3–5] Major blood vessel injury coupled with severe soft tissue and bony injury remains an indication for primary amputation.[8]

Severe bony destruction or bone loss may on occasion be an indication for amputation (Fig. 21–1). However, various bone grafting techniques, autogenous free-vascularized bone transplant, or bone transport to bridge defects and gain length are now being utilized for the reconstruction of some of these injuries.[3,4,10–16] (Fig. 21–2).

Major nerve injury remains the principal insoluble problem, at the present time, in the salvage of these severely injured extremities. Although traumatized limbs with sciatic nerve lacerations can be salvaged, they are generally functionally less useful than a well fitting prosthesis with a good stump of optimal length. A simple femur fracture compounded by an isolated sciatic laceration is probably best treated by routine fracture methods and nerve repair. Late muscle transfers or a knee fusion can be done later if necessary to improve function. However, when these major nerve injuries occur in conjunction with other severe bony and soft tissue trauma to the leg, an amputation is usually indicated.[5,9]

Injury to lesser peripheral nerves generally do not warrant primary amputation. For example, amputation in the face of a completely disrupted posterior tibial nerve has been recommended due to the skin breakdown which occurs in insensate feet.[3] Amputation for this reason is best deferred and the limb observed for several months, as protective sensation

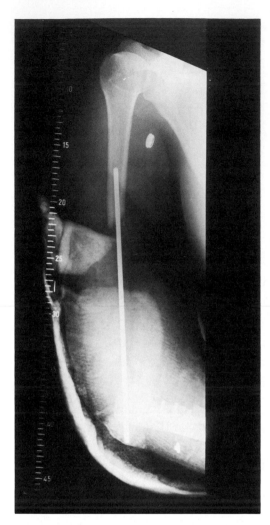

Figure 21–1.   Loss of distal half of humerus secondary to open injury. Temporary stabilization with intramedullary pin between humerus and olecranon is being used to keep soft tissues out to length prior to bony reconstruction.

to the plantar surface of the foot is often maintained by the sural and saphenous nerves. If so, the patient may never need an amputation.

Although isolated skin, muscle, vessel, bone, or nerve injury are rarely severe enough to warrant primary amputation, when they occur together in a patient compromised by other systemic injuries they may result in an extremity that is best treated by amputation due to the poor prospect of salvaging a functional extremity.

Today, absolute indications for primary amputation include a Grade IIIc open fracture of the tibia with an associated posterior tibial nerve disruption or any Grade IIIc open fractures with such severe tissue damage that even if the extremity is salvaged, marked loss of function would persist. A relative indication is any Grade IIIc open fracture which has not been treated within the first eight hours following injury.[8]

In an attempt to better quantify which fractures are best served by primary amputation, the Mangled Extremity Severity Score has been developed. Generally, patients scoring less

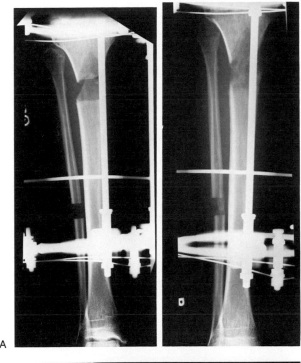

A   B

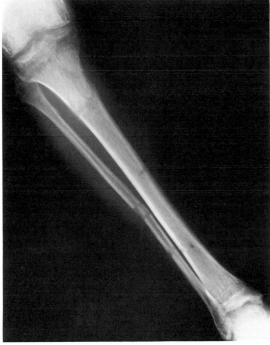

Figure 21–2. Bone transport used for osteoneogenesis to make up bone defect. **A:**
Lengthening of tibia for patient with posttraumatic shortening from malunion. **B:** Osteoneogenesis forming in lengthened areas.
C: Consolidation of bone in lengthened area.

C

Table 21–1   MESS
(Mangled Extremity Severity Score)

A. Skeletal and soft tissue injury	
Low energy (stabs, simple fracture, low energy GSW)	1
Medium energy (open or multiple fractures, dislocation)	2
High energy (close range shotgun, high energy GSW, crush injuries)	3
Very high energy (gross contamination, tissue avulsion)	4
B. Limb ischemia	
Pulse reduced or absent, perfusion normal	1*
Pulseless, parasthesias, diminished capillary refill	2*
Cool, paralyzed, insensate, numb	3*
*Double score for ischemia > 6 hrs	
C. Shock	
Systolic BP always above 90 mm Hg	0
Transient hypotension	1
Persistent hypotension	2
D. Age	
0–30	0
30–50	1
50+	2

Score less than 7 = salvageable extremity.
Score 7 or greater = nonsalvageable extremity.

than 7 will have salvageable extremities (Table 21–1), while those scoring 7 or more have limbs that are not salvageable and should be amputated primarily.[19]

As regards the upper extremity, cervical nerve root injuries and extensive brachial plexus injuries which result in a flail extremity have poor prognosis for recovery. A difficult decision is entailed when the outcome of treatment will be a flail extremity, because, as opposed to the lower extremity, any return of function is better than amputation.

Finally, amputation to reduce invalidism is done on a delayed basis for many trauma victims after the attempt for limb salvage has failed due to poor circulation, or semiacutely in the face of an open fracture in which infection cannot be controlled due to the loss of vascularity. An initially successful revascularization that subsequently fails may also precipitate a delayed or late amputation.

ASSESSMENT

The initial evaluation of the extremity in the trauma victim involves assessment of soft tissue injury, bony abnormalities, neurologic function, and the vascularity to determine the severity of injury. In the amputated or near-amputated limb, a decision must be made as to whether the probability of successful repair of the neurologic, vascular, soft tissue, and bony injuries will result in a useful extremity. Assessment of the patient with a complete amputation is straightforward. The decision whether or not to attempt limb salvage can be very difficult when there is a near amputation.

There are three types of traumatic amputation. These are classified as 1) the complete amputation, 2) the near or partial amputation, and 3) the segmental amputation.

A complete amputation is self-explanatory. No connection is left between the extremity and the patient. The decision with these injuries simply involves whether attempted replantation is warranted.

The partial amputation consists of severe open fractures (usually Grade III) with variable amounts of soft tissue, nerve, vascular, and bony connection between the body and the limb. The initial judgement involves whether vascular integrity can be obtained and maintained, whether there is a potential for sufficient nerve function to render the salvaged limb useful, and whether bony connection can be re-established without undue morbidity or mortality.

The complete and near amputations leave no question as to the diagnosis. More difficult to diagnose and assess is the segmental amputation. In these cases, the internal structures (bone, muscle, vasculature, nerves) have been badly crushed or severed, but the enveloping skin is intact, although it is usually contused or abraded. A typical example of a segmental amputation is a tibia caught between two automobile bumpers where the force is so great that everything is crushed with only the skin remaining intact, hiding the underlying damage (Fig. 21–3A,B).

The segmental amputation can be difficult to diagnose, but is recognized when one can palpate defects in the soft tissues under the badly contused and angry-looking skin. Massive swelling can occur on a delayed basis, in which case a compartment syndrome is common. The tell-tale sign of the segmental amputation is seen when a skin incision is made and a total lack of integrity of the internal structures is noted.

These segmental amputations cannot be safely treated surgically as simple fractures, but must be approached more along the lines of severe open fractures and initially stabilized through external fixation, skeletal traction, or percutaneous pinning until the soft tissue injury declares itself or resolves. After the soft tissues are in good condition, open surgery may safely be performed if indicated. If the acute segmental amputation is opened for primary internal fixation, there is a high risk of skin slough and soft tissue necrosis. This converts the closed injury into an open one, and often precipitates loss of the extremity.

TREATMENT

The complete amputation involving the lower extremity is generally best treated in the adult by making no attempt at replantation. Regeneration of lower extremity nerves following repair is not comparable to that seen in the upper extremity.[18] Sciatic nerve repairs have very poor return of function[4,18]—so even if a replanted leg survives, the neurologic deficit may be such that a good prosthesis will be more functional for the patient.

An exception to replantation surgery in the lower extremity is traumatic amputation in the child or infant. Due to their remarkable regenerative ability, if the replanted limb remains viable, it may have surprisingly good function. Also, the young child will adapt much better to an impaired extremity than an adult. In these instances, an attempted replant is worthwhile if the amputated part is not otherwise damaged by crush or contusion.

The results of upper extremity replantation have been much more successful. Shoulder disarticulation injuries if replanted will not be functionally useful, but may be more cosmetically acceptable to some patients than a prosthesis. The more distal the replant, the better the return of neurologic function.[1,4,5,18] For this reason, finger replants are more successful than upper arm replants. Also, muscle is not as tolerant to ischemia as the

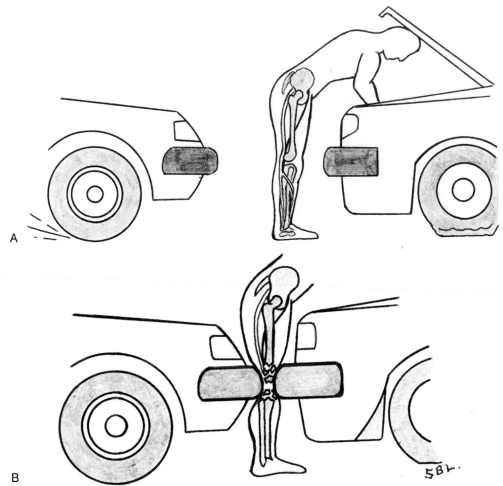

Figure 21–3.   A, B: Bumper injury. Leg is crushed between two bumpers leading to transection of neurovascular structures, comminuted fractures, and extensive soft tissue damage and stripping. The leg remains attached to the body only through the enveloping skin.

tendinous, fibrous, and bony structures such as are found in the digits. With increasingly proximal levels, muscle mass increases, contributing to a poorer result.

A more difficult judgement decision is involved in the near amputation. The key factors are the potential status of nerve function and the viability of the extremity. Complete nerve root or brachial plexus lesions have a poor prognosis for recovery, but injuries at these levels are often isolated to but one or two nerve roots or cords. Muscle and tendon transfers can be used subsequently to provide function in denervated areas.

The ability to successfully restore vascular function is often critical to initial success. The loss of vascular integrity for more than 6 to 8 hours usually results in death of muscle tissue despite subsequent restoration of blood flow in main channels. Amputation must then be carried out at the site of ischemic demarcation.

If an attempt is to be made to save these near complete amputations, maintain hemostasis by sterile pressure dressings. Tourniquets should not be used—either initially in the emergency department or subsequently in the operating room. These limbs are hypercoagulable and pressure applied, even for short periods, will result in thrombosis of arterial blood supply and venous drainage. Once bleeding is controlled and the patient is properly stabilized, treat the patient with antibiotics, irrigation, and debridement as for an open fracture (see Chapter 7); this is followed by vascular repair, fracture stabilization, nerve repair, and tendon and muscle reapproximation. The wound is left open and subsequent after-care including debridements, antibiotic therapy, and eventual wound closure are handled the same as for an open fracture.

In cases of severe multiple trauma, even though a partial amputation may be salvageable, the patient may be unable to tolerate the lengthy procedures necessary to do so and require completion of the amputation.

AMPUTATION

The basic principles of amputation surgery are followed for the traumatic amputation and in cases where a partial amputation is completed. These include preserving length, fashioning sufficient soft tissue flaps for eventual stump contouring and padding of the bone ends for subsequent prosthesis wear, sharp division of nerves under tension to allow retraction back into areas padded by muscle to prevent painful neuroma formation at the stump, prevention of postoperative contractures, and stump shrinking and maturation techniques once the wound is healed for prosthesis fitting.[4,5]

The single most important factor leading to a good result is the maintenance of length, as energy expenditure for prosthetic ambulation decreases with longer stumps. In order to keep energy expenditure within normal limits, the prosthesis-wearing amputee will adjust his walking speed. Traumatic below knee amputees modify their walking speed to 87% and above knee amputees to 63% of normal in order to maintain normal oxygen consumption.[20] When a below knee stump is at least 50% of the length of the remaining limb, oxygen consumption is only 10% higher than prior to amputation. If the stump is less than or equal to 25% of the length of the opposite leg, oxygen consumption is increased by 40%.[7] Energy expenditure and oxygen consumption increases dramatically with amputations above the knee and for bilateral amputees. With a longer stump, prosthetic fitting is also easier.

Ideally, a longer posterior flap is fashioned for below knee amputations due to the muscle tissue available for padding the end of the bone and better vascular supply to this area. Often, flaps will be dictated by the nature of the traumatic wounds. Medial and lateral flaps work well also,[14] as this technique will allow the maximum possible length to the stump.[21]

The level of amputation will be determined by the nature of the patient's injury, the presence of any infection, and the location of the wounds and any necrotic musculature. For these reasons, an ideal stump may not always be possible to fashion for traumatic amputations. Every attempt should be made to salvage greater than 5 cm of distal tibia, as below knee amputations shorter than this function as an above knee amputation.[4] Amputations distal to the myotendinous junction of the gastrocnemius-soleus muscle group do not provide enough soft tissue coverage for adequate stump coverage. The ideal bone length of the residual stump is 12 to 17 cm depending on the height of the patient.[3] This can be determined by allowing 2.5 cm of bone length for each 30 cm of body height.[4]

The level for optimal amputation is more easily determined by the technique of Wagner.[13] The tibia is divided into four equal segments between the knee joint line and the gastroc-soleus myotendinous junction. The posterior flap is marked by the myotendinous junction, and the bone cut is made at the proximal end of the most distal quarter.

Through knee amputations once were difficult prosthesis fitting challenges. However, with recent improvements, good prostheses for these levels are now available. The large surface area of the distal femur is a natural weight-bearing surface.[17] Either anterior-posterior or medial-lateral flaps may be used. The femoral condyles (especially the medial) is shaved down for a better contoured stump and improved prosthesis fitting. The articular cartilage of the femur and patella is not disturbed. The infrapatellar ligament and gastrocnemius muscle remnants are sutured to the cruciate ligament stubs and soft tissues in the intercondylar notch.

Above knee amputations are performed with the same general principles as below knee amputations. The amputation must be 9 to 10 cm proximal to the knee joint to allow for the prosthetic knee joint.[4] If the patient's contralateral and prosthetic knees are at different heights it may be cosmetically unacceptable, especially during sitting, even though function will not be affected. Amputations within 5 cm of the lesser trochanter will function as hip disarticulations,[4] as femoral length is necessary for good sitting balance.[15] A myoplastic closure must be performed to keep the femur centralized within its cuff of musculature. If not, the femur will migrate anterolaterally and become subcutaneous.

Upper extremity amputations should likewise preserve as much length as possible, as function increases with length. Only 50% of adult upper extremity amputees will be rehabilitated with a functional prosthesis, but this number can be increased to 90% with early prosthesis fitting within the first month following amputation.[12]

If it is necessary to maintain as much length as possible in open injuries undergoing amputation, little or no bone shortening is done after the debridement of the open wound. A circular or "guillotine" type of amputation is performed, the wound is left open and treated with dressing changes.[4] Skin traction is applied with tincture of benzoin and stockinette to prevent flap retraction.

For far distal wounds or in situations where the patient cannot tolerate open treatment, some length must be sacrificed with revision of the traumatic amputation level to a higher level where good intact tissues are present. In these instances, primary closure can be obtained so long as a thorough irrigation and debridement has been performed, and there is good vascularity with normal tissues at the chosen level.

Once the definitive amputation is completed, a rigid postoperative dressing will help prevent contracture, decrease swelling and pain, and promote healing. In addition, the lower extremity amputee can be fitted with pilon attached to the cast for early weight bearing if desired.

REFERENCES

1. Beasley RW. *Hand Injuries*. Philadelphia, Pa: WB Saunders; 1981.
2. Bondurant FJ, et al. The medical and economic impact of severely injured lower extremities. *J Trauma*. 1988; 28:1270–1273.
3. Chapman MW, ed. *Operative Orthopaedics*. Philadelphia, Pa: JB Lippincott; 1988.

4. Crenshaw AH, ed. *Campbell's Operative Orthopaedics*. 7th ed. St. Louis, Mo: CV Mosby; 1987.
5. Evarts CM, ed. *Surgery of the Musculoskeletal System*. Edinburgh, Scotland: Churchill Livingstone; 1983.
6. Garrison FH. *An Introduction to the History of Medicine*. 4th ed. Philadelphia, Pa: WB Saunders; 1929.
7. Gonzalez E, et al. Energy expenditure in below knee amputations: correlation with stump length. *Arch Phys Med Rehabil*. 1974;55:111.
8. Gustillo RB, et al. The management of open fractures. *J Bone Joint Surg*. 1990;72-A:299–304.
9. Hansen ST Jr. Overview of the severely traumatized lower limb. Reconstruction versus amputation. *Clin Orthop*. 1989;243:17–19.
10. Ilizarov GA. The tension-stress effect on the genesis and growth of tissues: Part I. The influence of stability of fixation and soft-tissue preservation. *Clin Orthop*. 1989;238:249–281.
11. Ilizarov GA. The tension-stress effect on the genesis and growth of tissues: Part II. The influence of the rate and frequency of distraction. *Clin Orthop*. 1989;239:263–285.
12. Malone J, et al. Immediate, early and late postsurgical management of upper limb amputation. *J Rehabil R and D*. 1984;21:33.
13. Mooney V, et al. The below the knee amputation for vascular disease. *J Bone Joint Surg*. 1976;58-A:365.
14. Persson BM. Sagittal incision for below-knee amputation in ischaemic gangrene. *J Bone Joint Surg*. 1974; 56-B:110.
15. Pinzur MS, et al. Selection of patients for through-the-knee amputation. *J Bone Joint Surg*. 1988;70-A: 746–750.
16. Rockwood CA Jr, Green DP, eds. *Fractures in Adults*. 2nd ed. Philadelphia, Pa: JB Lippincott; 1975.
17. Rogers SP. Amputation at the knee joint. *J Bone Joint Surg*. 1940;22:973.
18. Sunderland S. *Nerves and Nerve Injuries*. Edinburgh, Scotland: Churchill Livingstone; 1978.
19. Swiontkowsky MF. Limb reconstruction or primary amputation in massive lower extremity trauma? The development of a decision making scale. *AO/ASIF*. 1990;3:1–4.
20. Waters RL, et al. Energy cost of walking of amputees: the influence of level of amputation. *J Bone Joint Surg*. 1976;58-A:42–46.
21. Yamanaka M, Kwong PK. The side-to-side flap technique in below-the-knee amputation with long stump. *Clin Orthop*. 1985;201:75–79.

Index

Abrasion, 18
Acetabular fractures, 240–252
    assessment, 242–243
    history, 240
    treatment, 243–252
Acromioclavicular joint dislocation, 130–132
Ala fractures, 223, 227 (*illus.*), 230, 237 (*illus.*)
Allen test, 46
Allis technique, 255, 256 (*illus.*)
Aluminum splints, 31, 32 (*illus.*)
Amputation
    hand or arm, 208–210
        degloving injuries, 209
        indications for, 208
        management of stump, 209–210
        replantation, 210
        thumb, 209
    lower extremity vascular injury, 68, 80, 81
    and open fractures, 102
    traumatic, 358–366
    upper extremity vascular injury, 58
Anastomosis, 74, 77
Anesthesia, 124, 192
Ankle injuries, 322–329
    assessment, 324–326
    dislocation, 323, 328–329
    fractures and sprains, 322–324
    history, 322
    management, 327
    radiology, 327
    treatment, 327–329
Anterior horn cells, 85
Anterior sacroiliac ligament, 215, 216 (*illus.*), 218
    (*illus.*)
Anterior tibial artery, 63, 65–66, 72–74, 78
Anterior tibial pulse, 2
Anterior ulnar collateral artery, 44
Arterial hematoma, 7
Arteriography, 9, 14, 297 (*illus.*)
Arthrotomy, traumatic, *see* Traumatic arthrotomy
Articular fractures, 170
Avascular necrosis, 129, 268, 331
Aviator's astragalus, 330
Avulsions, 21, 95, 157, 199, 215, 228 (*illus.*), 288,
    289 (*illus.*), 290, 291 (*illus.*), 292 (*illus.*)
    see also specific types
Axillary artery, 41–43, 49–50, 56

Axillary vein, 43, 56
Axonotmesis, 86
Axons, 84, 85, 87

Backfire fracture, 169–170
Bag-of-bones technique, 144
Barton's fracture, 168–169
Baseball finger, *see* Mallet finger
Basilic vein, 43–44
Benett's intra-articular fracture, 205
Beverage can position, 33, 34 (*illus.*)
Bipartite patella, 290
Bleeding, 2, 7, 79, 190, 232
Blood pressure, 46
Blow-out fractures, 248, 250 (*illus.*)
Blunt trauma, 8
    dislocations, 10
    fractures, 9–10, 14
    hand injuries, 10–11
    lower extremity vascular injury, 67, 70
    manifestations of, 47
    neurologic, 9, 90
    upper extremity vascular injuries, 41, 46, 47
    vascular, 8–9
Bone grafting, 144, 271, 299, 301, 314–315
Boutonniere deformity, *see* Buttonhole deformity
Brachial artery, 43, 50–51, 52 (*illus.*), 54–55, 56
    (*illus.*), 143
Brachial plexus, 43, 50, 88, 89 (*illus.*), 90, 91, 95,
    96
Buck's traction, 36, 267, 269
Buttonhole deformity, 202–203

Calcaneal pins 37, 307, 308 (*illus.*)
Calcaneus fracture, 333–335
Calf, 348, 350
Cancellous bone, 232, 334
Capitate, 165 (*illus.*), 176, 178 (*illus.*), 180 (*illus.*)
Cardboard box "U" splint, 31, 32 (*illus.*)
Carpal canal (carpal tunnel), 186, 188 (*illus.*)
Carpal fractures, 174
Carpal instability patterns, 175–182
Carpal tunnel syndrome, 166
Carpometacarpal joint dislocations, 183
Casts, 83
Catheters, 78
Cephalad-caudad migration, 221 (*illus.*), 222

Cephalic vein, 44
Chauffeur's fracture, 169–170
Chip avulsion fractures, 335
Circulatory system, 2, 196
Clavicle injuries, 130, 132
Closed reduction, 268, 334
Clot, 777
Codivilla technique, 36
Collateral, 58, 77
Colles' fracture, 167, 171 (*illus.*)
Comminuted fractures, 170, 171, 172 (*illus.*), 173
  (*illus.*), 288
Common femoral artery, 62, 68–69, 74, 81
Compartment syndrome, 24, 57, 79, 83, 84, 101,
  158, 305, 344–356
  assessment, 347–351
  diagnosis, 347
  etiology, 345–346
  history, 344
  location, 344–345
  pathophysiology, 346
  pressure measurements, 349 (*illus.*), 351–352
  treatment, 352–356
Compression injuries, 199, 211
Computerized tomographic (CT) scan, 91, 220,
  221 (*illus.*), 227 (*illus.*), 245 (*illus.*), 247–248
  (*illus.*), 251 (*illus.*), 335 (*illus.*)
Condyle fractures, 296, 298 (*illus.*), 299, 300
  (*illus.*)
Contusion, 18–19, 199
Coronoid fractures, 157
Cross-locking intramedullary nails, 273
Crush injuries, 211
C-spine series, 4
CT scan, *see* Computerized tomographic (CT)
  scan

Danis-Weber classification, 323
Dashboard injuries, 5, 6 (*illus.*), 264, 288, 289
  (*illus.*)
Debridement, 105, 106 (*illus.*), 193
Decompression, 12, 352–355
Deformity, 3–4, 157, 180, 202
Degloving injuries, 209
Dislocation
  ankle, 323, 328–329
  hand, 206–207
  hip, 10, 252–259
  joint, 12, 13
    acromioclavicular, 130–132
    assessment, 4
    carpometacarpal, 183
    sternoclavicular, 131–132
  knee, 10, 293–296
  lower extremity, 14, 84
  open, 13, 112–113
  patellar, 292–293
  perilunate, 176, 179 (*illus.*), 181 (*illus.*)
  scapulothoracic, 133, 134 (*illus.*)
  shoulder, 115–124
  subtalar, 332–333
  upper extremity, 14
  wrist, 162–166, 183

Displaced fractures, 127, 128 (*illus.*)
Distal humerus fractures, 142–145
  assessment, 143
  treatment, 143–145
Distal median nerve, 88
Distal phalangeal fractures, 205–206
Distal pulses, 2
Distal radioulnar joint (DRUJ), 172, 174
Distal radius fractures, 166–172, 173 (*illus.*)
Distal ulna injuries, 172, 174–175
Doppler velocity wave form, 47
Dorsalis pedis pulse, 2
Dorsal root ganglion, 85, 86 (*illus.*)
Dressings, 195, 196
DREZ, *see* Spinal cord dorsal root entry zone
DRUJ, *see* Distal radioulnar joint
Duverney's fracture, 228, 229 (*illus.*)

Edema, 205
Elbow, 151
  dislocation, 146, 148, 149 (*illus.*)
    evaluation, 146
    treatment, 146–148
  radial head and neck fractures, 148–150
  stiffness, 144
Elective injuries, 12, 13
Electromyography (EMG), 90, 91, 94
Emergent injuries, 12
EMG, *see* Electromyography
Endoneurial sheath, 84, 87
Endoneurium, 84 (*illus.*), 85
Endosteum, 14
Epineurial repair, 91–92
Epineurium, 84 (*illus.*), 85
Eskimo technique, 123
Essex-Lopresti fracture, 150, 152–153, 154 (*illus.*),
  157, 174, 334
Evaluation
  history, 1
  initial survey, 2
  secondary survey-specific, 2–4
    dislocation assessment, 4
    fracture assessment, 3–4
    neurologic assessment, 4
    vascular assessment, 2–3
  see also specific conditions
Extensor retinaculum 187, 188 (*illus.*)
Extensor tendons, 187, 200–203
External fixation, 9, 10, 311–313
External iliac artery, 74
Extra-articular fracture, 156
Extrinsic flexor tendons, 186

Fascicles, 84, 85
Fasciotomies, 352–355
Femoral artery, 61–63, 68–71
Femoral head, 255 (*illus.*), 262 (*illus.*), 264–266
Femoral shaft, 67
Femur fractures, 9, 276–285
  history, 276–277
  indication for nailing, 280
  initial evaluation, 277–280

open, 281, 284
technique, 281, 282–284 (*illus.*)
timing of surgery, 280–281
Fibular fractures, 315–316
Fifth-degree nerve injury, 87
Fingers, 186, 187 (*illus.*), 201–210
amputation, 208–210
dislocation, 206–207
mallet, 201–202
First-degree nerve injury, 86
Flap avulsions, 21
Flexor tendon, 203–204
Fogarty catheter, 78
Forearm
and compartment syndrome, 350, 351 (*illus.*),
352, 353 (*illus.*)
fractures, 157–160
evaluation, 157–158
nightstick, 158, 160
treatment, 158
injury, 150–151
Forefoot, 337–342
Foreign bodies, 210–211
Fourth-degree nerve injury, 87
Fracture
acetabular, 240–252
articular, 170
assessment, 3–4
blisters, 24
blunt trauma, 9–10, 14
clavicle, 132
closed, 9
comminuted, 170, 171, 172 (*illus.*), 288
compound, 9
distal humerus, 142–145
elbow radial head and neck, 148–150
elective, 13
femoral, 9, 67, 276–285
fibular, 315–316
forearm, 150–154, 157–160
hand, 204–206
hip, 261–274
humerus shaft, 136–141
intra-articular, 107, 142, 156, 205, 296–303
knee, 287, 296–303
lower extremity, 14, 15
major, 47
nonarticular, 170
nondisplaced, 127, 128 (*illus.*)
occult, 5
olecranon, 154–157
open, *see* Open fractures
patella, 287–292
pediatric, 11, 262, 268, 274
pelvic, 13, 214–238
prioritization of, 11–13
proximal humerus, 125–127
scapular, 132–133
upper extremity, 14
wrist, 162–175
see also specific fractures
Frykman classification, 168
Functional position, 34

Galleazi fracture, 152, 153 (*illus.*), 157
Goyrand's fracture, 167–168
Grasping, 189
Greater saphenous vein, 66
Gunshot wounds, 67, 108–112

Hamstring avulsions, 225, 228 (*illus.*)
Hand injuries, 10–11, 185–197
amputation, 208–210
anatomy, 185–189
contusion and compression, 199
dislocations, 206–207
dressing and splints, 195–196
evaluation, 190–192
examination, 190
foreign bodies, 210–211
fractures, 204–206
history, 185, 198
incidence of, 185
injection, 211–212
ligamentous, 207
management of specific, 198–213
medical history, 190
nerve, 204
physiology, 189
postinjury and postoperative care, 196–197
preoperative preparation, 192
priorities, 190
rehabilitation, 213
skin avulsions, 199
surgical techniques, 193–195
tendon, 199–204
trauma, 212
Hare splint, 31
Harmon's approach, 355
Harris axial views, 333, 334 (*illus.*)
Hawkins technique, 127
Hemarthrosis, 23–24
Hematoma, 7, 19, 231, 232
Hemorrhage, *see* Bleeding
Heterotopic ossification, 25–27
Hill-Sachs lesion, 117–118, 119, 127, 129
Hindfoot injuries, 330–335
Hip, 242
Hip dislocation, 10, 252–259
assessment, 252–253
treatment, 253–259
Hip fracture, 261–274
anatomy, 264
femoral head, 264–266
assessment, 265
treatment, 265–266
history, 261–262
intertrochanteric, 263 (*illus.*), 268–271
intracapsular neck, 267–268
subtrochanteric, 263 (*illus.*), 271–273
in young, 262, 268, 274
Hippocratic method, 123
Humeral head, 122 (*illus.*), 125, 126 (*illus.*), 127,
129 (*illus.*)
Humeral head impaction fracture, *see* Hill-Sachs
lesion
Humerus shaft fracture, 136–142

assessment, 137
  history, 136
  operative technique, 141–142
  treatment, 137–141
Hunter's canal, 70
Hutchinson's fracture, 169–170
Hybrid pin, 37

Iliac artery, 74
Iliac wing, 228, 229 (*illus.*)
Iliolumbar ligament, 215, 217 (*illus.*), 224 (*illus.*)
Immobilization, *see* Splinting and immobilization
Indomethacin, 26
Infection, 102, 107, 195
Inferior profunda artery, 43
Injection injuries, 211–212
Interfascicular repair, 92–93
Internal fixation, 9, 107, 127, 129 (*illus.*), 156,
  171, 236, 237 (*illus.*), 247, 266, 269 (*illus.*)
Interosseous scapholunate ligament, 176, 177
  (*illus.*)
Intertrochanteric fractures, 263 (*illus.*), 268–271
Intra-articular avascular fragments, 125
Intra-articular foreign body, 111
Intra-articular fractures, 107, 142, 156, 205, 296–
  303
Intracapsular neck fractures, 267–268
Intracondylar fractures, 143, 144 (*illus.*), 145
  (*illus.*)
Intramuscular hematoma, 19
Irrigation, 193
Ischemia
  and compartment syndrome, 345
  irreversible, 208
  lower extremity vascular injury, 80
  tourniquet, 192
  vascular, 12, 14
Ischemic fibrosis, 199
Isolated ulnar shaft fracture, *see* Nightstick
  fracture

Joy-stick technique, 171

Knee dislocation, 10, 293–296
  assessment, 293–294
  treatment, 294–296
  see also Patellar dislocation
Knee fracture
  history, 287
  intra-articular, 296–303
  assessment, 297–298
  treatment, 298–303
  see also Patellar fracture
Knife wounds, 67
K-wires, 171

Laceration, 19–20
  of brachial artery, 143
  complex, 55
  of nerves, 83
  over patella, 17
  simple, 55 (*illus.*), 56
Lag screw fixation, 299–300 (*illus.*)

Laparotomy, 231
Lateral thoracic artery, 42
Leg, lower, 350 (*illus.*), 353, 354 (*illus.*)
Lesser saphenous vein, 66
Ligamentous injuries, 207
Limb loss, *see* Amputation
Lisfranc's joints, 336–337, 338–341 (*illus.*)
Longitudinal incision, 68
Lower extremity vascular injury
  anatomy of, 62–66
  assessment, 67–68
  complications and postoperative management,
    79–80
  exposure, 68–74
  history, 60–61
  incidence and location, 61
  preoperative management, 68
  principles of repair, 74, 77–78
  results, 80–81
Lunate, 165 (*illus.*), 176, 177 (*illus.*), 178 (*illus.*),
  180 (*illus.*)

Maissoneuve injury, 324, 326
Malgaigne fracture, 230, 231 (*illus.*), 235 (*illus.*)
Mallet finger, 201–202
Mangled Extremity Severity Score, 360, 362
Massive tissue trauma, 12
Medial femoral condyle, 298 (*illus.*)
Median nerve, 44, 187, 191
Mesoneurium, 85
Metatarsal head, 339, 341–342 (*illus.*)
Metatarsal-phalangeal joints, 338
Metatarsals, 337–338 (*illus.*)
Midfoot injuries, 335–337
  fractures, 336
  ligamentous, 335–336
  Lisfranc's, 336–337
Monteggia fracture, 151–152, 157
Mortise, 323, 325 (*illus.*), 326 (*illus.*)
Motor vehicle accidents, 242, 364 (*illus.*)
  see also Dashboard injuries; specific injuries
Multiple pin/screw technique, 268, 269 (*illus.*)
Muscle
  and compartment syndrome, 347
  function, 94
  laceration, 20
  spasm, 123
Musculoskeletal injuries, 12
Myositis ossificans, 19

Nails, 141–142, 143 (*illus.*), 313
  see also specific types
Neck fractures, 148–150
Nerve action potentials (NAP), 90
Nerve function, 140
Nerve graft, 93, 94 (*illus.*)
Nerve injury, *see* Neurologic injury
Nerve regeneration, 87
Neurapraxia, 86
Neurologic assessment, 4
Neurologic blunt trauma, 9
Neurologic injury, 15, 18, 58, 82–96
  anatomy and physiology, 84–87

assessment, 88
complications, 95
of hand, 204
history, 82
and humerus fractures, 137
incidence and mechanism of, 83–84
initial management, 88, 90–91
postoperative care and follow-up, 93–94
repair, 90–93
results, 95–96
Neurologic lesion, 13, 117
Neurologic penetrating trauma, 8
Neuropraxia, 117
Neurotmesis, 86
Nightstick fracture, 158, 160
Nonarticular fractures, 170
Nondisplaced fractures, 127, 128 (*illus.*)
Non-reamed nails, 141–142, 143 (*illus.*), 313, 314
    (*illus.*)

Olecranon fractures, 154–157
    assessment, 155
    management, 155–157
Open book type pelvic fracture, 222, 224 (*illus.*),
    230
Open fractures, 3, 9, 10, 13, 46, 98–112, 140
    classification, 99–101
    decision making, 102
    evaluation, 101–102
    femur, 281, 284
    gunshot wounds, 108–112
    history, 98–99
    knee, 301
    operative fixation, 107–108
    operative treatment, 104–107
    pelvic, 219, 232–238
    protocol, 102–104
    tibial, 310–314
Open reduction, 146
Orthopaedic injuries, 8
Osteoneogenesis, 361 (*illus.*)

Pain, 95, 150, 196, 197, 347
Palmar flexion, 182
Paradox of reduction, 182
Paralysis, 197
Parona's space, 186
Patellar dislocation, 292–293
Patellar fracture
    assessment, 288, 290
    history, 287
    treatment, 290–292
Pediatric fractures, 11, 274
Pelvic fracture, 12, 214–238
    anatomy, 215–218
    evaluation and management, 230–232
    history, 214–215
    major, 228
    minor, 223, 225, 228
    open, 232–238
    physical exam, 218–223
    types of, 229–230
    see also Acetabular fractures

Penetrating trauma, 5, 7
    lower extremity vascular injury, 67
    neurologic, 8, 83
    orthopaedic, 8
    upper extremity vascular injury, 47
    vascular, 7–8
Perilunate dislocations, 176, 179 (*illus.*), 181 (*illus.*)
Perineurium, 84, 85
Periosteum, 14
Peripheral nerve injury, 83, 87, 89
Peroneal artery, 63, 64 (*illus.*), 66, 74, 78
Peroneal nerve, 96, 316
Pins, 36–38, 238, 311–312
Plate and screw fixation, 141, (*illus.*), 158, 159
    (*illus.*), 171, 314
Popliteal artery, 61, 63–64, 67, 70–71, 72 (*illus.*),
    77, 80, 81, 295 (*illus.*), 297 (*illus.*)
Popliteal fossa, 295 (*illus.*)
Popliteal space, 71, 72
Popliteal vein, 64–65
Posterior approach to popliteal artery, 70
Posterior ligamentous complex, 215, 216 (*illus.*)
Posterior splints, 57
Posterior tibial artery, 63, 64 (*illus.*), 66, 74, 75–
    76 (*illus.*), 78
Posterior tibial nerve, 66
Postganglionic injuries, 86
Pouteau fracture, 167
Preganglionic fibers, 85–86
Preganglionic injuries, 86
Profunda brachial artery, 43
Profunda femoral artery, 61, 63, 69–70, 74
Profunda femoral vein, 63
Proximal humerus fracture, 125–129
    classification, 125, 127
    evaluation, 127
    treatment, 127–129
Proximal major pulses, 2
Proximal median nerve, 88
Proximal ulna, 151, 157

Radial artery, 45–46, 51, 53 (*illus.*), 53–54
Radial nerve, 84, 137, 138 (*illus.*), 139 (*illus.*),
    140, 151, 187, 191
Radial pulse, 2
Radial styloid, 163, 164 (*illus.*), 170
Radiation, 26
Radiology
    and ankle injuries, 327
    evaluation, 4–5
    immobilization for, 30, 31
    pelvic, 219–223
    and shoulder dislocation, 117–121
    upper extremity vascular trauma, 8
    wrist, 163, 164 (*illus.*), 165 (*illus.*)
Radius, 146, 148–150, 151
Rami fractures, 223, 227 (*illus.*)
Reamed nailing, 307, 308 (*illus.*), 309 (*illus.*)
Rectus femoris avulsions, 225, 228 (*illus.*)
Reperfusion syndrome, 80
Resting position, 33
Revascularization, 14
Reverse Colles' fracture, 167–168

Rigid nails, 141–142, 143 (*illus.*)
Ring avulsions, 209
Robert Jones dressing, 34, 35 (*illus.*), 309, 327, 328
Roentgenograms, 191
Root avulsion, 91
Rule of Threes, 149

Sacral ala, 230, 237 (*illus.*)
Sacroiliac, 215, 216–218 (*illus.*), 220, 221–222 (*illus.*), 224 (*illus.*)
Sacrospinous ligaments, 216, 218 (*illus.*)
Sacrotuberous ligament, 215, 217 (*illus.*), 224 (*illus.*)
Saline dump, 101, 103
Saphenous vein, 66, 74
Sartorius avulsions, 225, 228 (*illus.*)
Saturday-night syndrome, 345, 353 (*illus.*)
Scaphoid, 165 (*illus.*), 175, 180, 181–182 (*illus.*)
Scapholunate, 165 (*illus.*), 176, 180
Scapular injuries, 132–134
Scapular manipulation, 124
Scapular Y x-ray, 118, 119–121 (*illus.*)
Schwann cells, 85
Sciatic nerve, 96, 242 (*illus.*), 255 (*illus.*)
Second-degree nerve injury, 86–87
Semielective injuries, 13
Semirigid nonreamed nails, 141
Sensibility, hand, 189
Shotgun wounds, 111
Shoulder dislocation, 115–121
   anterior, 116, 117, 124
   classification, 116
   evaluation, 117
   history, 115
   inferior (luxatio erecta), 116
   mechanism, 116
   posterior, 116, 117, 118 (*illus.*), 119, 122 (*illus.*), 124
   radiology, 117–121
   treatment, 121, 123–124
Shoulder fracture, *see* Proximal humerus fracture
Skin, 186, 191, 199, 211
Smith's fracture, 167–168
Smooth pins, 36
Soft tissue injury, 16–27
   abrasion, 18
   avulsion, 21
   contusion, 18–19
   examination, 17–18
   hemarthrosis, 23–24
   heterotopic ossification, 25–27
   history, 16
   laceration, 19–20
   sprains and strains, 25
   swelling syndromes, 24–25
   traumatic arthrotomy, 22–23
Soupy pins, 238
Spasm, 2
Spinal cord dorsal root entry zone (DREZ), 95
Splinting and immobilization, 29–39
   ankle injuries, 327
   application, 33–34

   hand injuries, 195–196
   history, 29–30
   neurologic injuries, 93–94
   shoulder dislocation, 124
   types of splints, 31–33
Sprains, 25, 180, 322–324
Steinmann pin, 36, 37(*illus.*), 38 (*illus.*)
Sternoclavicular joint dislocation, 131–132
Stimson maneuver, 123–124, 255, 256 (*illus.*)
Strains, 25
Stretch type injury, 8, 46, 84, 96
Styloid fracture, 172–174
Subluxation, 182
Subtalar dislocation, 332–333
Subtrochanteric fractures, 263 (*illus.*), 271–273
Sugar-tong splint, 33, 138, 139 (*illus.*)
Superficial femoral artery, 63, 70, 71 (*illus.*), 74, 77, 80, 81
Superficial femoral vein, 63
Supracondylar femoral fracture, 299, 300 (*illus.*)
Supracondylar humeral fracture, 142, 145 (*illus.*)
Sural nerve, 93
Suture, 20, 200
Swan-neck deformity, 202
Swelling syndromes, 24–25
Symphisis pubis, 223 (*illus.*)

Talo-calcaneal joint, 332
Talus fractures, 330–332, 333 (*illus.*)
Tendon injuries, 199–204
   extensor, 200–203
   flexor, 203–204
   pelvic avulsion fracture, 225
Tenorrhapy, 200, 201 (*illus.*), 204
Terry Thomas sign, 180, 182 (*illus.*)
TFCC, *see* Triangular fibrocartilaginous complex
Third-degree nerve injury, 87
Thoracoacromial artery, 42
Threaded pin, 37
Thrombosis
   complications, 57, 79
   of repairs, 58
   of side branches of major arteries, 77
   and stretch type injury, 46
   and vascular blunt trauma, 8
Thumb, 189, 209
Tibial fracture, 9, 304–320
   history, 304
   pilon, 316–320
      assessment and goals, 316–317
      mechanism, 316
      treatment, 319–320
   plateau, 299, 301, 302 (*illus.*)
   tibia shaft, 305–315
      anatomy, 305
      assessment, 305–306
      bone grafting, 314–315
      management considerations, 307
      open, 310–314
      treatment, 307–310
Tibial pin traction, 271, 272 (*illus.*)
Tibial-talar joint, 328
Tinel's sign, 94

Tourniquets, 83, 104, 192, 319
Traction, 14, 35–36, 39
  injuries, 83
  principles, 36–38
  and shoulder dislocation, 121
Transcervical fracture, 263 (*illus.*)
Transverse arch, 337 (*illus.*)
Trauma, blunt, *see* Blunt trauma
Trauma, hand, 212
Traumatic amputation, 358–366
  assessment, 362–363
  history, 358
  indications, 359–362
  surgery, 365–366
  treatment, 363–365
Traumatic arthrotomy, 13, 22–23
Triangular fibrocartilaginous complex (TFCC), 172, 174–175
Triceps aponeurosis, 156
Triceps mechanism, 155
Triceps tendon, 157
Triquetrolunate joint, 176, 178 (*illus.*)
Tuberosity avulsions, 117

Ulna, 146, 149, 151, 157
Ulnar artery, 44–45, 52, 53–55
Ulnar bursa, 186
Ulnar nerve, 84, 88, 187, 191
Ulnar pulse, 2
Upper extremity vascular injury, 40–58
  anatomy of, 41–46, 48
  assessment, 46–48
  complications, 57–58
  history, 40
  incidence, 41
  operative exposure, 48–52

  postoperative care, 57
  preoperative management, 48
  results, 58
  vascular repair, 52–57
Urgent injuries, 12–13

Vascular assessment, 2–3
Vascular blunt trauma, 8–9
Vascular injury, lower extremity, *see* Lower extremity vascular injury
Vascular injury, upper extremity, *see* Upper extremity vascular injury
Vascular ischemia, 12, 14
Vascular penetrating trauma, 7–8
Venous injuries, 8
Vessel inury, 2
Volar ligaments, 175, 176 (*illus.*)
Volar plate, 186, 187 (*illus.*)
Volkmann's contracture, 346

Watson-Jones exposure, 271
Weber fibular fracture, 323–325 (*illus.*)
Wringer injuries, 211
Wrist
  carpal instability patterns, 175–182
  dislocations and fractures, 162–183, 206
    assessment, 163–165, 180
    carpometacarpal joint dislocations, 183
    distal radius fractures, 166–172
    history, 162
    treatment, 165–166, 170–172, 180, 182
  injury, 151
    distal ulna, 172, 174–175
  pain, 150

X-rays, *see* Radiology